Electrophysi
Testing

Pos Lead 1
Neg Lead arf = LAD

Electrophysiologic Testing

FIFTH EDITION

Richard N. Fogoros, MD
Pittsburgh, PA

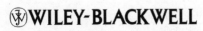
A John Wiley & Sons, Ltd., Publication

This edition first published 2012, © 2012 by John Wiley & Sons Ltd.

Wiley-Blackwell is an imprint of John Wiley & Sons, formed by the merger of Wiley's global Scientific, Technical and Medical business with Blackwell Publishing.

Registered office: John Wiley & Sons, Ltd, The Atrium, Southern Gate, Chichester, West Sussex, PO19 8SQ, UK

Editorial offices: 9600 Garsington Road, Oxford, OX4 2DQ, UK
The Atrium, Southern Gate, Chichester, West Sussex, PO19 8SQ, UK
111 River Street, Hoboken, NJ 07030-5774, USA

For details of our global editorial offices, for customer services and for information about how to apply for permission to reuse the copyright material in this book please see our website at www.wiley.com/wiley-blackwell

Designations used by companies to distinguish their products are often claimed as trademarks. All brand names and product names used in this book are trade names, service marks, trademarks or registered trademarks of their respective owners. The publisher is not associated with any product or vendor mentioned in this book. This publication is designed to provide accurate and authoritative information in regard to the subject matter covered. It is sold on the understanding that the publisher is not engaged in rendering professional services. If professional advice or other expert assistance is required, the services of a competent professional should be sought.

The contents of this work are intended to further general scientific research, understanding, and discussion only and are not intended and should not be relied upon as recommending or promoting a specific method, diagnosis, or treatment by physicians for any particular patient. The publisher and the author make no representations or warranties with respect to the accuracy or completeness of the contents of this work and specifically disclaim all warranties, including without limitation any implied warranties of fitness for a particular purpose. In view of ongoing research, equipment modifications, changes in governmental regulations, and the constant flow of information relating to the use of medicines, equipment, and devices, the reader is urged to review and evaluate the information provided in the package insert or instructions for each medicine, equipment, or device for, among other things, any changes in the instructions or indication of usage and for added warnings and precautions. Readers should consult with a specialist where appropriate. The fact that an organization or Website is referred to in this work as a citation and/or a potential source of further information does not mean that the author or the publisher endorses the information the organization or Website may provide or recommendations it may make. Further, readers should be aware that Internet Websites listed in this work may have changed or disappeared between when this work was written and when it is read. No warranty may be created or extended by any promotional statements for this work. Neither the publisher nor the author shall be liable for any damages arising herefrom.

Library of Congress Cataloging-in-Publication Data

Fogoros, Richard N.
  Electrophysiologic testing / Richard N. Fogoros. – 5th ed.
    p. ; cm.
  Includes index.
  ISBN 978-0-470-67423-9 (pbk.)
  I. Title.
  [DNLM: 1. Arrhythmias, Cardiac–diagnosis. 2. Arrhythmias, Cardiac–therapy.
  3. Electrophysiologic Techniques, Cardiac. WG 330]
  616.1'2807547–dc23

                                                      2012016779

A catalogue record for this book is available from the British Library.

Wiley also publishes its books in a variety of electronic formats. Some content that appears in print may not be available in electronic books.

Cover design by Steve Thompson. Courtesy of Max Delson / iStockphoto.

Set in 9.25/12pt Meridien by Thomson Digital, Noida, India.
Printed and bound in Singapore by Markono Print Media Pte Ltd

4   2015

To Anne, Emily and Joe

Contents

Preface

This book always has been aimed at demystifying electrophysiology for non-electrophysiologists who find themselves wanting to (or perhaps more often, having to) learn something about this difficult and often intimidating field. From the beginning I wanted very much to write a book that was readable and easy to understand for the students, residents, cardiology fellows, cardiologists, primary care physicians, nurses, technicians, and other non-electrophysiologists who need a solid grounding in this information in order to do their jobs well. For this work to have continued to find its intended audience through four editions has been very gratifying to me.

Accordingly, my chief goal in writing the Fifth Edition of *Electrophysiologic Testing* has been to update what needed updating without losing sight of that underlying purpose. While minor corrections and additions have been made throughout, the chief revisions have been made in Chapters 7 (ventricular arrhythmias) and 8 (ablation therapy), where the field has advanced significantly over the past few years. Also, a new chapter has been added (Chapter 11) on the dysautonomias—a group of broadly misunderstood disorders whose sufferers (like it or not) often wind up these days being referred to the electrophysiologist. These patients come in without a diagnosis and often without much hope. A basic understanding of their condition will make life a lot easier for both doctor and patient.

I would like to thank the many readers who have taken the time to let me know that this volume has made a difference in their professional lives. Their words have made all the effort that has gone into this project, a project which has now spanned nearly a quarter century, more than worthwhile.

Acknowledgements

I would like to thank the three people from Wiley-Blackwell who are most responsible for shepherding me through this fifth edition: Thomas Hartman, Senior Editor; Ian Collins, Senior Editorial Assistant to Mr Hartman; and Kate Newell, Senior Developmental Editor.

And as always, I want to thank my beloved wife, Anne, for her endless patience while I worked on this book, and of course, for tolerating a lot more besides.

I DISORDERS OF THE HEART RHYTHM: BASIC PRINCIPLES

1 The Cardiac Electrical System

The heart spontaneously generates electrical impulses, and these electrical impulses are vital to all cardiac functions. On a basic level, by controlling the flux of calcium ions across the cardiac cell membrane, these electrical impulses trigger cardiac muscle contraction. On a higher level, the heart's electrical impulses organize the sequence of muscle contraction during each heartbeat, important for optimizing the cardiac stroke volume. Finally, the pattern and timing of these impulses determine the heart rhythm. Derangements in this rhythm often impair the heart's ability to pump enough blood to meet the body's demands.

Thus, the heart's electrical system is fundamental to cardiac function. The study of the electrical system of the heart is called cardiac electrophysiology, and the main concern of the field of electrophysiology is the mechanisms and therapy of cardiac arrhythmias. The electrophysiology study is the most definitive method of evaluating the cardiac electrical system. It is the subject of this book.

As an introduction to the field of electrophysiology and to the electrophysiology study, this chapter reviews the anatomy of the cardiac electrical system and describes how the vital electrical impulse is normally generated and propagated.

The anatomy of the heart's electrical system

The heart's electrical impulse originates in the sinoatrial (SA) node, located high in the right atrium near the superior vena cava. The impulse leaves the SA node and spreads radially across both atria. When the impulse reaches the atrioventricular (AV) groove, it encounters the "skeleton of the heart," the fibrous structure to which the valve rings are attached, and which separates the atria from the ventricles. This fibrous structure is electrically inert and acts as an insulator—the electrical impulse cannot cross this

Electrophysiologic Testing, Fifth Edition. Richard N. Fogoros.
© 2012 John Wiley & Sons, Ltd. Published 2012 by John Wiley & Sons, Ltd.

structure. Thus the electrical impulse would be prevented from crossing over to the ventricular side of the AV groove if not for the specialized AV conducting tissues: the AV node and the bundle of His (Figure 1.1).

As the electrical impulse enters the AV node, its conduction is slowed because of the electrophysiologic properties of the AV nodal tissue. This slowing is reflected in the PR interval on the surface electrocardiogram (ECG). Leaving the AV node, the electrical impulse enters the His bundle, the most proximal part of the rapidly conducting His–Purkinje system. The His bundle penetrates the fibrous skeleton and delivers the impulse to the ventricular side of the AV groove.

Once on the ventricular side, the electrical impulse follows the His bundle as it branches into the right and left bundle branches.

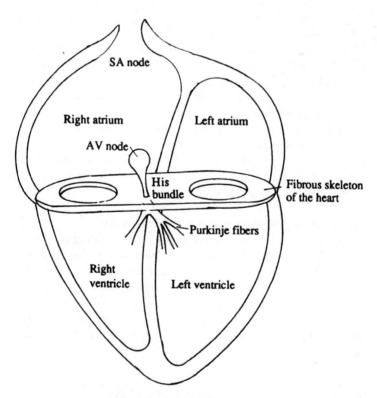

Figure 1.1 Anatomy of the electrical system of the heart.

Branching of the Purkinje fibers continues distally to the furthermost reaches of the ventricular myocardium. The electrical impulse is thus rapidly distributed throughout the ventricles.

Hence, the heart's electrical system is designed to organize the sequence of myocardial contraction with each heartbeat. As the electrical impulse spreads over the atria toward the AV groove, the atria contract. The delay provided by the AV node allows for complete atrial emptying before the electrical impulse reaches the ventricles. Once the impulse leaves the AV node, it is distributed rapidly throughout the ventricular muscle by the Purkinje fibers, providing for brisk and orderly ventricular contraction.

We next consider the character of the electrical impulse, its generation, and its propagation.

The cardiac action potential

The cardiac action potential is one of the most despised and misunderstood topics in cardiology. The fact that electrophysiologists claim to understand it is also a leading cause of the mystique that surrounds them and their favorite test, the electrophysiology study. Because the purpose of this book is to debunk the mystery of electrophysiology studies, we must confront the action potential and learn to understand it. Fortunately, this is far easier than legend would have it.

Although most of us would like to think of cardiac arrhythmias as an irritation or "itch" of the heart (and of antiarrhythmic drugs as a balm or a salve that soothes the itch), this conceptualization of arrhythmias is wrong and leads to the faulty management of patients with arrhythmias. In fact, the behavior of the heart's electrical impulse and of the cardiac rhythm is largely determined by the shape of the action potential; the effect of antiarrhythmic drugs is determined by how they change that shape.

The inside of the cardiac cell, like all living cells, has a negative electrical charge compared to the outside of the cell. The resulting voltage difference across the cell membrane is called the *transmembrane potential*. The resting transmembrane potential (which is -80 to $-90\,\text{mV}$ in cardiac muscle) is the result of an accumulation of negatively charged molecules (called ions) within the cell. Most cells are happy with this arrangement and live out their lives without considering any other possibilities.

Cardiac cells, however, are excitable cells. When excitable cells are stimulated appropriately, tiny pores or channels in the cell membrane open and close sequentially in a stereotyped fashion.

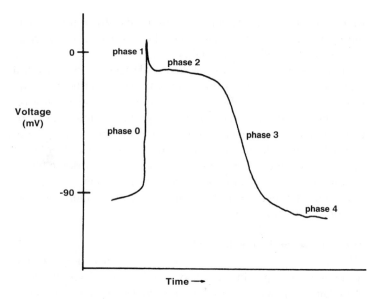

Figure 1.2 The cardiac action potential.

The opening of these channels allows ions to travel back and forth across the cell membrane (again in a stereotyped fashion), leading to patterned changes in the transmembrane potential. When these stereotypic voltage changes are graphed against time, the result is the cardiac action potential (Figure 1.2). The action potential is thus a reflection of the electrical activity of a single cardiac cell.

As can be seen in Figure 1.2, the action potential is classically divided into five phases. However, it is most helpful to consider the action potential in terms of three general phases: depolarization, repolarization, and the resting phase.

Depolarization

The depolarization phase (phase 0) is where the action of the action potential is. Depolarization occurs when the rapid sodium channels in the cell membrane are stimulated to open. When this happens, positively charged sodium ions rush into the cell, causing a rapid, positively directed change in the transmembrane potential. The resultant voltage spike is called *depolarization*. When we speak of the heart's electrical impulse, we are speaking of this depolarization.

Depolarization of one cell tends to cause adjacent cardiac cells to depolarize, because the voltage spike of a cell's depolarization causes the sodium channels in the nearby cells to open. Thus, once a cardiac cell is stimulated to depolarize, the wave of depolarization (the electrical impulse) is propagated across the heart, cell by cell.

Further, the speed of depolarization of a cell (reflected by the slope of phase 0 of the action potential) determines how soon the next cell will depolarize, and thus determines the speed at which the electrical impulse is propagated across the heart. If we do something to change the speed at which sodium ions enter the cell (and thus change the slope of phase 0), we therefore change the speed of conduction (the conduction velocity) of cardiac tissue.

Repolarization

Once a cell is depolarized, it cannot be depolarized again until the ionic fluxes that occur during depolarization are reversed. The process of getting the ions back to where they started is called *repolarization*. The repolarization of the cardiac cell roughly corresponds to phases 1 through 3 (i.e. the width) of the action potential. Because a second depolarization cannot take place until repolarization occurs, the time from the end of phase 0 to late in phase 3 is called the *refractory period* of cardiac tissue.

Repolarization of the cardiac cells is complex and poorly understood. Fortunately, the main ideas behind repolarization are simple: 1) repolarization returns the cardiac action potential to the resting transmembrane potential; 2) it takes time to do this; and 3) the time that it takes to do this, roughly corresponding to the width of the action potential, is the refractory period of cardiac tissue.

There is an additional point of interest regarding repolarization of the cardiac action potential. Phase 2 of the action potential, the so-called plateau phase, can be viewed as interrupting and prolonging the repolarization that begins in phase 1. This plateau phase, which is unique to cardiac cells (e.g. it is not seen in nerve cells), gives duration to the cardiac potential. It is mediated by the slow calcium channels, which allow positively charged calcium ions to slowly enter the cell, thus interrupting repolarization and prolonging the refractory period. The calcium channels have other important effects in electrophysiology, as we will see.

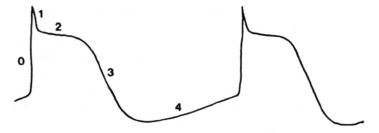

Figure 1.3 Automaticity. In some cardiac cells, there is a leakage of ions across the cell membrane during phase 4, in such a way as to cause a gradual, positively directed change in transmembrane voltage. When the transmembrane voltage becomes sufficiently positive, the appropriate channels are activated to automatically generate another action potential. This spontaneous generation of action potentials due to phase 4 activity is called automaticity.

The resting phase

For most cardiac cells, the resting phase (the period of time between action potentials, corresponding to phase 4) is quiescent, and there is no net movement of ions across the cell membrane.

For some cells, however, the so-called resting phase is not quiescent. In these cells, there is leakage of ions back and forth across the cell membrane during phase 4, in such a way as to cause a gradual increase in transmembrane potential (Figure 1.3). When the transmembrane potential is high enough (i.e. when it reaches the threshold voltage), the appropriate channels are activated to cause the cell to depolarize. Because this depolarization, like any depolarization, can stimulate nearby cells to depolarize in turn, the spontaneously generated electrical impulse can be propagated across the heart. This phase 4 activity, which leads to spontaneous depolarization, is called *automaticity*.

Automaticity is the mechanism by which the normal heart rhythm is generated. Cells in the SA node (the pacemaker of the heart) normally have the fastest phase 4 activity within the heart. The spontaneously occurring action potentials in the SA node are propagated as described earlier, resulting in normal sinus rhythm. If, for any reason, the automaticity of the sinus node should fail, there are usually secondary pacemaker cells (often located in the AV junction) to take over the pacemaker function of the heart, but at a slower rate.

Thus, the shape of the action potential determines the conduction velocity, refractory period, and automaticity of cardiac tissue. Later we shall see how these three electrophysiologic characteristics directly affect the mechanisms of cardiac rhythms, both normal and abnormal. To a large extent, the purpose of the electrophysiology study is to assess the conduction velocities, refractory periods, and automaticity of various portions of the heart's electrical system.

Localized variations in the heart's electrical system

In understanding cardiac arrhythmias, it is important to consider two issues involving localized differences in the heart's electrical system: variations in the action potential and variations in autonomic innervation.

Localized differences in the action potential

The cardiac action potential does not have the same shape in every cell of the heart's electrical system. The action potential we have been using as a model (see Figure 1.2) is a typical Purkinje fiber action potential. Figure 1.4 shows representative action potentials from several key locations of the heart—note the differences in shape.

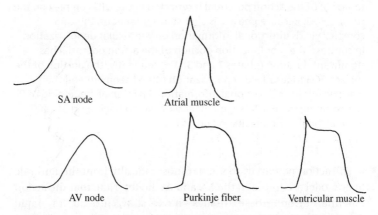

Figure 1.4 Localized differences in the cardiac action potential. Cardiac action potentials from different locations within the heart have different shapes. These differences account for the differences seen in the electrophysiologic properties of various tissues within the heart.

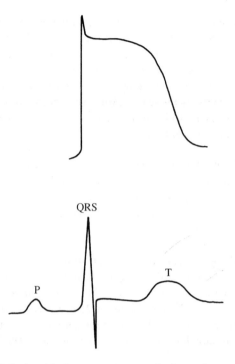

Figure 1.5 Relationship between the ventricular action potential (*top*) and the surface ECG (*bottom*). The rapid depolarization phase (phase 0) of the action potential is reflected in the QRS complex on the surface ECG. Because phase 0 is almost instantaneous, the QRS complex yields directional information on ventricular depolarization. In contrast, the repolarization portion of the action potential has significant duration (phases 2 and 3). Consequently, the portion of the surface ECG that reflects repolarization (the ST segment and the T wave) yields little directional information. PR interval, beginning of P to beginning of QRS; ST segment, end of QRS to beginning of T; QT interval, beginning of QRS to end of T.

The action potentials that differ most radically from the Purkinje fiber model are found in the SA and AV nodes. Note that the action potentials from these tissues have slow instead of rapid depolarization phases (phase 0). This slow depolarization occurs because SA and AV nodal tissues lack the rapid sodium channels responsible for the rapid depolarization phase (phase 0) seen in other cardiac tissues. In fact, the SA and AV nodes are thought to be entirely dependent on the slow calcium channel for depolarization.

Because the speed of depolarization determines conduction velocity, the SA and AV nodes conduct electrical impulses slowly. The slow conduction in the AV node is reflected in the PR interval on the surface ECG (see Figure 1.5).

Localized differences in autonomic innervation   Fast

In general, an increase in sympathetic tone causes enhanced automaticity (pacemaker cells fire more rapidly), increased conduction velocity (electrical impulses are propagated more rapidly), and decreased action-potential duration and thus decreased refractory periods (cells become ready for repeated depolarizations more quickly). Parasympathetic tone has the opposite effect (i.e. depressed automaticity, decreased conduction velocity, and increased refractory periods).

Sympathetic and parasympathetic fibers richly innervate both the SA and the AV node. In the remainder of the heart's electrical system, while sympathetic innervation is abundant, parasympathetic innervation is relatively sparse. Thus, changes in parasympathetic tone have a relatively greater effect on the SA and AV nodal tissues than on other tissues of the heart. This fact has implications for the diagnosis and treatment of some heart-rhythm disturbances.

Relationship between action potential and surface ECG

The cardiac action potential represents the electrical activity of a single cardiac cell. The surface ECG reflects the electrical activity of the entire heart—essentially, it represents the sum of all the action potentials of all cardiac cells. Consequently, the information one can glean from the surface ECG derives from the characteristics of the action potential (Figure 1.5).

For most cardiac cells, the depolarization phase of the action potential is essentially instantaneous (occurring in 1–3 msec) and occurs sequentially, from cell to cell. Thus, the instantaneous wave of depolarization can be followed across the heart by studying the ECG. The P wave represents the depolarization front as it traverses the atria, and the QRS complex tracks the wave of depolarization as it spreads across the ventricles. Changes in the spread of the electrical impulse, such as occur in bundle branch block or in transmural myocardial infarction, can be readily diagnosed. Because the depolarization phase of the action potential is relatively instantaneous, the P wave and the QRS complex can yield specific directional information (i.e. information on the sequence of depolarization of cardiac muscle).

In contrast, the repolarization phase of the action potential is not instantaneous—indeed, repolarization has significant duration. Thus, while depolarization occurs from cell to cell sequentially, repolarization occurs in many cardiac cells simultaneously. For this reason, the ST segment and T wave (the portions of the surface ECG that reflect ventricular repolarization) give little directional information, and abnormalities in the ST segments and T waves are most often (and quite properly) interpreted as being nonspecific. The QT interval represents the time of repolarization of the ventricular myocardium and reflects the average action-potential duration of ventricular muscle.

2 Abnormal Heart Rhythms

Abnormalities in the electrical system of the heart result in two general types of cardiac arrhythmia: heart rhythms that are too slow (bradyarrhythmias) and heart rhythms that are too fast (tachyarrhythmias). To understand the use of the electrophysiology study in evaluating cardiac arrhythmias, one needs a basic understanding of the mechanisms of these arrhythmias.

Bradyarrhythmias

There are two broad categories of abnormally slow heart rhythms— the failure of pacemaker cells to generate appropriate electrical impulses (disorders of automaticity) and the failure to propagate electrical impulses appropriately (heart block).

Failure of impulse generation

Failure of SA nodal automaticity, resulting in an insufficient number of electrical impulses emanating from the SA node (i.e. sinus bradycardia (Figure 2.1)), is the most common cause of bradyarrhythmias. If the slowed heart rate is insufficient to meet the body's demands, symptoms result. Symptomatic sinus bradycardia is called *sick sinus syndrome*. If sinus slowing is profound, subsidiary pacemakers located near the AV junction can take over the pacemaker function of the heart. The electrophysiology study, as we will see in Chapter 5, can be useful in assessing SA nodal automaticity.

Failure of impulse propagation

The second major cause of bradyarrhythmias is the failure of the electrical impulses generated by the SA node (or by subsidiary atrial pacemakers) to conduct normally to the ventricles. This condition, known as *heart block* or *AV block*, implies an abnormality of conduction velocity and/or refractoriness in the conducting system.

Electrophysiologic Testing, Fifth Edition. Richard N. Fogoros.
© 2012 John Wiley & Sons, Ltd. Published 2012 by John Wiley & Sons, Ltd.

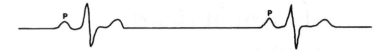

Figure 2.1 Sinus bradycardia.

Because conduction of the electrical impulse to the ventricles depends on the function of the AV node and the His–Purkinje system, heart block is virtually always due to AV nodal or His–Purkinje disease.

Heart block is classified into three categories based on severity (Figure 2.2). First-degree AV block means that, while all atrial impulses are transmitted to the ventricles, intraatrial conduction, conduction through the AV node, and/or conduction through the His bundle is slow (manifested on the ECG by a prolonged PR interval). Second-degree AV block means that conduction to the ventricles is intermittent; that is, some impulses are conducted and some are blocked. Third-degree AV block means that block is complete and no atrial impulses are conducted to the ventricles.

If third-degree AV block is present then sustaining life depends on the function of subsidiary pacemakers distal to the site of block.

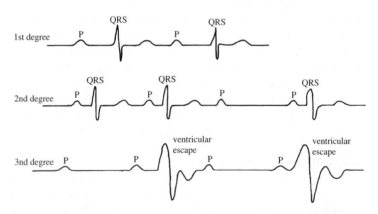

Figure 2.2 Three categories of heart block. In first-degree block (*top tracing*), all atrial impulses are conducted to the ventricles, but conduction is slow (the PR interval is prolonged). In second-degree block (*middle tracing*), some atrial impulses are conducted and some are not. In third-degree block (*bottom tracing*), none of the atrial impulses are conducted to the ventricles.

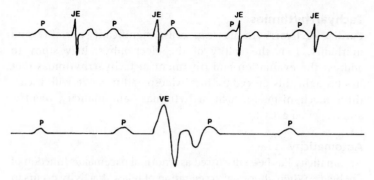

Figure 2.3 Examples of escape pacemakers. When block is localized to the AV node (*top tracing*), junctional escape pacemakers (JE) are usually stable enough to prevent hemodynamic collapse. When block is located in the distal conducting tissues (*bottom tracing*), escape pacemakers are usually located in the ventricles (VE) and are slower and much less stable.

The competence of these subsidiary pacemakers, and therefore the patient's prognosis, depends largely on the site of block (Figure 2.3). When block is within the AV node, subsidiary pacemakers at the AV junction usually take over the pacemaker function of the heart, resulting in a relatively stable, non-life-threatening heart rhythm, with a rate often in excess of 50 beats/min. On the other hand, if block is distal to the AV node, the subsidiary pacemakers tend to produce a profoundly slow (usually less than 40 beats/min) and unstable heart rhythm.

If heart block is less than complete (i.e. first- or second-degree), it is still important to pinpoint the site of block to either the AV node or the His–Purkinje system. First- or second-degree block in the AV node is benign and tends to be nonprogressive. Thus, implanting a permanent pacemaker is rarely required. First- and especially second-degree block distal to the AV node, on the other hand, tends to progress to a higher degree of block; prophylactic pacing is often indicated.

Differentiating the site of heart block requires careful evaluation. This evaluation can usually be made noninvasively by studying the surface ECG and taking advantage of the fact the AV node has rich autonomic innervation and the His–Purkinje system does not. Sometimes, however, the electrophysiology study is useful in locating the site of block. Chapter 5 considers heart block in detail.

Tachyarrhythmias

Cardiac tachyarrhythmias can cause significant mortality and morbidity. It is the ability of the electrophysiology study to address the evaluation and treatment of tachyarrhythmias that has brought this procedure into widespread use. We will discuss three mechanisms for tachyarrhythmias—automaticity, reentry, and triggered activity.

Automaticity

Automaticity has been discussed as a normal pacemaker function of the heart. When abnormal acceleration of phase 4 activity occurs in some location of the heart, an automatic tachyarrhythmia is said to occur (Figure 2.4). Such an abnormal automatic focus can appear in the atria, the AV junction, or the ventricles (thus leading to automatic atrial, junctional, or ventricular tachycardia).

Automaticity is not a common cause of tachyarrhythmias, probably accounting for less than 10% of all abnormal tachyarrhythmias. Automatic tachyarrhythmias are usually recognizable by their characteristics and the settings in which they occur.

In gaining an understanding of the automatic tachyarrhythmias, it is helpful to consider the characteristics of sinus tachycardia, which is a *normal* automatic tachycardia. Sinus tachycardia usually occurs as a result of appropriately increased sympathetic tone (for instance, in response to increased metabolic needs during exercise). When sinus tachycardia develops, the heart rate gradually increases from the basic (resting) sinus rate; when sinus tachycardia subsides, the rate likewise decreases gradually.

Similarly, automatic tachyarrhythmias often display a warm-up and warm-down in rate when the arrhythmia begins and ends. Analogous to sinus tachycardia, automatic tachyarrhythmias also

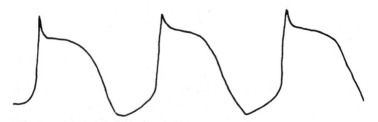

Figure 2.4 Abnormal automaticity causes the rapid generation of action potentials and thus inappropriate tachycardia.

often have metabolic causes, such as acute cardiac ischemia, hypoxemia, hypokalemia, hypomagnesemia, acid–base disorders, high sympathetic tone, and the use of sympathomimetic agents. Therefore, automatic arrhythmias are often seen in acutely ill patients, often in the intensive-care setting, with all the attendant metabolic abnormalities. For example, acute pulmonary disease can lead to multifocal atrial tachycardia, the most common type of automatic atrial tachycardia. Induction of, and recovery from, general anesthesia can cause surges in sympathetic tone, and automatic arrhythmias (both atrial and ventricular) can result. In addition, acute myocardial infarction is often accompanied by early ventricular arrhythmias that are most likely automatic in mechanism.

Of all tachyarrhythmias, automatic arrhythmias most closely resemble an "itch of the heart," and it is tempting to apply the salve of antiarrhythmic drugs. Antiarrhythmic drugs can sometimes decrease automaticity; automatic arrhythmias, however, should be treated primarily by identifying and reversing the underlying metabolic cause.

Automatic tachyarrhythmias cannot be induced by programmed pacing techniques, so these arrhythmias are generally not amenable to provocative study in the electrophysiology laboratory.

Reentry

Reentry is the most common mechanism for tachyarrhythmias; it is also the most important, because reentrant arrhythmias cause the deaths of hundreds of thousands of people every year. Fortunately, reentrant arrhythmias lend themselves nicely to study in the electrophysiology laboratory. It was the recognition that most tachyarrhythmias are reentrant in mechanism and that the electrophysiology study can help significantly in assessing reentrant arrhythmias that led to widespread proliferation of electrophysiology laboratories from the early 1980s onward.

Unfortunately, the mechanism of reentry is not simple to explain or to understand, and the prerequisites for reentry seem on the surface to be unlikely at best. The failure to understand (and possibly to believe in) reentry has helped keep the electrophysiology study an enigma to most people in the medical profession. The following explanation of reentry therefore errs on the side of simplicity and might offend some electrophysiologists. If the reader can keep an open mind and accept this explanation for now, we hope to show later (in Chapters 6 and 7) that reentry is a compelling explanation for most cardiac tachyarrhythmias.

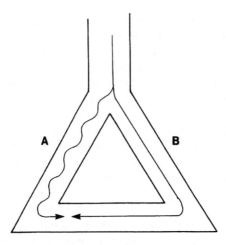

Figure 2.5 Prerequisites for reentry. An anatomic circuit must be present in which two portions of the circuit (pathways A and B in the figure) have electrophysiologic properties that differ from one another in a critical way. In this example, pathway A conducts electrical impulses more slowly than pathway B, while pathway B has a longer refractory period than pathway A.

Reentry requires that the following criteria be met (Figure 2.5). First, two roughly parallel conducting pathways (shown as pathways A and B) must be connected proximally and distally by conducting tissue, thus forming a potential electrical circuit. Second, one of the pathways (pathway B in our example) must have a refractory period that is substantially longer than that of the other pathway. Third, the pathway with the shorter refractory period (pathway A) must conduct electrical impulses more slowly than the other pathway.

If all these seemingly implausible prerequisites are met, reentry can be initiated when an appropriately timed premature impulse is introduced to the circuit (Figure 2.6). The premature impulse must enter the circuit at a time when pathway B (the one with the long refractory period) is still refractory from the previous depolarization and at a time when pathway A (the one with the shorter refractory period) has already recovered and is able to accept the premature impulse. While pathway A slowly conducts the premature impulse, pathway B has a chance to recover. By the time the impulse reaches pathway B from the opposite direction, pathway B is no longer

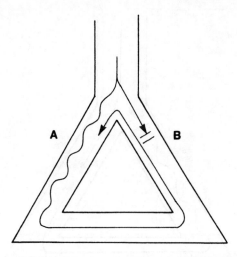

Figure 2.6 Initiation of reentry. If the prerequisites in Figure 2.5 are present, an appropriately timed premature impulse can block in pathway B (which has a relatively long refractory period) while conducting down pathway A. Because conduction down pathway A is slow, pathway B has time to recover, allowing the impulse to conduct retrogradely up pathway B. The impulse can then reenter pathway A. A continuously circulating impulse is thus established.

refractory and is able to conduct the beat in the retrograde direction (upward in the figure). If this retrograde impulse reenters pathway A and is conducted antegradely (as it is likely to be, given the short refractory period of pathway A), a continuously circulating impulse is established, spinning around and around the reentrant loop. All that remains in order for this reentrant impulse to usurp the rhythm of the heart is for the impulse to exit from the circuit at some point during each lap and thereby depolarize the myocardium outside of the loop.

Just as reentry can be initiated by premature beats, it can be terminated by premature beats (Figure 2.7). An appropriately timed impulse can enter the circuit during reentry and collide with the reentrant impulse, thus abolishing the reentrant arrhythmia.

Because reentry depends on critical differences in conduction velocities and refractory periods in the various pathways of the reentrant circuit, and because conduction velocity and refractory periods are determined by the shape of the action potential, it should be obvious that the action potentials in pathway A and

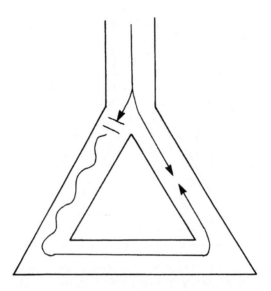

Figure 2.7 Termination of reentry. An appropriately timed premature impulse can enter the circuit during a reentrant tachycardia, collide with the reentrant impulse as shown, and terminate reentry.

pathway B are different from one another. This means furthermore that drugs that change the shape of the action potential might be useful in the treatment of reentrant arrhythmias.

Reentrant circuits occur with some frequency in the human heart. Some reentrant circuits are present at birth, especially those causing supraventricular tachycardias (e.g. reentry associated with AV bypass tracts or with dual SA and AV nodal tracts). More malignant forms of reentrant circuit, however, are usually not congenital but are acquired as cardiac disease develops during life. In reentrant ventricular tachyarrhythmias, the reentrant circuits arise in areas where normal cardiac tissue is interspersed with patches of scar tissue, forming many potential anatomic circuits. Thus, ventricular reentrant circuits usually occur only when scar tissue develops in the ventricles (such as during a myocardial infarction or with cardiomyopathic diseases).

Theoretically, if all the anatomic and electrophysiologic criteria for reentry are present, any impulse that enters the circuit at the appropriate time will induce a reentrant tachycardia. The time from the end of the refractory period of pathway A to the end of the refractory period of pathway B, during which reentry can be induced, is called the *tachycardia zone*. Treating reentrant arrhythmias sometimes involves trying to narrow or abolish the tachycardia zone (by increasing the refractory period of pathway A or decreasing the refractory period of pathway B).

Because reentrant arrhythmias can be reproducibly induced and terminated with appropriately timed impulses, reentrant arrhythmias are ideal for study in the electrophysiology laboratory. In fact, it is mainly the inducibility of reentrant arrhythmias that distinguishes them from automatic arrhythmias in the electrophysiology lab. By inducing reentrant arrhythmias in a controlled setting, the location of the anatomic circuit can be mapped and the effect of various therapies assessed.

Triggered activity

Electrophysiologists try to divide the universe of tachyarrhythmias into two parts—automatic arrhythmias (which cannot be induced in the laboratory) and reentrant arrhythmias (which can be induced). This is a useful and practical way of thinking about tachyarrhythmias. Simple and convenient classification systems are usually wrong, however, and this classification system is no exception.

There are other mechanisms for tachyarrhythmias, no doubt including some that have not yet been identified. While most of these other mechanisms can safely be ignored, at least one appears commonly in the clinical setting—triggered activity.

Triggered activity has some features of both automaticity and reentry and can be difficult to distinguish in the electrophysiology laboratory. Like automaticity, triggered activity involves the leakage of positive ions into the cardiac cell, leading to a bump on the action potential (Figure 2.8a) in late phase 3 or early phase 4. This bump is called an *afterdepolarization*. If these afterdepolarizations are of sufficient magnitude to engage the rapid sodium channels (i.e. if they reach the threshold voltage), another action potential can be generated (Figure 2.8b). Thus, triggered activity resembles automaticity in that new action potentials can be generated by leakage of positive ions into the cell. Many electrophysiologists classify triggered activity as a subgroup of automaticity.

Unlike automaticity (and like reentry), however, triggered activity is not always spontaneous (and therefore not truly automatic). Triggered activity can be provoked by premature beats. Thus, triggered activity, like reentry, can be induced with programmed pacing techniques.

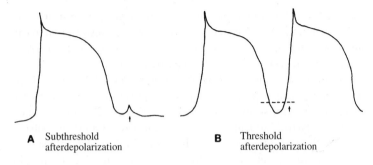

A Subthreshold
afterdepolarization

B Threshold
afterdepolarization

Figure 2.8 Triggered activity. (a) In some circumstances, premature cardiac action potentials will display a late bump (called an afterdepolarization). (b) If the afterdepolarization is of sufficient magnitude, the rapid sodium channels are engaged and a second action potential is generated.

Theoretically, because it can be induced during electrophysiologic testing, triggered activity poses a potential threat to the use of the inducibility of an arrhythmia as the major criterion for diagnosing a reentrant mechanism. If an arrhythmia is induced, the following have been proposed as ways of differentiating between reentry and triggered activity: triggered activity resembles automaticity in displaying warm-up and warm-down; triggered activity is felt to depend on calcium channels and thus may respond to calcium-channel blockers; in distinction to most reentrant arrhythmias, inducing arrhythmias due to triggered activity may require introducing a pause into the sequence of paced beats used for induction (such arrhythmias, called "pause-dependent" arrhythmias, will be discussed in Chapter 7); reentry is the more likely mechanism in the presence of underlying structural cardiac disease.

The clinical significance of triggered activity has become more clear in recent years. Triggered activity is most likely the mechanism for digitalis-toxic supraventricular and ventricular arrhythmias, as well as for some of the rare cases of ventricular tachycardia that respond to calcium-blocking agents. More importantly, triggered activity is now thought to be the mechanism of torsades de pointes—the polymorphic, pause-dependent ventricular arrhythmias often associated with the use of certain antiarrhythmic drugs.

Triggered activity as a cause of ventricular arrhythmias will be discussed more fully in Chapter 7.

3 Treatment of Arrhythmias

Pharmacologic therapy

Antiarrhythmic drugs are not arrhythmia suppressants in the same way that menthol is a cough suppressant. They do not work by soothing irritable areas. In fact, most antiarrhythmic drugs work merely by changing the shape of the cardiac action potential. By changing the action potential, these drugs alter the conductivity and refractoriness of cardiac tissue. Thus, it is hoped, the drugs will change the critical electrophysiologic characteristics of reentrant circuits to make reentry less likely to occur.

Channels and gates

Antiarrhythmic drugs are thought to affect the shape of the action potential by altering the channels that control ionic fluxes across the cardiac cell membrane. The class I antiarrhythmic drugs, which affect the rapid sodium channel, provide the clearest example (Figure 3.1).

The rapid sodium channel is controlled by two gates: the m gate and the h gate. In the resting state (a), the m gate is closed and the h gate is open. When an appropriate stimulus occurs, the m gate opens (b) and positively charged sodium ions rush into the cell rapidly, causing the cell to depolarize (phase 0 of the action potential). After a few milliseconds, the h gate slams shut (c), closing the sodium channel and ending phase 0.

Class I antiarrhythmic drugs work by binding to the h gate, making it behave as if it were partially closed (d). In this case, when the m gate is stimulated to open, the opening through which sodium ions enter the cell is narrower (e). Consequently, it takes longer to depolarize the cell (i.e. the slope of phase 0 is decreased). Because the speed of depolarization determines how quickly adjacent cells will depolarize (and therefore the speed of impulse propagation),

Electrophysiologic Testing, Fifth Edition. Richard N. Fogoros.
© 2012 John Wiley & Sons, Ltd. Published 2012 by John Wiley & Sons, Ltd.

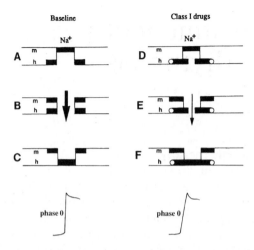

Figure 3.1 The effect of class I drugs on the rapid sodium channel. (a) through (c) display the baseline (drug-free) state. In (a), the resting state, the m gate is closed and the h gate is open. The cell is stimulated in (b), causing the m gate to open, thus allowing positively charged sodium ions to enter the cell rapidly (*large arrow*). In (c), the h gate shuts and sodium transport stops (i.e. phase 0 ends). (d) and (e) display the effect of adding a class I antiarrhythmic drug (*open circles*). (d) shows the class I drug binding to the h gate, making it behave as if it were partially closed. When the cell is stimulated in (e), the m gate still opens normally, but the channel through which sodium ions enter the cell is narrower and sodium transport is slower. It subsequently takes longer to reach the end of phase 0 (f), and the slope of phase 0 is decreased.

class I drugs as a group tend to decrease the conduction velocity of cardiac tissue.

Although their precise sites of action have not all been worked out, most antiarrhythmic drugs act in a similar fashion: that is, by altering the function of the various channels that control transport of ions across cardiac cell membranes. The resultant changes in the cardiac action potential (Figure 3.2) cause changes in the conduction velocity, refractoriness, and automaticity of cardiac tissue, and also provide the basis for the classification of antiarrhythmic drugs.

Classification of antiarrhythmic drugs

Table 3.1 lists the most frequently used classification system for antiarrhythmic drugs.

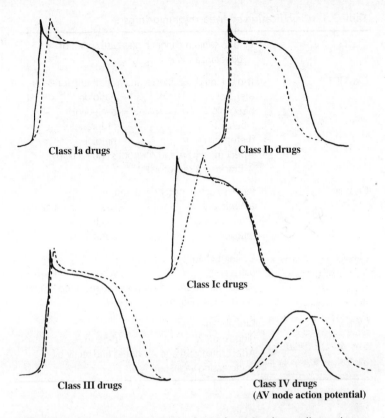

Figure 3.2 The effect of antiarrhythmic drugs on the cardiac action potential. The solid lines represent the baseline action potential and the dotted lines represent the changes that result in the action potential when various classes of antiarrhythmic drug are given. The Purkinje fiber action potential is shown, except in the case of class IV drugs, for which the AV nodal action potential is depicted.

Class I is reserved for drugs that block the rapid sodium channel (as shown in Figure 3.1). Because drugs assigned to class I block the sodium channel in varying degrees and also have varying effects on action-potential duration, class I is currently broken down into three subgroups (Table 3.2). Class Ia drugs (quinidine, procainamide, and disopyramide) slow conduction velocity and increase refractory periods. Class Ib drugs (lidocaine, tocainide, mexiletine, and phenytoin) actually have little effect on depolarization when used in systemic doses (although in high concentrations these drugs

Table 3.1   Classification of antiarrhythmic drugs

Class I	Bind to sodium channel, decrease speed of depolarization
Class II	β-blocking drugs, decrease sympathetic tone
	atenolol nadolol
	bisoprolol carvedilol
	labetolol propranolol
	metoprolol timolol
	Affect mainly SA and AV nodes (indirectly by blocking β receptors)
Class III	Increase action potential duration
	amiodarone N-acetylprocainamide
	dronedarone sotalol
	ibutilide dofetilide
Class IV	Calcium-channel blockers
	diltiazem verapamil
	Affect mainly SA and AV nodes (direct membrane effect, see Figure 3.2)
Class V	Digitalis agents
	digitoxin digoxin
	Affect mainly SA and AV nodes (indirectly by increasing vagal tone)

Table 3.2   Subclassification of class I antiarrhythmic agents

Class Ia	Quinidine, procainamide, disopyramide
	Slow upstroke of action potential + +
	Prolong duration of action potential + +
	Decrease conductivity, increase refractoriness
Class Ib	Lidocaine, phenytoin, tocainide, mexiletine
	Minimal effect on upstroke of action potential
	Shorten duration of action potential
	Decrease refractoriness
Class Ic	Flecainide, encainide, propafenone, moricizine[a]
	Marked slowing of upstroke of action potential + + + +
	Minimal effect on action potential duration +
	Marked decrease in conductivity, little effect on refractoriness

[a]The classification of moricizine is controversial, and some place it in class Ib. It is placed in class Ic here to emphasize its class Ic-like proarrhythmic potential.

too can block sodium transport—this is why lidocaine is an excellent local anesthetic agent). In systemic doses, class Ib drugs decrease action-potential duration and shorten refractory periods but have little effect on conduction velocity. Class Ic drugs (flecainide, encainide, and propafenone) have a pronounced depressant effect on conduction velocity, with relatively little effect on refractory periods.

β-blocking agents are assigned to class II. These drugs have little direct effect on the action potential and work mainly by decreasing the sympathetic tone.

Class III drugs (amiodarone, dofetilide, dronedarone, ibutilide, N-acetylprocainamide, and sotalol) increase the action-potential duration and therefore refractory periods, and have relatively little effect on the conduction velocity.

Class IV includes the calcium-channel blockers. They mainly affect the SA and AV nodes, because these structures are almost exclusively depolarized by the slow calcium channels.

Class V includes digitalis agents, whose antiarrhythmic effects are related to the increase in parasympathetic activity caused by these drugs.

Effect of antiarrhythmic drugs

Most antiarrhythmic drugs are felt to ameliorate automatic tachyarrhythmias to some extent, although it must again be stressed that the primary treatment for automatic arrhythmias is to remove the underlying cause. Many antiarrhythmic drugs slow the phase 4 ionic fluxes that are responsible for automaticity.

Figure 3.3 shows two examples of how antiarrhythmic drugs may affect reentrant circuits. Figure 3.3a shows a reentrant circuit with the same characteristics as described in Chapter 2. Figure 3.3b illustrates the changes that can occur if a class Ia drug is administered. These drugs increase refractory periods. By further lengthening the already long refractory period of pathway B, the class Ia drugs can convert unidirectional block to bidirectional block, thus chemically amputating one pathway of the reentrant circuit. Figure 3.3c shows what happens if a class Ib drug is given. These drugs shorten the duration of the action potential, thus decreasing the refractory period. In this example, a class Ib drug shortens the refractory period of pathway B, thus rendering the refractory periods in pathways A and B relatively equal. (In other words, the *tachycardia zone* is significantly narrowed.) Without a difference in refractory

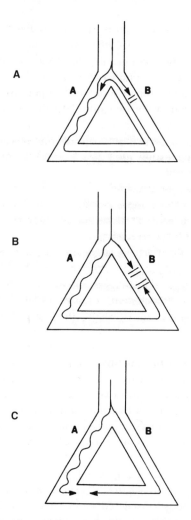

Figure 3.3 Effect of antiarrhythmic drugs on a reentrant circuit. (a) A prototype reentrant circuit (the same as that described in Figures 2.5 and 2.6). (b) Changes that may occur with administration of a class Ia drug. The refractory period of pathway B may be sufficiently prolonged by the drug to prevent reentry from occurring. (c) Changes that may occur with administration of a class Ib drug. The refractory period of pathway B may be shortened, so that the refractory periods of pathways A and B are nearly equal. A premature impulse would then be more likely to either conduct or block down both pathways, thus preventing the initiation of reentry.

periods between the two pathways of the anatomic circuit, reentry cannot be initiated.

The drug effects illustrated in Figure 3.3 should not be taken literally. The key point in understanding how drugs affect reentry is this: because reentry requires a critical relationship between the refractory periods and the conduction velocities of the two pathways of the reentrant circuit, and because antiarrhythmic drugs alter the refractory periods and conduction velocities, these drugs can make reentry less likely to occur.

Proarrhythmia

Unfortunately, there is another side to that coin. Consider the following scenario: a patient with a previous myocardial infarction and complex ventricular ectopy (but no sustained tachyarrhythmias) has an anatomic circuit whose electrophysiologic characteristics are like those shown in Figure 3.3b. In other words, while the anatomic circuit is present, the electrophysiologic characteristics necessary to activate the circuit are not present. If this patient is placed on a class Ib drug, it is possible to selectively decrease the refractory period of pathway B, giving this circuit the characteristics shown in Figure 3.3a. In other words, the antiarrhythmic drug may make a sustained tachycardia more likely to occur. A similar scenario may develop if a class Ia drug is used in a patient with a circuit resembling the one shown in Figure 3.3c. By increasing the refractory period of pathway B, the benign circuit may be converted to a potentially malignant one. To put it another way, when we administer an antiarrhythmic drug, we may be just as likely to increase as to decrease the tachycardia zone within a potential reentrant circuit—and thus make a sustained arrhythmia more likely instead of less likely.

The phenomenon just described is *proarrhythmia*, or arrhythmia exacerbation. Although proarrhythmia is a common occurrence, for many years it was only poorly recognized by many physicians who used antiarrhythmic drugs. Failure to recognize that drug therapy is actually worsening arrhythmias frequently leads to inappropriate therapy (such as increasing or adding to the offending drug) and sometimes to death. Herein lies the problem with considering antiarrhythmic drugs to be simply arrhythmia suppressants. Proarrhythmia is an inherent property of antiarrhythmic drugs: the mechanism that controls reentrant arrhythmias is the same as that which can worsen arrhythmias.

Unfortunately, whether a drug will improve or worsen an arrhythmia is difficult to predict before actually administering it.

Proarrhythmia, therefore, is a possibility for which one must be vigilant whenever using antiarrhythmic drug therapy.

Drug toxicity

Proarrhythmia is probably the most important, and is certainly the most universal, type of toxicity seen with antiarrhythmic drugs. The form of proarrhythmia just mentioned—that is, the worsening of reentrant arrhythmias—can be seen with any class of antiarrhythmic drug.

In addition, certain antiarrhythmic drugs can produce a second type of proarrhythmia called *torsades de pointes*. Torsades de pointes (which is discussed in more detail in Chapter 7) is a polymorphic, pause-dependent ventricular tachycardia that is associated with prolongation of the QT interval and the subsequent development of triggered activity. (Triggered activity was described briefly in Chapter 2.) Torsades commonly causes syncope and can cause sudden death. It is seen in a subset of otherwise normal individuals—probably 3–4% of the population at large—who are prone to develop triggered activity whenever something acts to prolong their cardiac action potentials. Thus, antiarrhythmic drugs in classes Ia and III tend to cause torsades in such individuals. Table 3.3 lists the

Table 3.3   Relative risk of drug-induced proarrhythmia

Drug	Risk of Exacerbation of Reentry	Risk of Torsades de Pointes
Class Ia		
Quinidine	++	++
Procainamide	++	++
Disopyramide	++	++
Class Ib		
Lidocaine	+	0
Mexiletine	+	0
Phenytoin	+	0
Class Ic		
Flecainide	+++	0
Propafenone	+++	0
Moricizine	+++	+
Class III		
Amiodarone	+	+
Dronedarone	+	+
Sotalol	+	+++
Ibutilide	+	+++
Dofetilide	+	+++

relative risk of drug-induced proarrhythmia of both types for the various antiarrhythmic drugs. Even aside from proarrhythmia, antiarrhythmic drugs as a group are relatively toxic and poorly tolerated. Table 3.4 lists some of the common side effects of antiarrhythmic drugs.

Amiodarone, a class III drug, deserves special recognition as a drug that is uniquely toxic not only among antiarrhythmic drugs but also among all drugs used legally in the United States. Amiodarone has a singular spectrum of toxicities that can be subtle in onset and difficult to recognize and to treat: it can affect virtually every organ system, it is accumulated slowly in many organs (toxicity may be related to cumulative lifetime dose), and its half-life may be

Table 3.4 Common side effects of antiarrhythmic drugs

Hypotension	Negative Inotropy	Bradycardia
IV procainamide	β-blockers	β-blockers
IV quinidine	flecainide	calcium blockers
IV phenytoin	disopyramide	amiodarone
IV bretylium		
CNS Effects	*GI Effects*	*Hepatic Effects*
all class Ib	all drugs, especially quinidine, procainamide & class Ib	amiodarone
amiodarone		phenytoin
β-blockers		dronedarone
flecainide		
Pneumonitis	*Blood Dyscrasias*	*Autonomic Effects*
amiodarone	quinidine	disopyramide
tocainide	tocainide	quinidine
	phenytoin	β-blockers
		digitalis
		sotalol

Other Notable Toxicities
procainamide—drug-induced lupus
amiodarone—peripheral neuropathy, proximal myopathy, skin discoloration, skin photosensitivity, hypothyroidism, hyperthyroidism
disopyramide—urinary hesitancy
dronedarone—increases mortality with heart failure

CNS, central nervous system; GI, gastrointestinal.

as long as 100 days. The only reason amiodarone is used, given this toxic potential, is that it is the most efficacious drug yet developed for the treatment of serious cardiac arrhythmias. In carefully selected patients, the use of amiodarone is appropriate and quite helpful.

Because of the problems associated with the use of antiarrhythmic drugs, as a general rule they should be used only when arrhythmias are significantly symptomatic or life-threatening.

Nonpharmacologic therapy

Reversing the underlying cause for arrhythmias

The treatment of cardiac arrhythmias should always begin with an attempt to identify and treat reversible etiologies for the arrhythmias. To those etiologies already listed (including electrolyte and acid–base disturbances, ischemia, and pulmonary disorders), we must now add antiarrhythmic drugs. A patient with recurrent arrhythmias who is on antiarrhythmic drug therapy should be regarded in the same way as a patient with fever of unknown origin who is on antibiotic therapy—strong consideration should be given to stopping the drug and reassessing the baseline state. Stopping antiarrhythmic drugs will often improve the frequently recurring arrhythmias.

Surgical and ablation therapy

Surgical procedures are frequently helpful in the treatment of arrhythmias. Arrhythmias due to cardiac ischemia often respond to coronary artery bypass surgery. The location of reentrant circuits can be mapped (especially those due to AV bypass tracts and to ventricular tachycardias associated with a discrete ventricular aneurysm) and the reentrant circuit can be disrupted surgically. Transcatheter ablation in the electrophysiology laboratory has largely supplanted most types of arrhythmia surgery and is extremely useful in the management of many supraventricular tachyarrhythmias and some ventricular arrhythmias. (Transcatheter ablation will be discussed in detail in Chapter 8.) All these procedures carry at least some risk of complications.

Device therapy

Permanent artificial pacemakers are the mainstay of treatment for bradyarrhythmias. Permanent pacemakers consist of a source of electrical current that is attached to cardiac muscle (usually to ventricular muscle) by a wire (lead) and is under the control of an integrated circuit (a small computer). If the heart is not generating intrinsic electrical impulses often enough, the pacemaker sends an electrical current down the lead to stimulate it. The current depolarizes the cardiac cells at the tip of the lead (i.e. an action potential is generated) and that depolarization propagates across the myocardium in the normal fashion.

Pacemakers today are increasingly sophisticated and complex. Many features are now programmable, such as the rate of pacing and the energy used with each impulse. Pacemakers are available that guarantee the normal sequence of AV contraction with each heartbeat. Other pacemakers can use some physiologic variable (such as the patient's level of exercise) to judge the optimal heart rate from moment to moment and vary the rate of pacing accordingly. Selecting the appropriate pacemaker for a patient requires extensive knowledge of the technology available.

Devices are also useful for patients with tachyarrhythmias. Many patients with malignant ventricular tachyarrhythmias are now being offered the automatic implantable cardioverter–defibrillator (ICD). This device monitors the heart rhythm constantly and, if a potentially lethal tachyarrhythmia occurs, automatically delivers a large defibrillating current (shock) to the heart to terminate the arrhythmia. The implantable defibrillator has prevented sudden death in thousands of patients who have lethal ventricular arrhythmias. The use of this device, however, can be difficult and patient selection is less straightforward than it might be. (This is discussed in detail in Chapter 7.)

Note: The term decrement to describe rate dependent prolongation of conduction.

The term is used to mean progressive loss of action potential strenth as conduction progresses over a structure until it is insufficient to excite further tissue.

II THE ELECTROPHYSIOLOGY STUDY IN THE EVALUATION AND THERAPY OF CARDIAC ARRHYTHMIAS

4 Principles of the Electrophysiology Study

Read →

The electrophysiology study can be helpful in evaluating a broad spectrum of cardiac arrhythmias. It can help with assessing the function of the SA node, the AV node, and the His–Purkinje system; with determining the characteristics of reentrant arrhythmias; with mapping the location of arrhythmogenic foci for potential ablation; and with evaluating the efficacy of antiarrhythmic drugs and devices.

One might expect a test that can accomplish all this to be extraordinarily complex. On the contrary (although electrophysiologists may not like to admit it), the electrophysiology study is performed by doing two simple things: recording the heart's electrical signals and pacing from localized areas within the heart. Using the information obtained from these relatively simple tasks and keeping in mind the concepts outlined in Part I, one can assess and decide on treatment for a wide array of heart-rhythm disturbances.

In this chapter, we introduce the principles used in performing the electrophysiology study.

Recording and pacing

To discuss intracardiac recording and pacing, we need to introduce two terms that are used by electrophysiologists relating to time measurements. Time measurements are reported in milliseconds (msec, one thousandth of a second), the basic unit of time in electrophysiology.

Cycle length

When electrophysiologists talk about heart rate, they typically speak in terms of cycle length—the length of time between each heartbeat (Figure 4.1a). Thus, the faster the heart rate, the shorter the cycle length: an arrhythmia with a rate of 100 beats/min has a

Electrophysiologic Testing, Fifth Edition. Richard N. Fogoros.
© 2012 John Wiley & Sons, Ltd. Published 2012 by John Wiley & Sons, Ltd.

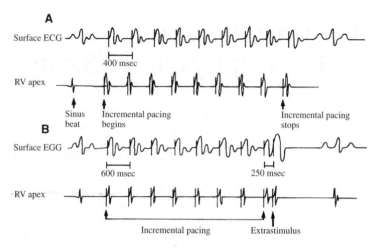

Figure 4.1 Time measurements in the electrophysiology laboratory. This figure depicts pacing from the right ventricular apex. (a) *Cycle length* is the interval of time between heartbeats during either incremental pacing (as in this figure) or a spontaneous rhythm. The cycle length of the incrementally paced beats in (a) is 600 msec. (b) *Coupling interval* is the interval of time between the last normal beat and a premature impulse. In this figure, the normal beats are represented by eight incrementally paced beats at a cycle length of 600 msec. Following the last incrementally paced beat, a single premature stimulus is delivered with a coupling interval of 250 msec.

cycle length of 600 msec, while an arrhythmia with a rate of 300 beats/min has a cycle length of 200 msec. Non-electrophysiologists must pay close attention when discussing heart rate with electrophysiologists, to avoid some amusing miscommunications.

Coupling interval

When using a pacemaker to introduce a premature impulse, the coupling interval is the time between the last normal impulse and the premature impulse (Figure 4.1b). With earlier premature impulses, the coupling interval is shorter; with later premature impulses, the coupling interval is longer.

The electrode catheter

The electrophysiology study is performed by inserting electrode catheters into blood vessels and positioning these catheters in strategic locations within the heart. Once in position, the catheters

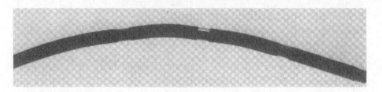

Figure 4.2 The tip of a quadripolar electrode catheter. The electrodes are numbered 1 through 4, the distal (tip) electrode being number 1. The spacing between electrodes is 1 cm.

can be used to perform the two essential tasks of the electrophysiology study: recording the heart's electrical signals and pacing.

Electrode catheters consist of insulated wires; at the distal tip of the catheter (the end inserted into the heart (Figure 4.2)), each wire is attached to an electrode, which is exposed to the intracardiac surface. At the proximal end of the catheter (the part not inserted into the body (Figure 4.3)), each wire is attached to a plug, which can be connected to an external device (such as a recording device or an external pacemaker). Apart from the fact that they usually have more than two electrodes, these catheters are similar to many temporary pacemaker catheters used in emergency rooms and coronary care units. The catheter shown in Figures 4.2 and 4.3 is a quadripolar electrode catheter, the type most commonly used in electrophysiology studies.

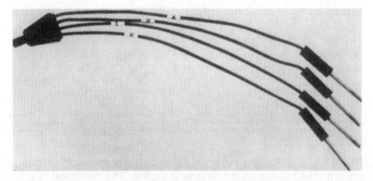

Figure 4.3 The proximal end of a quadripolar electrode catheter. The number on each plug corresponds to the appropriate electrode at the tip of the catheter.

Recording intracardiac electrograms

The recording made of the cardiac electrical activity from an electrode catheter placed in the heart is called an *intracardiac electrogram*. The intracardiac electrogram is essentially an ECG recorded from within the heart. The major difference between a body-surface ECG and an intracardiac electrogram is that the surface ECG gives a summation of the electrical activity of the entire heart, whereas the intracardiac electrogram records only the electrical activity of a localized area of the heart—the cardiac tissue located near the electrodes of the electrode catheter. In general, the intracardiac electrogram records the electrical activity between two of the electrodes (i.e. an electrode pair) at the tip of the catheter. This is called a *bipolar recording configuration*.

The intracardiac electrogram is filtered electronically, so that in general only the rapid depolarization phase of the cardiac tissue (corresponding to phase 0 of the action potential) is recorded. Figure 4.4 shows an intracardiac electrogram recorded from a catheter in the right atrium during normal sinus rhythm. As the wave of depolarization spreading outward from the SA node passes by the catheter, a discrete high-frequency, high-amplitude signal is recorded. This signal indicates the precise moment at which myocardial depolarization occurs at the electrode pair which is being

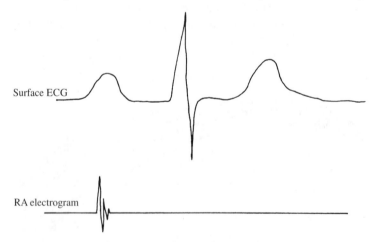

Figure 4.4 Surface ECG and intracardiac electrogram recorded from the high right atrium (RA) during sinus rhythm. The deflection recorded on the RA electrogram reflects the precise moment at which the portion of the right atrium at the tip of the electrode catheter is being depolarized.

used for recording. By having catheters positioned in several different intracardiac locations, one can accurately measure the conduction time from one location to another. Further, if enough catheter positions are used, one can map the sequence of myocardial depolarization as an electrical impulse traverses the heart.

In summary, the deflection recorded from the electrode catheter represents depolarization of the cardiac tissue in the immediate vicinity of the catheter's electrodes. Thus, the intracardiac electrogram gives precise, localized data on the heart's electrical impulse.

Pacing

The electrode catheter is also used for pacing. To pace, a pulse of electrical current is carried by the electrode catheter from an external pacemaker to the intracardiac surface, where it causes cardiac cells near the catheter's electrodes to depolarize. The depolarization of these cardiac cells is then propagated across the heart, just as an electrical impulse arising in the SA node is propagated. Thus, to pace is to artificially generate a cardiac impulse. By careful positioning of the electrode catheter, one can initiate electrical impulses from almost any desired intracardiac location.

During the electrophysiology study, pacing is used to introduce premature electrical impulses, delivered in predetermined patterns and at precisely timed intervals. Such pacing is called *programmed stimulation*.

There are several reasons for performing programmed stimulation. Precisely timed premature impulses allow us to measure the refractory periods of cardiac tissue. By introducing premature impulses in one location and recording electrograms in other locations, one can assess the conduction properties of the intervening cardiac tissue and the pattern of myocardial activation. Programmed stimulation can also help to assess the automaticity of an automatic focus and to study the presence and characteristics of reentrant circuits.

Programmed stimulation consists of two general types of pacing: incremental and extrastimulus (Figure 4.5).

Incremental pacing (or burst pacing) consists of introducing a train of paced impulses at a fixed cycle length. The incremental train may last for a few beats or for several minutes.

The *extrastimulus* technique consists of introducing one or more premature impulses (called extrastimuli), each at its own specific coupling interval. The first extrastimulus is introduced at a coupling interval timed either from an intrinsic cardiac impulse or from the last of a short train of incrementally paced impulses. (This train is

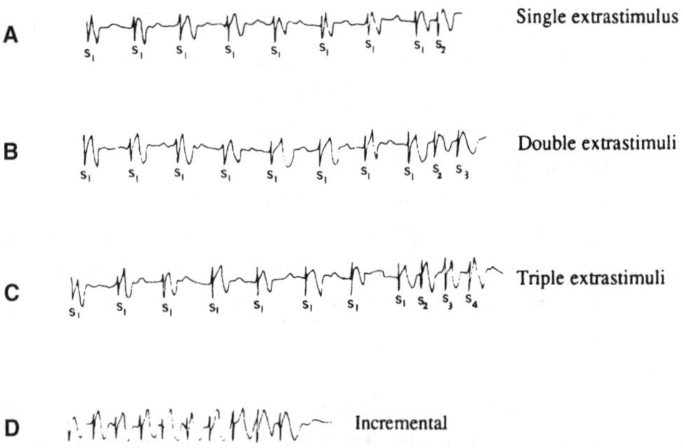

Figure 4.5 Extrastimulus and incremental pacing. Right ventricular pacing is depicted. (a) Extrastimulus pacing involves introducing one or more extrastimuli either during the patient's spontaneous rhythm or (as depicted here) following a train of impulses delivered at a fixed cycle length. This panel shows a single extrastimulus. The fixed-cycle-length impulses from which the extrastimuli are timed are referred to as the S1 beats. The first extrasimulus is labeled S2. (b) Same as in (a), except that a second extrastimulus is delivered (labeled S3). (c) Same as in (a) and (b), except that a third extrastimulus is delivered (labeled S4). (d) Incremental pacing consists of a train of paced impulses at a fixed cycle length. The S1 beats in (a) through (c) are incrementally paced impulses.

usually eight beats in duration, owing to tradition rather than to scientific reasons.) The generally accepted nomenclature for the extrastimulus technique is illustrated in Figure 4.5. The term "S1" (stimulus 1) is used for the incrementally paced impulses or the intrinsic beat from which the first extrastimulus is timed; "S2" is used for the first programmed extrastimulus; "S3" stands for the second programmed extrastimulus; and so on. This nomenclature (in which, for example, the number 2 is attached to the first extra-stimulus) causes a lot of confusion among the uninitiated.

Performance of the electrophysiology study

The physical setup of the electrophysiology laboratory
The electrophysiology study is a type of heart catheterization, and much of the equipment necessary for electrophysiologic testing can be found in a general cardiac catheterization laboratory. This includes a fluoroscopic unit, a radiographic table, a physiologic

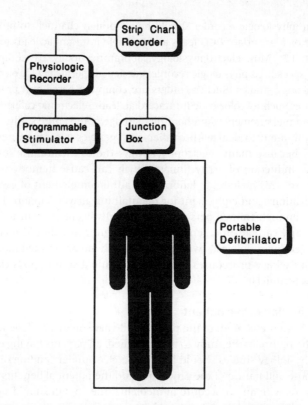

Figure 4.6 Schematic for the layout of a typical electrophysiology laboratory.

recorder, oscilloscopes, instrumentation for gaining vascular access, and emergency equipment. Equipment required specifically for electrophysiologic testing includes a programmable stimulator, a multichannel lead switching box (a junction box), and electrode catheters. An arrangement for a typical electrophysiology laboratory is shown in Figure 4.6.

The programmable stimulator is a specialized pacing unit built especially for electrophysiology studies. It has the capability to introduce complex sequences of paced beats with an accuracy of within 1 msec. It can also synchronize pacing to the intrinsic heart rhythm and can pace multiple intracardiac sites simultaneously.

The junction box allows the laboratory personnel to control the connections from the electrode catheters to the various recording and pacing devices. With a series of switches, multiple electrode pairs from multiple catheters can be sorted out for recording and pacing.

The physiologic recorder should have enough channels to process three or four surface ECG leads and multiple intracardiac leads (often up to 12). Most electrophysiology laboratories today are equipped with specialized physiologic recorders designed specifically for electrophysiology studies. Such recorders are computer-based and provide features such as color-coded intracardiac leads, electronic calipers for precise measurements, and hard-disk storage of the entire study.

Equipment to deal with cardiac emergencies is essential, especially because many electrophysiology studies include the intentional induction of arrhythmias, which can cause hemodynamic collapse. This includes a defibrillator, a full complement of cardiac medications, and equipment for maintaining airway support. Likewise, enough trained personnel should always be present to deal with any cardiac emergency. As a minimum, this should include the electrophysiologist, two cardiac nurses who are trained in electrophysiologic procedures (or one nurse and a second physician), and a technician.

Preparation of the patient

Although preparation of the patient will vary somewhat depending on the nature of the study to be performed, all patients having electrophysiology studies should be given a clear understanding of the purpose and nature of the procedure and the potential benefits and risks. As with any procedure in medicine, the patient should sign a statement of informed consent prior to the study.

Ideally, the electrophysiologic evaluation should be performed while the patient is in a baseline state—non-essential drugs should be withdrawn (especially antiarrhythmic agents), any cardiac ischemia or heart failure maximally treated, electrolytes controlled, and every effort made to prevent excessive anxiety, which can cause excessive sympathetic tone. Anxiety is most easily kept to an acceptable level by adequately preparing the patient for what to expect in the electrophysiology laboratory.

Any cardiac catheterization procedure can cause potentially dangerous arrhythmias, but patients having electrophysiology studies need to be especially aware of this possibility. In particular, patients who are having studies for known or suspected ventricular tachyarrhythmias should be psychologically prepared for the possibility that induction of an arrhythmia might produce loss of consciousness and require defibrillation. Fortunately, the efficacy of electrophysiologic testing and the remarkable safety record achieved in most laboratories go a long way toward allaying the fears of most patients and their families. Detailed discussions with the patient serve not only to guarantee truly informed consent but also to alleviate the patient's anxiety and build his or her confidence in the electrophysiologist.

Insertion and positioning of electrode catheters

The patient is brought to the catheterization laboratory in the fasting state, and the catheterization sites are prepared and draped. The majority of electrophysiology studies can be performed from the venous side of the vascular system, thus precluding the necessity of catheterizing the arterial tree. Under sterile conditions and after local anesthesia is given, catheters are inserted in most instances percutaneously by the modified Seldinger technique (a needle-stick technique that does not require a cutdown). Only extremely rarely do patients need to be placed under general anesthesia to perform an electrophysiology study; however, premedication with a benzodiazepine is sometimes used in patients who are extremely anxious. Most often, catheters are inserted into the femoral veins (two catheters can safely be inserted into the same femoral vein). Catheters may be inserted from the upper extremities for one of several reasons: for more complicated studies, which require multiple catheters; when there is a contraindication to the use of the femoral veins; when a catheter will be left in place at the end of the procedure; or when positioning of the catheter is easier from the upper extremities (such as in coronary sinus catheterization). In these cases, the internal or external jugular veins, the subclavian veins, or the brachial veins may be used. In those instances where access to the left ventricle is required, the femoral-arterial approach is used most often. In many laboratories, a small catheter is routinely inserted into an artery for continuous monitoring of blood pressure.

Under fluoroscopic guidance, the catheters are placed into the proper intracardiac positions. For a simple diagnostic study, generally one catheter is positioned in the high right atrium and the second catheter is placed in the His position (described later). One of these catheters can later be moved to the right ventricle if ventricular pacing is required. For studies of supraventricular tachycardias, additional catheters are commonly placed in the right ventricle and the coronary sinus (thus allowing recordings from all four major cardiac chambers and from the His position).

In the right atrium, catheters are most commonly positioned in the high lateral wall, near the junction of the superior vena cava. This position approximates the location of the SA node and is the region of the atrium that is depolarized earliest during normal sinus rhythm. Pacing from this area results in P wave configurations that are similar to normal sinus beats.

Pacing and recording from the left atrium are usually accomplished by inserting an electrode catheter into the coronary sinus (Figure 4.7). The os of the coronary sinus lies posterior and slightly

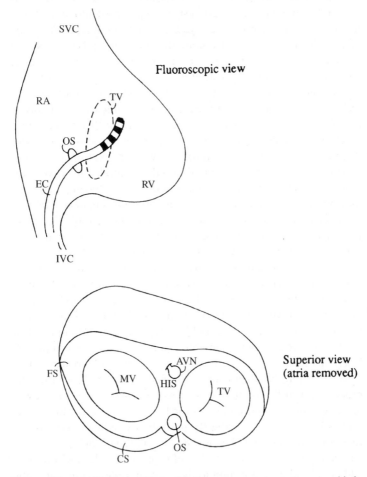

Figure 4.7 A catheter positioned in the coronary sinus can record left atrial and left ventricular electrograms because the coronary sinus lies in the AV groove between the left atrium and the left ventricle. AVN, AV node; CS, coronary sinus; EC, electrode catheter; FS, fibrous skeleton of the heart; HIS, His bundle; IVC, inferior vena cava; MV, mitral valve; OS, os of the coronary sinus; RA, right atrium; RV, right ventricle; SVC, superior vena cava; TV, tricuspid valve.

inferior to the tricuspid valve and is most easily entered from a superior approach (i.e. from the upper extremities). The coronary sinus itself lies in the AV groove—that is, between the left atrium and the left ventricle. Thus, deflections from both the left atrium and the left ventricle are easily recorded from a catheter positioned in the coronary sinus. Pacing the left atrium from the coronary sinus is accomplished routinely—only rarely can the left ventricle be paced from this position. Although a patent foramen ovale will sometimes allow direct entry into the left atrium, we prefer to use the coronary sinus to avoid the slight possibility of causing an embolus in the systemic circulation.

Electrode catheters in the right ventricle are usually positioned in the apex for recording and the apex or the outflow tract for pacing.

Placing electrode catheters in the left ventricle is not part of the standard electrophysiology study. When it is necessary to do so (e.g. when ablation procedures require access to the left ventricle or left atrium), vascular access is usually gained through one of the femoral arteries, although some electrophysiologists have become adept at entering the left side of the heart transseptally from the right atrium.

The *His-bundle electrogram* is the recording that gives the most information about AV conduction. To record the His-bundle electrogram, an electrode catheter is passed across the posterior aspect of the tricuspid valve (near the penetration of the His bundle into the fibrous skeleton (Figure 4.8)). The catheter is maneuvered while continuously recording electrograms from several electrode pairs (so that the best pair for recording can be selected), until an electrogram similar to the one shown in Figure 4.8 is seen. The electrode pair that records the His electrogram is thus placed in a strategic location. It straddles the important structures of the AV conduction system and allows one to record the electrical activity of the low right atrium, the AV node, the His bundle, and a portion of the right ventricle—all from one electrode pair.

Once the catheters are in position, the various electrode pairs are set up for recording and pacing. The leads recorded include various surface ECG leads and intracardiac electrograms from each electrode catheter. Figure 4.9 shows a typical baseline recording for a typical baseline electrophysiology study, displaying surface ECG leads I, II, and V_1 (thus providing a lateral, an inferior, and an anterior lead from which to assess the QRS axis), as well as leads from two intracardiac catheters (high right atrium and His positions). For ventricular recording and pacing, the right atrial catheter is moved to the right ventricle after atrial pacing is completed.

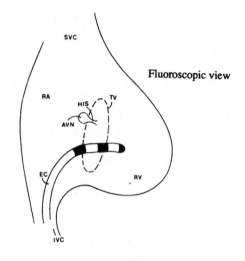

Fluoroscopic view

His electrogram

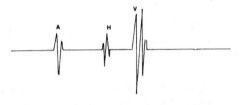

Figure 4.8 Positioning of the His-bundle catheter. The His-bundle electrogram is recorded from a catheter that lies across the posterior aspect of the tricuspid valve. Abbreviations are the same as in Figure 4.7. See Chapter 5 for a description of "A," "H," and "V" spikes on the His electrogram.

Read

The basic electrophysiology protocol

The protocol used in electrophysiology studies varies according to the specific type of procedure being performed, but most electrophysiologic procedures follow the same general outline:

1. Measurement of baseline conduction intervals.
2. Atrial pacing:
   a. assessment of SA nodal automaticity and conductivity;
   b. assessment of AV nodal conductivity and refractoriness;

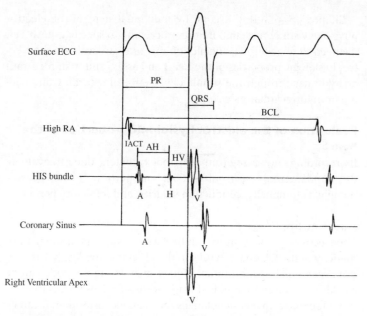

Figure 4.9 Typical baseline recording of intracardiac electrograms. In this figure, one surface ECG lead is shown, as well as intracardiac electrograms from the high right atrium (RA), His bundle, coronary sinus, and right ventricular apex. Conduction intervals are as follows: BCL (basic cycle length) is the interval between successive A waves (measured from the RA catheter); PR interval is the time from the beginning of the P wave to the beginning of the QRS complex (measured from the surface ECG); QRS duration is the width of the QRS complex on the surface ECG; IACT (intraatrial conduction time) is the interval from the SA node to the AV node and is measured from the beginning of the P wave on the surface ECG to the A deflection on the His-bundle electrogram. The AH and HV intervals are discussed in detail in Chapter 5.

    c. assessment of His–Purkinje system conductivity and refractoriness;
    d. induction of atrial arrhythmias.
3. Ventricular pacing:
    a. assessment of retrograde conduction;
    b. induction of ventricular arrhythmias.
4. Drug testing.

Chapters 5, 6 and 7 discuss the individual steps of the electrophysiology study in detail. Before proceeding to specifics, however, we need to review the principles of how one can evaluate the electrophysiologic properties of the heart and assess and treat reentrant arrhythmias through the simple expediency of recording and pacing from intracardiac electrodes.

Evaluation of the electrophysiologic properties of the heart

By recording and pacing from electrode catheters, one can evaluate the fundamental electrophysiologic properties of the heart— namely, automaticity, conduction velocity, and refractory periods.

Automaticity

The electrophysiology study can be used to assess the normal automaticity of the SA node, thanks to the phenomenon known as *overdrive suppression*. An automatic focus such as the SA node can be overdriven by a more rapidly firing pacemaker. This means that the more rapid pacemaker depolarizes the SA node faster than it can be depolarized by its intrinsic automaticity. When the overdriving pacemaker stops, there is often a relatively long pause before the SA node recovers and begins depolarizing spontaneously again. The pause induced in an automatic focus by a temporarily overdriving pacemaker is called overdrive suppression.

Overdrive suppression of the SA node is accomplished in the electrophysiology laboratory by pacing the atrium rapidly (thus overdriving the SA node), then suddenly turning off the pacemaker, and measuring how long it takes for the SA node to recover. A diseased SA node tends to have a grossly prolonged recovery time after overdrive pacing. The evaluation of SA nodal dysfunction is covered in detail in Chapter 5.

Overdrive suppression of automatic foci is also clinically relevant when patients are dependent on subsidiary escape pacemakers to sustain life (e.g. patients with complete heart block and ventricular escape rhythms). These subsidiary pacemakers are automatic foci like the SA node and are thus subject to overdrive suppression. If such a patient receives a temporary pacemaker and after a time the temporary pacemaker suddenly loses capture (as temporary pacemakers sometimes do), the patient may be left with a prolonged, possibly fatal asystolic episode due to overdrive suppression of the escape pacemaker. In such patients, careful positioning of the temporary pacemaker to guarantee excellent pacing thresholds in a very stable location is essential, and every precaution must be taken to keep the temporary lead stable (such as enforced bed rest) until a permanent pacemaker can be inserted.

Tachyarrhythmias due to abnormal automaticity (such as automatic ventricular tachycardia due to ischemia) do not lend themselves well to study in the electrophysiology laboratory. Overdrive suppression of such abnormal automatic foci is not a prominent feature and usually cannot be demonstrated. Also, as we have already discussed, automatic arrhythmias cannot be induced during electrophysiologic testing. Thus, the evaluation of automatic tachyarrhythmias is not an indication for an electrophysiology study.

Conduction velocity

Conduction velocity refers to the speed of conduction of an electrical impulse across the heart and, as we have noted, is related to the rate of rise (i.e. the slope) of the depolarization phase (phase 0) of the action potential. By measuring the time it takes for an electrical impulse to travel from one intracardiac location to another (referred to as a *conduction interval*), one can use electrode catheters to assess the conduction velocities of various portions of the cardiac electrical system.

The best example of measuring conduction velocity from intracardiac electrograms is given by the His-bundle electrogram. As noted previously, this electrogram contains signals from all the critical structures of the AV conducting system. Figure 4.8 represents the His-bundle electrogram of a patient in normal sinus rhythm. As shown, the His electrogram contains three major deflections. The first deflection is the A spike. This represents depolarization of the tissue in the low right atrium, just as the electrical impulse enters the AV node. Once in the AV node, the impulse encounters tissue that depolarizes slowly. (As discussed in Chapter 1, the slow depolarization of the AV nodal tissue is a result of the lack of rapid sodium channels in AV nodal cells). Because the depolarization of the AV node is slow, no high-frequency signal is generated, and the passage of the impulse through the AV node does not produce a deflection on the His-bundle electrogram. When the impulse exits the AV node and zips down the His bundle (again encountering rapidly depolarizing cells), the His-bundle deflection (i.e. the H spike) is produced on the electrogram. As the impulse passes distally through the bundle branches and on to the farther reaches of the Purkinje system, it moves away from the recording electrode pair. Because of their distance from the recording electrodes, the Purkinje-fiber depolarizations are not recorded on the His electrogram (although the right bundle branch depolarization is sometimes seen). Finally, as the impulse is spread to the ventricular myocardium, the depolarization of the ventricular muscle near the His catheter produces the V deflection on the His electrogram.

By analyzing the deflections on the His-bundle electrogram, the conduction properties of the major structures of the AV conduction system can be deduced. The conduction interval from the beginning of the A deflection to the beginning of the H deflection (the AH interval) represents the conduction time through the AV node (normally 50–120 msec). The interval from the beginning of the H deflection to the beginning of the V deflection (the HV interval) represents the conduction time through the His–Purkinje system (normally 35–55 msec). Disease in the AV node will often produce a prolongation in the AH interval, whereas disease in the distal conducting system produces a prolongation in the HV interval.

The AH and HV intervals are two of the basic conduction intervals measured at the beginning of the electrophysiology study. Other basic conduction intervals (shown in Figure 4.9) include the basic cardiac cycle length, the QRS duration, the PR interval, and the intraatrial conduction interval. The basic cycle length is the interval between successive atrial impulses as measured in the right atrial catheter (in order to approximate the basic rate of depolarization of the SA node). The PR interval is measured from the surface ECG leads and is defined as the interval from the beginning of the P wave to the beginning of the QRS complex. The QRS duration, the interval from the beginning of the QRS complex to the end of the QRS complex, is also measured from the surface ECG leads. The intraatrial conduction interval approximates the conduction time from the sinus node to the AV node and is measured from the beginning of the P wave on the surface ECG to the beginning of the A spike on the His-bundle electrogram. Note that the intraatrial conduction interval, the AH interval, and the HV interval are the three basic components of the PR interval.

Depending on the type of electrophysiology study being performed and the type of information needed, other conduction intervals may be measured, such as retrograde conduction intervals (from the ventricle to the atrium).

Refractory periods

Thus far, we have defined the refractory period as the period of time after depolarization during which a cell cannot be depolarized again, and we have related the refractory period of a cell to the duration of the action potential. Because we cannot measure a cell's action-potential duration in the electrophysiology laboratory, the refractory period must be redefined in such a way as to make it meaningful in the laboratory setting. Thus, the refractory period of cardiac tissue is defined in terms of the tissue's response to premature paced impulses. Here, electrophysiologists have outdone themselves by defining three different kinds of refractory period: the effective refractory period, the relative refractory period, and the functional refractory period.

The *effective refractory period* (*ERP*; Figure 4.10) is the definition that most closely coincides with our original definition of the refractory period. When introducing a premature impulse, that impulse will fail to propagate through tissue that is refractory. The ERP of a tissue is the longest coupling interval for which a premature impulse fails to propagate through that tissue. In other words, the ERP refers to the latest early impulse that is blocked—if the premature impulse were any later, the tissue would be recovered and would propagate the impulse. In general, the end of ERP occurs sometime during the last third of phase 3 of the action potential.

The *relative refractory period* (*RRP*; Figure 4.10) requires the introduction of a new concept. Recovery from refractoriness turns out to

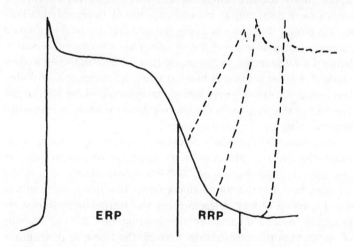

Figure 4.10 Effective and relative refractory periods. During the effective refractory period (ERP), the cell cannot be depolarized. During the relative refractory period (RRP), the cell can be depolarized, but the resultant action potential displays slower phase 0 activity (*dotted lines*).

be a gradual process instead of an instantaneous one. As shown, the end of the ERP occurs during phase 3, before a cell is fully repolarized (that is, before phase 4 begins). If a cardiac cell is stimulated after the end of the ERP but before the cell is fully repolarized, the resulting action potential has a slower upstroke (phase 0) and therefore propagates at a slower conduction velocity. The period of time from the end of the ERP to the beginning of phase 4 is called the RRP. Formally, the RRP of a tissue is the longest coupling interval for which a premature impulse results in slowed conduction through that tissue. At the end of the RRP, the tissue is fully recovered.

At least the ERP and RRP can be related in some way to the duration of the action potential. The *functional refractory period (FRP)* loses even that relationship to our original notion of "refractory period." The FRP of a tissue is the smallest possible time interval between two impulses that can be conducted through that tissue. The FRP is a measure of the output of a tissue. Think of a tiny electrophysiologist standing on the His bundle with a stopwatch, determined to measure the FRP of the AV node. A larger electrophysiologist is pacing the atrium with progressively earlier (i.e. more premature) impulses. The only thing our miniature friend can detect, however, is each electrical impulse exiting the AV node and zipping down the His bundle (don't worry—he is wearing rubber-soled shoes). Each time an impulse exits the AV node and stimulates the His bundle, the tiny electrophysiologist records the time interval since the previous impulse. Eventually, premature impulses stimulating the AV node are so premature that the ERP of the AV node is reached (i.e. the impulse is blocked when it reaches the AV node), and therefore no more impulses are transmitted to the His bundle. The FRP of the AV node is the shortest interval between successive impulses observed by our tiny timer.

What possessed electrophysiologists to invent such a thing as the FRP? First, since the FRP of a tissue is determined by transmission of impulses through that tissue, FRP is a measurement of both the refractoriness and the conduction velocity of a tissue. As shown in the discussion of RRP, refractoriness and conduction velocity are intimately related at narrower coupling intervals. The FRP is a way of quantifying this relationship. Second, the FRP may be clinically relevant more often than the more straightforward types of refractory periods. The best example is in atrial fibrillation, in which much effort is often spent in slowing the ventricular response. The drugs used for this purpose tend both to increase refractoriness and to slow conduction in the AV conducting system. One of the best measures of effective therapy, then, is the narrowest interval between successive QRS complexes (i.e. the FRP of the AV conducting system). Third, when inventing a list of anything (such as types of refractory period), it is best to have at least three items on the list.

The effect of cycle length and autonomic tone on refractory periods and conduction velocity

The refractory period of cardiac tissue is affected by the cycle length. For most tissue, shorter cycle lengths (i.e. faster heart rates) decrease refractory periods. The glaring exception to this general rule is the AV node, in which shorter cycle lengths increase refractory periods.

Autonomic tone affects both refractory periods and conduction velocity. An increase in sympathetic tone increases the conduction velocity and decreases the refractory periods throughout the heart. An increase in parasympathetic tone decreases the conduction velocity and increases the refractory periods. Here, again, there is a differential effect on the AV node, which is far more richly supplied by parasympathetic fibers than is most of the heart. Thus, parasympathetic tone has a disproportionate effect on the AV node.

Evaluation of reentrant arrhythmias

The ability to induce and terminate reentrant arrhythmias renders them amenable to detailed study. Consequently, the electrophysiology study has become vitally important in the evaluation and treatment of reentrant tachyarrhythmias. Although the techniques used to study different types of reentrant arrhythmia vary (this will be discussed in detail in Chapters 6 and 7), the principles behind the electrophysiologic evaluation of all types of reentry are the same.

Programmed stimulation in reentrant arrhythmias

The hallmark of the reentrant mechanism is the ability to induce and terminate the arrhythmia with programmed pacing techniques. Figure 2.6 shows the basic principle behind inducing a reentrant arrhythmia. A paced premature impulse enters the reentrant loop at a critical coupling interval, when pathway B is still refractory from the previous impulse (i.e. the premature impulse arrives during the ERP of pathway B)—but after the ERP of pathway A, which accepts the early impulse. Note that, if the impulse enters pathway A during its RRP, the requirement for slow conduction down pathway A may be met automatically (since by definition conduction is slow during the RRP). Because of the slow conduction down pathway A, pathway B has time to recover and accepts the premature impulse in the retrograde direction. Reentry is established.

Once a reentrant arrhythmia is established, premature paced impulses encountering the loop can do one of three things (Figure 4.11). First, the early impulse may encounter refractory tissue, which will prevent it from entering the circuit (Figure 4.11b). In this case, the premature beat will not affect the reentrant rhythm. Second, the early paced impulse may enter the loop and conduct down the slow pathway (pathway A) but collide with the reentrant impulse in the fast pathway (Figure 4.11b). In this case, the paced impulse resets the reentrant rhythm. Finally, the early impulse may enter the loop at just the right moment to encounter refractory tissue in pathway A and collide with the circulating wavefront in pathway B (Figure 4.11c). In this case, the reentrant rhythm is terminated.

A paced impulse must reach a reentrant circuit at a critical moment to start or stop an arrhythmia. The ability to arrive at such a critical moment is dependent on several factors, including the distance of the pacing electrode from the reentrant circuit and the refractoriness and conduction velocity of the tissue lying between the catheter and the circuit. If the catheter is far away from the reentrant circuit and if the intervening tissue has long refractory periods and slow conduction, it is less likely that a paced impulse will reach the reentrant circuit early enough to either induce or terminate an arrhythmia. For this reason, stimulation protocols usually call for pacing from more than one location, to improve the chances of finding a location near the reentrant circuit. In addition, most stimulation protocols call for coupling up to four premature impulses together. The resulting short cycle lengths reduce refractory periods and increase conduction velocity in the intervening tissue, giving subsequent impulses a better chance of reaching the reentrant circuit.

Pacing from various locations during supraventricular tachycardia can help to determine whether certain intracardiac locations are part of the reentrant loop. For instance, pacing from a right ventricular site which does not affect a narrow complex tachyarrhythmia is evidence against a macroreentrant tachycardia that includes both atrial and ventricular tissue in the reentrant loop. Chapter 6 discusses this concept in more detail.

Recording electrograms during reentrant arrhythmias
By recording intracardiac electrograms during reentrant tachycardias, it is possible to characterize the pathways of large reentrant

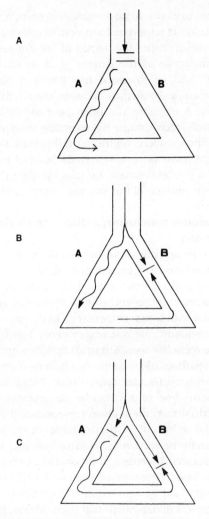

Figure 4.11 Effect of premature impulses on a reentrant arrhythmia. (a) A relatively late premature impulse may encounter refractory tissue that prevents penetration into the reentrant circuit. In this case, reentry is not affected. (b) An earlier premature impulse than that depicted in (a) may enter the reentrant circuit and abolish the reentrant impulse in one pathway (pathway B in this figure) but reestablish reentry by conducting down the opposite pathway (pathway A). In this case, the reentrant rhythm is reset. (c) A very early premature impulse may abolish the reentrant arrhythmia in pathway B while encountering refractory tissue in pathway A. In this case, reentry is terminated.

circuits (present in many supraventricular arrhythmias) or to map the general location of small reentrant circuits (present in most ventricular tachycardias). Especially helpful in the evaluation of supraventricular arrhythmias is the pattern of atrial activation during tachycardia. As will be discussed in Chapter 6, some types of reentrant supraventricular arrhythmia show characteristic patterns of atrial activation. A diagnosis can often be made by analyzing the intracardiac atrial electrograms. By recording multiple ventricular electrograms during induced ventricular tachycardia and looking for the earliest ventricular activation site, the general location of the reentrant circuit can be deduced. By thus mapping the ventricular activation pattern, ablation of the reentrant circuit can be attempted.

Effect of autonomic maneuvers, antiarrhythmic drugs, and devices on reentry

The electrophysiology study can help to determine the effect of autonomic maneuvers on reentrant arrhythmias. By manipulating autonomic tone and reassessing the inducibility of arrhythmias, one can determine whether reentrant arrhythmias are dependent on autonomic tone. In supraventricular arrhythmias, reentry which depends on autonomic tone is strong evidence that the AV node is involved in the reentrant loop. Stimulating the ventricle during the infusion of sympathomimetic agents can help to diagnose catecholamine-dependent ventricular tachycardia. Diagnosing this relatively infrequent type of ventricular tachycardia is important because this arrhythmia almost always responds to β-blockers.

Likewise, the effect of antiarrhythmic drugs on reentrant arrhythmias can be assessed in the electrophysiology laboratory. As discussed in Chapter 3, drugs can ameliorate, exacerbate, or not affect reentrant loops. Programmed stimulation offers a way of predicting the effect of a drug on a reentrant loop before committing a patient to long-term therapy with that drug. Ideally, if a drug has a favorable effect on a reentrant circuit, it will render a previously inducible arrhythmia noninducible. This is the rationale behind serial drug testing in the electrophysiology laboratory.

By studying the characteristics of an induced arrhythmia, one can assess the feasibility of using implantable antitachycardia devices to terminate spontaneous arrhythmias. Several factors may be important before considering implantable devices. How many different types of arrhythmia are inducible? What are their cycle lengths? What pacing sequences reliably terminate the induced arrhythmias? Does pacing ever degenerate a hemodynamically stable arrhythmia to an unstable one? Are there benign tachyarrhythmias (such as sinus tachycardia) that might fool a device into delivering inappropriate therapy? How do drugs affect the inducibility, rate, morphology, and terminability of arrhythmias? All these questions can be addressed through careful study in the electrophysiology laboratory.

Complications of electrophysiologic testing

On first learning about the electrophysiology study—especially when the purpose of that study is to induce lethal ventricular arrhythmias—many physicians assume that a test that sounds so barbaric must be dangerous. On the contrary: the electrophysiology study is remarkably safe, often much safer than the standard cardiac catheterization.

The electrophysiology study is a form of heart catheterization, and it necessarily carries the qualitative risks of a heart catheterization. These include cardiac perforation, hemorrhage, thromboembolism, phlebitis, and infection. Because the most common complications of a general heart catheterization involve damage to the arterial tree, and because most electrophysiology studies do not require arterial puncture, the statistical risk of serious vascular damage is actually substantially less with the electrophysiology study than with a standard cardiac catheterization. In most laboratories, the cumulative risk of thromboembolism or phlebitis, bacteremia, or hemorrhage requiring transfusion is well below 1%.

One might think that a procedure that sometimes intentionally induces lethal arrhythmias would entail significant mortality. In fact, the risk of death during an electrophysiology study approaches zero. Reentrant ventricular arrhythmias are induced in the electrophysiology laboratory under controlled circumstances. Immediate efforts are made to terminate hemodynamically unstable arrhythmias, and it turns out that these arrhythmias are readily terminable if they are attacked quickly. In most laboratories, the average length of time for which the patient remains in an induced ventricular tachycardia is less than 30 seconds. Only a small minority of patients with inducible ventricular tachyarrhythmias require DC shocks for termination, and the need to initiate cardiopulmonary resuscitation procedures is exceedingly rare.

5 The Electrophysiology Study in the Evaluation of Bradycardia: The SA Node, AV Node, and His–Purkinje System

As we saw in Chapter 2, the SA node, AV node, and His–Purkinje system are responsible for generating, propagating, and distributing the heart's electrical impulse, and thus for determining the cardiac rhythm and rate, and for optimizing hemodynamic performance. Specifically, the SA node continuously regulates the heart rate according to the body's fluctuating needs; the AV node and His bundle optimize the transmission of the electrical impulse from the atria to the ventricles; and the Purkinje system coordinates the contraction of the left and right ventricles.

In this chapter, we will discuss the electrophysiologic problems that produce bradycardia: disorders of the SA node, AV node, and His–Purkinje system, emphasizing how (and when) the electrophysiology study can help in their evaluation. We will also briefly review pacemaker therapy.

As we do so, the reader will note a recurring theme: while the electrophysiology study has provided us with detailed knowledge of how the SA node, AV node, and His–Purkinje system work, now that we have acquired this knowledge, we can usually evaluate patients with disorders of these cardiac structures without actually having to perform an electrophysiology study. Indeed, the original electrophysiologists were so successful in achieving their prime directive—understanding how the cardiac impulse is formed and propagated–that they nearly put themselves out of business. Fortunately, a second generation of electrophysiologists quickly figured

Electrophysiologic Testing, Fifth Edition. Richard N. Fogoros.
© 2012 John Wiley & Sons, Ltd. Published 2012 by John Wiley & Sons, Ltd.

out how to apply electrophysiologic testing to the tachyarrhythmias, thus rescuing the profession—but that's a story for later chapters.

Evaluation of SA nodal abnormalities

Anatomy of the SA node

The SA node can be thought of as a subendocardial, comma-shaped structure, approximately 3 mm in width and 10 mm in length, the head of which is located laterally to the right atrial appendage, near the junction of the atrium and the superior vena cava, on the crista terminalis. (The crista terminalis is an endocardial ridge extending like a narrow mountain chain from the superior to the inferior vena cava along the lateral right atrium.) The tail of the SA nodal "comma" extends downward along the crista terminalis, toward the inferior vena cava.

The SA node receives rich innervation from both sympathetic and parasympathetic fibers; accordingly, its function is strongly influenced by the autonomic nervous system. There is some evidence that autonomic tone helps to determine which portion of the SA node (i.e. the head or the tail) is "firing" at a given time— elevated sympathetic tone tends to trigger the head of the SA node, while elevated parasympathetic tone tends to trigger the tail.

SA nodal dysfunction

Disease of the SA node is the most common cause of bradycardia. The bradyarrhythmias that accompany SA nodal disease can manifest as intermittent or sustained sinus bradycardia, as sudden episodes of SA nodal arrest or exit block, or as sinus bradycardia alternating with paroxysms of atrial tachyarrhythmias (a condition referred to as "brady-tachy syndrome"). When sinus bradyarrhythmias are sufficient to produce symptoms, *sick sinus syndrome* is said to be present.

(Note that the "official" definition of sinus bradycardia can be misleading. While most textbooks define normal sinus rhythm as having a rate between 60 and 100 beats/min, this range is probably incorrect. Normal, healthy individuals often have resting sinus rates as low as 40; while resting heart rates in the upper 80s or 90s often indicate the presence of occult medical problems, such as anemia or cardiopulmonary or thyroid disorders.)

Clinical studies show that the bradycardia caused by SA nodal disease is usually benign. That is, people do not commonly die from sinus bradycardia. On the other hand, the presence of SA nodal disease is associated with increased mortality—but that excess mortality is often due to noncardiac causes.

Because sinus bradycardia is usually not lethal, the level of aggressiveness that ought to be used in evaluating and treating suspected SA nodal disease is solely dependent on whether any associated symptoms are thought to be present. If SA nodal disease is causing symptoms (i.e. if sick sinus syndrome is present), permanent pacing is indicated. If there are no symptoms, in general there is no indication for pacing.

By far the most common cause of SA nodal disease is simple fibrosis of the SA node; a condition that is associated with aging and often is also accompanied by diffuse fibrosis within the atria and the AV conducting system. Accordingly, most patients with SA nodal dysfunction are elderly. Other causes of SA nodal dysfunction include atherosclerotic disease involving the SA nodal artery; cardiac trauma, especially during surgical correction of congenital heart disease; cardiac infiltrative or inflammatory disorders; and thyroid disorders.

Brady-tachy syndrome deserves a special mention. This syndrome occurs because the diffuse atrial fibrosis that often accompanies SA nodal dysfunction can produce a propensity for atrial fibrillation or flutter. Individuals with brady-tachy syndrome thus will have intermittent episodes of atrial tachyarrhythmias, with intervening periods of sinus bradycardia. Importantly, because their diseased SA nodes often display exaggerated overdrive suppression (see Chapter 4 and later in this chapter), these patients tend to have very prolonged asystolic pauses when their tachyarrhythmias abruptly terminate. Quite often then, their presenting symptoms have little to do directly with either the tachycardia or the sinus bradycardia—instead they are frequently caused by this post-tachycardia asystole. Thus, patients with brady-tachy syndrome can have sudden and relatively severe episodes of lightheadedness, or even frank syncope. Furthermore, because the atrial fibrosis also commonly involves the AV conduction system, during their atrial tachyarrhythmias these patients may have surprisingly well-controlled (or even slow) ventricular responses. Seeing an unexpectedly slow ventricular response in a patient with atrial fibrillation should thus immediately raise the question of a generalized disorder of the conducting system—and the physician should be prepared to administer immediate pacing therapy if cardioversion is contemplated.

Patients with brady-tachy syndrome often end up with chronic atrial fibrillation accompanied by a reasonably well-controlled ventricular response. Indeed, one might be tempted to view this chronic atrial fibrillation as "God's way" of guaranteeing an adequate heart rate in the face of diffuse conducting system disease. While this may be so, in the intervening years patients are often very symptomatic, not to mention at risk for syncope-induced trauma, so sitting on one's hands and waiting for this final, relatively stable rhythm to occur does not constitute adequate therapy.

Although the electrophysiology study can help to document the presence of SA nodal dysfunction, it generally cannot help to assess whether such dysfunction is causing symptoms—or, therefore, whether pacing therapy is indicated. One is, however, occasionally faced with a patient who has symptoms suggesting significant bradycardia (such as lightheadedness or syncope), without clearly documented bradycardia. In such circumstances, the electrophysiology study can be helpful in determining whether or not the SA node is intrinsically normal.

Evaluating SA nodal function in the electrophysiology laboratory

Sinus node recovery time (SNRT)

A primary manifestation of SA nodal dysfunction is disordered automaticity, where the slope of phase 4 automaticity is reduced in the SA node, resulting in bradycardia.

The test designed to assess SA nodal automaticity in the electrophysiology laboratory is the "sinus node recovery time" (SNRT; Figures 5.1 and 5.2). Measurement of the SNRT is based on the phenomenon of overdrive suppression. Overdrive suppression is the temporary slowing of automaticity seen when an automatic focus is exposed to rapid, extrinsic electrical stimuli. When this overdriving stimulation stops, it takes the automatic focus a few cycles to recover its normal rate of discharge. Until it recovers, it fires more slowly than its original baseline rate; thus, the automatic focus has been transiently "suppressed" by overdrive stimulation. Overdrive suppression is a normal behavior of automatic foci; in SA nodal disease, however, overdrive suppression tends to be exaggerated.

In nature, as we have seen, overdrive suppression of the SA node is caused by atrial tachyarrhythmias. In the electrophysiology laboratory, we provoke it with a temporary pacemaker.

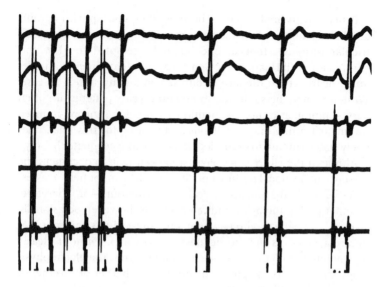

Figure 5.1 A normal sinus node recovery time (SNRT). This figure shows three surface ECG leads (*top three tracings*), a right atrial (RA) electrogram (*fourth tracing*), and a His-bundle electrogram (*fifth tracing*). In measuring the SNRT, only the RA electrogram needs to be examined. The first three impulses on the RA electrogram represent the final three paced beats during 30 seconds of incremental pacing. Pacing is stopped, and the interval from the last paced atrial complex to the first spontaneous atrial complex on the RA electrogram is measured. In this instance, the basic cycle length is 800 msec and the SNRT equals 1260 msec. This is a normal value.

Measuring SNRT   Measuring the SNRT is simple in concept and in practice, although interpreting the results can be more challenging. An electrode catheter is placed in the high right atrium near the SA node and pacing is initiated to overdrive the SA node. After a while, pacing is terminated and the ensuing "recovery" time from the last paced beat to the next spontaneous sinus beat is measured.

In the formal measurement of SNRT, several pacing sequences are tested, beginning with a pacing rate just slightly faster than the basic sinus rate, and generally ending with a cycle length of 300 msec (200 beats/min.) Each pacing sequence is maintained for at least 30 seconds to maximize overdrive suppression—and is then abruptly stopped. The first recovery interval (the interval from the

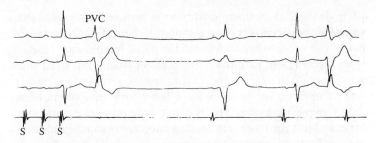

PVC

S S S

Figure 5.2 An abnormal sinus node recovery time (SNRT). This figure shows three surface ECG leads and the right atrial (RA) electrogram. The last three paced impulses are shown. The interval following termination of pacing (from the RA electrogram) is 2200 msec, an abnormally long SNRT. Note that during the recovery interval a premature ventricular complex (PVC) is seen. Because this PVC does not conduct retrogradely (this is obvious because no corresponding atrial activity is present on the RA electrogram), the PVC does not affect the sinus node and therefore does not affect measurement of the SNRT.

last paced atrial complex to the first spontaneous SA nodal depolarization) is normally longer than the pre-pacing baseline sinus interval, reflecting the degree of overdrive suppression induced by pacing. After pacing is stopped, the SA node gradually returns to its baseline rate over five to six beats. In SA nodal disease, two observations are commonly seen. First, the initial recovery interval can be longer than normal. Second, the gradual return to the baseline sinus rate can be interrupted during subsequent recovery intervals by marked "secondary pauses."

By the end of the study, several initial recovery intervals will have been measured: one at each pacing rate. In addition, one or more secondary pauses may have been observed. The official SNRT is deemed to be the longest recovery interval observed during the entire test, whether it is one of the initial recovery intervals or a secondary pause.

One might think that the longest post-pacing recovery times would always be seen after the more rapid pacing rates, but this is often not the case. Recovery times measured after slower pacing rates are frequently longer than those measured after faster pacing rates. This phenomenon—longer recovery times after slower overdrive suppression—is attributed to the conduction properties of the

SA node itself. If conduction within the perinodal cells (cells that surround the pacemaker cells) is abnormal then SA nodal "entrance block" can occur, wherein some of the paced impulses are blocked from reaching the pacemaker cells. Faster pacing rates can thus actually result in fewer impulses reaching the SA nodal pacemaker cells themselves, and hence in less-effective overdrive suppression, than slower pacing rates. This is why a wide range of pacing rates, instead of just the more rapid pacing rates, are used when measuring SNRT. (Assessment of the conduction properties of the SA node is discussed later in this chapter.)

In any case, determining the SNRT is easy enough; deciding whether that SNRT is normal or abnormal is a little more problematic. One difficulty is that overdrive suppression of the SA node, being a normal phenomenon, occurs in everybody. Unfortunately, there is wide variation in SNRTs among apparently normal individuals as well as considerable overlap in measured SNRTs between patients with apparently normal and clearly abnormal SA nodes.

Deciding on the upper normal values for the SNRT, then, is not dictated by nature, but by electrophysiologists. "Normal" values vary from laboratory to laboratory, depending on whether electrophysiologists want their measurements to err on the side of sensitivity (in which case a lower value would be used) or specificity (in which case a higher value would be used). A conservative upper limit of "normal" for the SNRT, above which most experts would agree that SA nodal dysfunction is present, is 1500 msec.

Another difficulty in interpreting SNRTs is the fact that the SNRT is related to the underlying heart rate (or the basic cycle length, BCL), such that at slower underlying heart rates, a longer recovery time is normally seen. An SNRT that is abnormal at a shorter BCL could be normal at a longer BCL.

To account for this relationship between SNRT and BCL, electrophysiologists have created two indices, one or both of which are now measured routinely during electrophysiology studies. The first is the corrected sinus node recovery time (CSNRT), which is calculated simply by subtracting the patient's BCL from the SNRT. Thus:

$$CSNRT = SNRT - BCL$$

By convention, the upper limit of "normal" for the CSNRT is 525 msec. In other words, the SNRT should be no more than 525 msec longer than the BCL.

The second index commonly used is the ratio of the SNRT to the BCL (SNRT/BCL × 100%). A ratio greater than 160% is usually considered abnormal.

Figure 5.1 demonstrates a normal SNRT. Here, the patient's BCL is 800 msec and the initial recovery interval is 1260 msec. Thus, the SNRT is 1260 msec, the CSNRT (SNRT − BCL) is 460 msec, and the ratio of the SNRT to the BCL is 158%. These values are all within normal limits.

An abnormal SNRT is demonstrated in Figure 5.2. The BCL in this example is also 800 msec. The longest recovery interval (and thus the SNRT) is 2200 msec. The CSNRT is 1400 msec, and the ratio of the SNRT to the BCL is 275%. All of these values are abnormal.

These two examples are straightforward in that all the SNRT measures—the SNRT itself, the CSNRT, and the ratio—are either normal (Figure 5.1) or abnormal (Figure 5.2). Not uncommonly, there will be divergence among these three measures. In such cases, the electrophysiologist must use his or her clinical judgment in interpreting the test. Given the relatively arbitrary nature of determining normal from abnormal SNRT values in the first place, this circumstance should not add appreciably to one's level of discomfort. Indeed, once you resort to the electrophysiology study for determining whether a patient's SA node is normal or not, you are signing up for a certain amount of arbitrariness.

Sinoatrial conduction time (SACT)

The sinoatrial conduction time (SACT) test is meant to assess how well the SA node is able to conduct the electrical impulses it produces out to surrounding atrial tissue. The idea that the SA node might not always allow generated impulses to reach the atria came from the observation of *SA nodal exit block* (see Figure 5.3). In exit block, a sudden sinus pause occurs with a duration that is exactly twice the normal sinus cycle length, suggesting that an impulse was indeed generated at the right time, but that it failed to conduct out of the SA node. Occasional episodes of exit block are relatively common in patients with SA nodal dysfunction. (SA nodal exit block is analogous to the entrance block we discussed in the section on SNRT, and reflects the same physiology.)

To understand how such an exit block might occur and how the SACT is measured, it is helpful to visualize the SA node as a small patch of pacemaker cells surrounded by a rim of specialized perinodal tissue that has electrophysiologic characteristics similar to those

Figure 5.3 This rhythm strip illustrates SA nodal exit block. Note the sudden sinus pause, with a duration that is almost exactly twice the normal sinus cycle length. Presumably, the SA nodal pacemaker cells fired at the appropriate time (indicated by the asterisk), but the impulse was blocked from exiting the SA node thanks to abnormal perinodal conduction. Patients with SA nodal dysfunction commonly display occasional episodes of exit block. These patients usually also have abnormal SACT measurements (*see text*).

of the AV node (Figure 5.4). To exit from the SA node, a generated impulse must pass through this rim of perinodal tissue; if conduction is abnormal, exit block may occur.

The SACT is a measure of the time it takes an impulse originating in the SA node to travel through the perinodal tissue and into the atria. Prolonged SACTs are thought to indicate abnormal conduction through this tissue, and thus a propensity for SA nodal exit block.

To measure SACT, an electrode catheter is placed in the high right atrium near the SA node and atrial pacing is performed to depolarize and thus reset the SA node. The subsequent return interval (i.e. the time from the last paced atrial depolarization to the first spontaneous SA nodal depolarization, as measured from the high right atrial electrode catheter) is assumed to reflect the sum of the time it takes for the paced impulse to penetrate into the SA node (at which time it resets the SA node) plus the basic sinus cycle length plus the time it takes for the subsequent spontaneous beat to penetrate out of the SA node. Assuming that the times of penetration into and out of the SA node are equivalent:

$$\text{Return interval} = \text{BCL} + 2\,\text{SACT}$$

Because the BCL is known and the return interval can be measured, the SACT can be calculated.

In Figure 5.5, the basic cycle length is 800 msec. The paced beat (A2) is assumed to penetrate and reset the SA node, and the return interval is 900 msec. From this formula, 900 msec = 800 msec + 2 SACT. The SACT is thus 50 msec. A normal SACT is considered to be approximately 50–125 msec.

SA Node

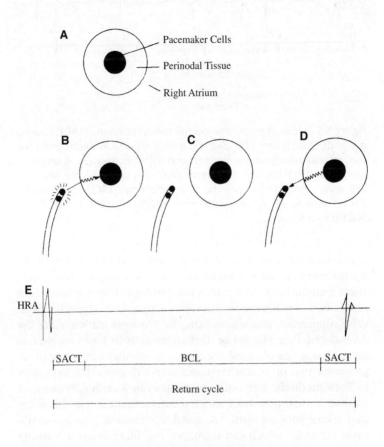

A

Pacemaker Cells

Perinodal Tissue

Right Atrium

B   C   D

E
HRA

SACT   BCL   SACT

Return cycle

Return cycle=BCL + 2SACT

Figure 5.4 Measurement of sinoatrial conduction time (SACT). (a) The SA node consists of a patch of pacemaker cells surrounded by a rim of perinodal tissue, which conducts electrical impulses slowly (similarly to the AV node). To measure SACT, an electrode catheter is positioned near the SA node and a premature impulse is delivered. The SACT can be deduced by measuring the interval from the premature paced impulse to the next spontaneous impulse (i.e. the return cycle). This return cycle consists of the conduction time into the SA node (b), the normal SA nodal depolarization time (i.e. the basic cycle length, BCL) (c), and the conduction time out of the SA node (d). (e) illustrates the resultant right atrial electrogram. The SACT is half the difference between the return cycle and the BCL.

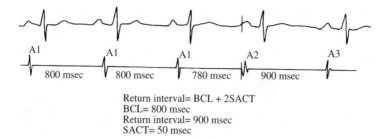

Return interval= BCL + 2SACT
BCL= 800 msec
Return interval= 900 msec
SACT= 50 msec

Figure 5.5 Measurement of sinoatrial conduction time (SACT, Strauss method). One surface ECG lead and a right artial (RA) electrogram are shown. Measurements are made from the RA electrogram. A single premature atrial impulse is delivered (A2) at a coupling interval of 780 msec: slightly faster than the basic cycle length (BCL) of 800 msec. The return interval (A2–A3) is 900 msec, which is the BCL + 2 SACT. The SACT is thus 50 msec.

Two methods have been developed for measuring SACT. In the Narula method, short trains of slow atrial pacing are used, barely faster than the basic sinus rate. A rate just faster than the basic sinus rate is used to minimize any overdrive suppression. (Inducing over-drive suppression would invalidate the SACT calculation, since the SA node would no longer be discharging at its BCL.) In the Strauss method, a series of single premature atrial impulses are used, to guarantee that no overdrive suppression will occur. The principles of both methods, however, are as described earlier. Whichever method is used to measure SACT, the main limitation of this test is that many patients with SA nodal dysfunction have modestly irregular BCLs, which can introduce considerable error into the SACT calculation.

Intrinsic heart rate (IHR)

As previously mentioned, the SA node is richly innervated by both sympathetic and parasympathetic fibers. Occasionally, it can there-fore be difficult to determine whether suspected SA nodal dys-function is actually intrinsic to the SA node, or whether it might be due to abnormal autonomic tone. In such cases it can be helpful to measure the intrinsic heart rate (IHR).

The IHR is assessed by administering drugs to block both branches of the autonomic nervous system then measuring the resultant heart rate. Classically, autonomic blockade is accomplished by giv-ing both propranolol (0.2 mg/kg) and atropine (0.04 mg/kg).

According to the formula devised by Jose, after autonomic blockade the normal IHR $= 118.1 - (0.57 \times age)$.

Patients presenting with sinus bradycardia but who turn out to have normal IHRs are considered to have normal intrinsic SA nodal function; their bradycardia is apparently due to autonomic influences. Patients with bradycardia and depressed IHRs are considered to have intrinsic SA nodal dysfunction. Alternately, patients with inappropriate sinus tachycardia (see Chapter 11) often have substantially elevated IHRs.

In clinical practice, it is rarely necessary to measure IHR in order to document intrinsic SA nodal disease. An exercise test, for instance, is a much simpler way to accomplish parasympathetic withdrawal in a patient presenting with sinus bradycardia, and a blunted heart-rate response to exercise (in the absence of drugs that cause bradycardia, such as β-blockers and calcium blockers) usually clinches the diagnosis of intrinsic SA nodal dysfunction.

Interpreting SA nodal tests: when to carry out electrophysiologic testing

When assessing patients for SA nodal dysfunction, several simple points bear keeping in mind. First, SA nodal dysfunction is generally not a lethal condition, and therapy is necessary only to the extent that it produces symptoms. Second, the best way to diagnose SA nodal dysfunction is to see it occurring spontaneously, because the specificity of such an observation is 100%. Thus, ambulatory cardiac monitoring (and not electrophysiologic testing) is the study of choice in assessing SA nodal dysfunction. Third, since the electrophysiology study can help to determine only whether SA nodal dysfunction is present (and not whether it causes symptoms), once unexplained sinus bradyarrhythmias are already known to occur, there is generally no reason to consider electrophysiologic testing. Fourth, while the electrophysiology study offers methods for evaluating both the automaticity (SNRT) and conductive properties (SACT) of the SA node, the specificities and sensitivities of these tests as usually applied are estimated to be only approximately 70%.

With these points in mind, we can confidently state the following guidelines in assessing SA nodal disease:

1. Asymptomatic sinus bradyarrhythmias need no evaluation or treatment.
2. Asymptomatic abnormal SNRTs or SACTs need no treatment.

3. Symptomatic sinus bradyarrhythmias should be treated with pacing, unless they are due to medications or to some other reversible cause.
4. The only inarguable indication for performing electrophysiology studies to assess SA nodal function is in the evaluation of patients who present with episodic symptoms suggestive of bradyarrhythmias (especially syncope), and for whom no significant bradycardia is documented during cardiac monitoring.

Evaluation of AV conduction disorders

AV conduction disorders are the second major cause of bradyarrhythmias. As with SA nodal disease, the clinician's chief concern with AV conduction disease is deciding whether the affected patient should receive a pacemaker. This decision is based on three essential pieces of data: whether the conduction disorder is producing *symptoms*; the *site* of the conduction disorder; and the *degree* of conduction block. Once again, thanks to what has been learned in the electrophysiology laboratory, we usually do not need to perform invasive testing to make this decision.

Symptoms of AV conduction disorders

The symptoms that occur with AV conduction disease are the same as those that occur with any bradyarrhythmia: lightheadedness, dizziness, presyncope, and syncope. Whatever the site or degree of block, AV block that produces any of these symptoms needs to be treated. Often, however, especially with first- or second-degree block, AV conduction disturbances are totally asymptomatic.

The site of the conduction disorder

Determining the site of the conduction disturbance is important for a simple reason: block that occurs in the AV node (proximal block) is usually benign, whereas block that occurs in the His–Purkinje system (distal block) is potentially lethal.

AV nodal block

Conduction disturbances in the AV node most often have acute, transient, and reversible causes. Ischemia or infarction involving the right coronary artery (which gives off the AV nodal artery in 90% of patients) can cause AV nodal block. Thus, heart block following an inferior myocardial infarction is usually localized to the AV node, and normal AV conduction almost always recovers (though block can persist for days or even weeks). Acute rheumatic fever and other cardiac inflammatory conditions can also produce transient AV nodal block. While drugs that affect AV nodal function—mainly digoxin, β-blockers and calcium blockers—may produce first-degree AV block, higher degrees of drug-induced AV nodal block suggest underlying intrinsic AV nodal dysfunction.

Complete heart block localized to the AV node is usually accompanied by the emergence of a relatively reliable escape pacemaker, located just distally to the AV node. This "high junctional" escape rhythm often yields a baseline heart rate of 40–55 beats/min, and responds at least moderately well to increases in sympathetic tone. Congenital complete heart block, which is usually localized to the AV node, illustrates the typical, relatively benign character of AV nodal block.

Since AV nodal block is usually reversible, it can frequently be managed simply by dealing with the underlying cause, although sometimes temporary pacing support is required in the meantime.

His–Purkinje block

In stark contrast to AV nodal block, block occurring distally to the AV node is potentially life-threatening. The potential lethal effect of distal heart block can largely be attributed to the unreliable, unstable, and slow escape pacemakers that tend to accompany this condition. These distal escape pacemakers usually discharge irregularly, 20 to 40 times per minute, and are prone to fail altogether. Thus, syncope, hemodynamic collapse, and death are much more likely to occur when AV block is located in the His–Purkinje system. Furthermore, distal AV block tends to be chronic and progressive in nature, instead of transient and reversible.

Distal AV block following myocardial infarction is almost always associated with occlusion of the left anterior descending artery, and thus with anterior myocardial infarctions. His–Purkinje block can also be seen with inflammatory and infiltrative cardiac disease, with myocardial fibrosis, and in association with aortic valve and mitral valve calcification.

The degree of AV block

First-degree AV block

In *first-degree AV block*, all atrial impulses are transmitted to the ventricles, but with prolonged conduction times (Figure 5.6). First-degree block is diagnosed from the ECG; all P waves are conducted,

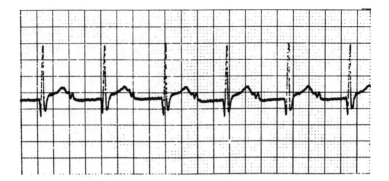

Figure 5.6 First-degree AV block. The PR interval in this figure is approximately 380 msec.

but the PR interval is prolonged (usually to between 0.20 and 0.40 seconds, but sometimes much longer.) In most patients with first-degree AV block, slow conduction is localized to the AV node; slow conduction in the His–Purkinje system can, however, occasionally cause first-degree block. First-degree AV block usually causes no symptoms.

Second-degree AV block: Mobitz classification

In *second-degree AV block*, intermittent AV block is seen; on the ECG, some P waves are followed by QRS complexes and others are not. Symptoms depend largely on the resultant ventricular rate.

When second-degree AV block is observed, one should attempt to classify the block as either Mobitz type I (also called Wenckebach block) or Mobitz type II. The Mobitz classification helps to localize the site of the second-degree AV block.

In Mobitz type I block, there is a gradual prolongation of the PR interval in the conducted beats immediately preceding a blocked beat (Figure 5.7). The site of Mobitz type I block is usually (but not always) localized to the AV node. (Note that Figure 5.7 shows the unusual case in which Mobitz type I block is due to distal conducting disease.) In Mobitz type II block, the blocked beat occurs suddenly, without any lengthening of the PR intervals in the conducted beats preceding the dropped beat (Figure 5.8). *Mobitz type II block always indicates distal block.*

When differentiating Mobitz I from Mobitz II block, a common mistake is to only compare the PR intervals of successive conducted beats. Sometimes the prolongation in the PR interval from one beat

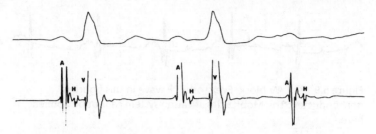

Figure 5.7 Mobitz I AV block. A surface ECG and a His-bundle electrogram from a patient with Mobitz I AV block are shown. On the surface ECG, progressive prolongation of the PR interval is seen prior to the nonconducted P wave. Although most instances of Mobitz I AV block are located in the AV node, this example illustrates that Mobitz I block occasionally can be seen with disease in the more distal conducting tissue. As seen in the His-bundle electrogram, PR prolongation occurs as a result of gradually slowing conduction beyond the His bundle (i.e. prolonging HV interval), and when block finally occurs, it occurs below the His bundle.

to the next is so subtle that it can be easily missed, in which case Mobitz II block may be mistakenly declared. The best way to tell that the Mobitz I pattern of PR interval prolongation is occurring is to compare the PR interval of the last conducted beat prior to the dropped beat with the PR interval of the first conducted beat after the dropped beat. That is, compare the "longest" conducted PR interval to the "shortest" conducted PR interval–a difference between these two PR intervals is almost always easily detectable with Mobitz I block.

It is important to realize that the Mobitz classification can only be used when you can find at least one instance in which two

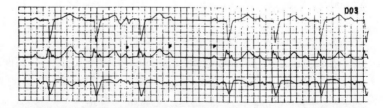

Figure 5.8 Mobitz II AV block. This figure shows three simultaneous surface ECG leads. The nonconducted P wave occurs suddenly, without progressive prolongation in the PR interval. Mobitz II block always indicates distal conducting system disease.

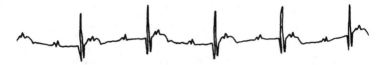

Figure 5.9 2 : 1 AV block. Every other P wave in this figure is nonconducted. The Mobitz classification system cannot be applied here.

consecutively conducted beats immediately precede a blocked beat. The reason for this limitation is simple—in order for there to be progressive prolongation in the PR interval prior to the dropped beat, at least two consecutively conducted beats must occur. Stating it another way: you cannot use the Mobitz classification with 2 : 1 AV block; by definition, it does not apply (Figure 5.9). Many clinicians make the mistake of automatically classifying 2 : 1 block as Mobitz II, thus misdiagnosing many cases of 2 : 1 AV nodal block as distal block. When 2 : 1 block is present, some means other than Mobitz classification must be used to deduce the site of block.

Third-degree AV block

In *third-degree AV block,* no atrial impulses are conducted to the ventricles—complete AV block is present (Figure 5.10). Maintaining a ventricular rhythm in the presence of third-degree AV block is totally dependent on subsidiary escape pacemakers. As noted earlier, the reliability of those escape pacemakers is related to the site of block. With AV nodal block, the escape pacemakers tend to be relatively reliable; with distal block, the escape pacemakers tend to be unreliable and slow. Distal third-degree AV block is much more likely to produce symptoms than third-degree block located in the AV node.

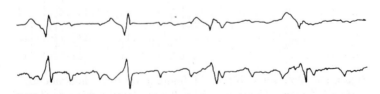

Figure 5.10 Complete heart block with a slow ventricular escape mechanism. Distal heart block is likely in this example.

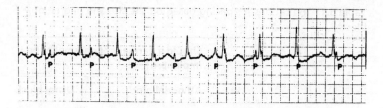

Figure 5.11 AV dissociation without complete heart block. In this tracing, the sinus rate is simply slower than the junctional escape rate. The fourth P wave conducts to the ventricles (since the following QRS complex occurs at a PR interval that is narrower than the escape interval of the junctional escape). Thus, not all AV dissociation is complete heart block.

AV dissociation The presence of AV dissociation can lead to confusion when attempting to discern whether third-degree AV block is present. AV dissociation simply means that the atria and the ventricles are each being controlled by their own independent pacemakers. While AV dissociation is present in all cases of complete heart block, complete heart block is *not* present in all cases of AV dissociation. Complete heart block is merely one variety of AV dissociation.

Figure 5.11 illustrates AV dissociation without complete heart block. Here, normal sinus rhythm is present at a rate of 65 beats/min; but an accelerated junctional pacemaker is also present with a rate of 78 beats/min. Thus, the atrial and ventricular rhythms are functioning independently—that is, they are dissociated. Note the fourth P wave in Figure 5.11. This P wave happens to occur at a time when the AV conducting system is no longer refractory from the previous junctional impulse, and it is conducted to the ventricles. Since an appropriately timed atrial complex is conducted, there is no heart block. As a general rule, when the atrial rate is faster than the ventricular rate and no atrial impulses are conducted, complete heart block is present. If the ventricular rate is higher than the atrial rate, AV dissociation without heart block should be suspected.

Treatment of AV block

Table 5.1 summarizes the treatment of AV block based on symptoms, the degree of block, and the site of block. In general, determining the presence or absence of symptoms and the degree of AV

Table 5.1 Indications for pacing based on the site and degree of AV block

	Should a permanent pacemaker be implanted?	
	AV nodal block	**Distal block**
First-degree AV block	No	No[a]
Second-degree AV block	No[b]	Yes
Third-degree AV block	No[b]	Yes

[a]Unless the HV interval is >100 msec.
[b]Unless symptomatic bradycardia is present.

block is simple. If there is a problem in deciding on therapy, it almost always lies in localizing the site of AV block.

Localizing the site of AV block

In most cases, localizing the site of block can be done noninvasively, by evaluating the ECG and performing selected autonomic maneuvers.

The ECG can be helpful in several ways. A wide QRS complex indicates the presence of distal conducting system disease and should raise suspicions of infranodal block. In cases of complete heart block, a wide-complex, slow (20–40 beats/min) escape pacemaker is a strong indicator of distal AV block; a narrow-complex and more rapid (40–55 beats/min) escape rhythm suggests AV nodal block (see Figure 2.3). If second-degree AV block is present, the Mobitz classification should be applied (unless the only conduction ratio seen is 2 : 1). Mobitz I block suggests AV nodal disease, whereas Mobitz II block always indicates distal block.

Autonomic maneuvers are useful because the AV node has rich autonomic innervation and the distal conducting system does not. Maneuvers that decrease vagal tone or increase sympathetic tone can be expected to improve AV nodal block but not distal block. Maneuvers that increase vagal tone or decrease sympathetic tone will worsen AV nodal block but not distal block.

Autonomic maneuvers are especially helpful when either Mobitz type I block or 2 : 1 second-degree AV block is present. In AV nodal block, exercise or atropine administration will improve or resolve the block. In distal block, these same maneuvers will not improve the AV block; in fact, the conduction ratio often worsens (e.g. 2 : 1

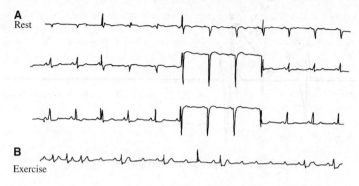

Figure 5.12 Exercise-induced worsening of AV conduction. (a) shows the resting 12-lead ECG of a patient who had intermittent 2:1 AV conduction. With exercise, (b), the conduction ratio is markedly worsened, strongly implying distal conducting system disease.

block may shift to 3:1 block; see Figure 5.12). Table 5.2 summarizes noninvasive techniques for localizing the site of AV block.

Occasionally, the site of block remains unclear even after a careful noninvasive evaluation. In these instances, the electrophysiology study virtually always resolves the issue.

The electrophysiology study in the evaluation of AV conduction disorders

The key to localizing AV conduction disorders in the electrophysiology laboratory is the His-bundle electrogram. The recording and interpretation of the His-bundle electrogram are described in detail in Chapter 4. In review, the His-bundle electrogram consists of three major deflections (Figure 5.13). The A deflection represents depolarization of atrial tissue proximate to the AV node. The H spike represents the depolarization of the His bundle itself. The V spike

Table 5.2 Noninvasive differentiation of AV nodal and infranodal block

	AV nodal	Infranodal
Exercise/isoproterenol	Improves	Conduction ratio may worsen
Atropine	Improves	Conduction ratio may worsen
Vagal maneuvers	Worsens	No change
β-blockers	Worsens	No change

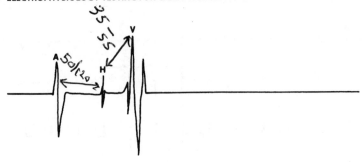

Figure 5.13   A typical His-bundle electrogram.

represents the depolarization of the ventricular myocardium. The AH interval is therefore an approximation of the conduction time through the AV node (normally 50–120 msec) and the HV interval is an approximation of the conduction time through the His–Purkinje system (normally 35–55 msec). Thus, the His-bundle electrogram reveals the function of all the major components of AV conduction.

Overt AV conduction disturbances

In the patient with overt AV conduction disturbances, the His-bundle electrogram immediately reveals the site of block.

When first-degree AV block is localized to the AV node, a prolonged AH interval will be seen (Figure 5.14a), while first-degree block below the AV node will produce a prolonged HV interval (Figures 5.14b and 5.15). It should be noted that significantly slowed conduction through the His–Purkinje structures can occur without overt first-degree AV block. For instance, a lengthening of the HV interval from 50 to 100 msec (a markedly abnormal value) may prolong the PR interval only from 140 to 190 msec (still within the normal range).

Occasionally, slowed conduction within the His bundle itself can be observed. The normal conduction time through the His bundle (measured by the duration of the H spike on the His-bundle electrogram) is less than 25 msec—a longer H spike duration reflects His-bundle conduction delay. Sometimes, a His-bundle conduction delay is sufficiently severe to produce an actual splitting of the His deflection (Figure 5.16).

While there is no general agreement on whether to treat patients with asymptomatic prolongations in the HV interval, most physicians agree that a permanent pacemaker is indicated if the HV

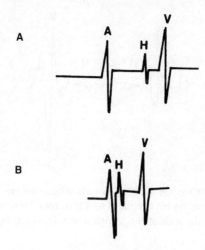

Figure 5.14 His-bundle electrogram patterns seen with first-degree AV block. (a) Prolonged conduction in the AV node (the AH interval is prolonged). (b) Prolonged conduction below the AV node (the HV interval is prolonged).

interval is very prolonged (i.e. greater than 100 msec) or if a split His is present.

With second-degree AV block of Mobitz type I (Figure 5.17), the intracardiac electrogram usually shows a progressive prolongation of the AH interval in the beats immediately prior to the dropped

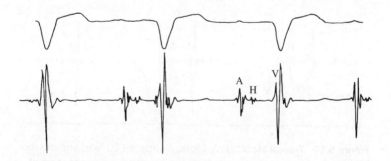

Figure 5.15 Distal first-degree AV block. A surface ECG lead and the His-bundle electrogram of a patient with first-degree AV block are shown. The conduction delay can be seen to occur in the distal structures because the AH interval is normal and the HV interval is prolonged.

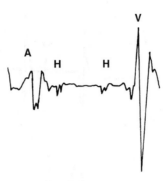

Figure 5.16 Split His. Conduction disease within the His bundle itself is present because the His bundle is split into two discrete components. A split His potential indicates significant distal conducting system disease.

atrial impulse (indicating a gradual slowing in conduction through the AV node before the dropped beat). With the dropped beat itself, the A deflection is not followed by an H spike, indicating block within the AV node. Again, while Mobitz type I block usually indicates AV nodal block, a Mobitz I pattern is occasionally seen with block in the His–Purkinje system (see Figure 5.7).

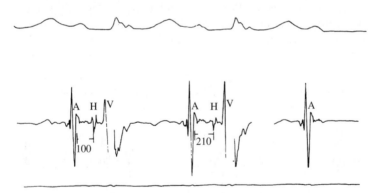

Figure 5.17 Typical Mobitz I AV block. A surface ECG lead and the His-bundle electrogram are shown. Note the progressive prolongation of the AH interval (and the PR interval) prior to the nonconducted P wave. The blocked beat occurs when the impulse fails to exit the AV node (the A complex is not followed by an H spike in the blocked beat). This is much more typical for Mobitz I AV block than the example shown in Figure 5.7.

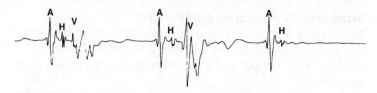

Figure 5.18 Mobitz II AV block. The His-bundle electrogram is shown. The beat is dropped after the H spike and has no prior prolongation in either the AH or the HV interval.

Mobitz type II block (Figure 5.18) is always located in the His–Purkinje system. Thus, the His-bundle electrogram shows a normal AH interval and a stable HV interval in all the conducted beats, but in the dropped beat there is suddenly no ventricular depolarization after the H spike.

With third-degree block within the AV node, the A spikes are not followed by H spikes. Further, since the escape pacemaker is usually proximal to the His bundle, escape pacemaker complexes are usually preceded by His potentials (Figure 5.19a). With third-degree block occurring in the His–Purkinje system, the A spike is followed by an H spike, but there is no V spike after the H. The escape ventricular electrogram is not preceded by a His potential, since these escape pacemakers are distal to the His bundle (Figure 5.19b).

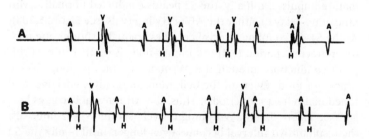

Figure 5.19 His-bundle electrograms in complete heart block. (a) With block in the AV node, H spikes are seen prior to the escape V complexes, indicating a high junctional escape pacemaker. No H spikes are seen after the blocked A complexes, indicating block in the AV node. (b) With distal AV block, an H spike follows each nonconducted A complex. The distal ventricular escape complexes are not preceded by H spikes.

Inapparent AV conduction disturbances

Patients may present with symptoms compatible with AV conduction disease but show no conduction abnormalities on either ECG or monitoring. In such cases the electrophysiology study can be quite helpful.

The goal in electrophysiologic testing is to stress AV conduction by pacing the right atrium, while recording the His electrogram to see what happens. Two primary pacing methods are used, as described in Chapter 4: the extrastimulus technique (in which a single atrial premature stimulus is introduced, after a drive train of stimuli at a fixed cycle length) and incremental pacing.

The extrastimulus technique   This technique is illustrated in Figure 5.20. Following a drive train of several (usually eight) incrementally paced beats (the S1 beats) at a fixed cycle length (usually 600 msec), a single premature atrial stimulus is introduced (the S2 beat). The coupling interval between the last S1 beat and the S2 beat is initially relatively long (usually 500 msec), but with each subsequent pacing sequence it is progressively shortened. The goal is to determine *when* AV block first occurs and *where* it first occurs (i.e. in or distal to the AV node) in response to the S2 impulses.

The normal sequence of events is shown in Figure 5.20. The AH interval and HV interval measured during the S1 drive train are considered to represent the baseline AV node and His–Purkinje conduction times. Any prolongations in AH and HV intervals observed with the S2 beat then reflect slowed conduction in response to premature impulses. Initially, the S2 beat is conducted normally, with little or no delay in either the AH or HV intervals (see Figure 5.20a). As the S1–S2 coupling interval becomes gradually shorter, the relative refractory period (RRP) of the AV node is reached (i.e. at this point conduction through the AV node becomes prolonged—see Chapter 4 for a review of the definitions of relative, effective, and functional refractory periods). Thus, the AH interval becomes longer (see Figure 5.20b). With progressively shorter S1–S2 intervals, the resultant AH interval becomes even longer, until finally the S2 beat is so early that block occurs in the AV node (see Figure 5.20c). The coupling interval that produces block in the AV node is the effective refractory period (ERP) of the AV node. By measuring the H1–H2 intervals that result with each pacing sequence, the functional refractory period (FRP) of the AV node can be determined (the FRP of the AV node is the shortest H1–H2 interval attained). The His–Purkinje ERP is usually significantly shorter than the AV nodal FRP, so that the

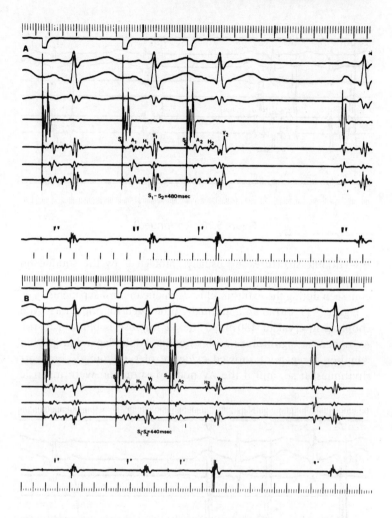

Figure 5.20 A typical response to the atrial extrastimulus technique. Three surface ECG leads, one right atrial electrogram, three His-bundle electrograms, and one right ventricular electrogram are shown. (a) The S1–S2 coupling interval of 480 msec is followed by a minimal prolongation of the AH interval. (b). With further shortening of the S1–S2 coupling interval (to 440 msec), progressive prolongation in the AH interval is seen (compare this A2–H2 interval to that in (a)). (c). With an S1–S2 coupling interval of 320 msec, the S2 stimulus is blocked in the AV node (the A2 complex is not followed by an H spike).

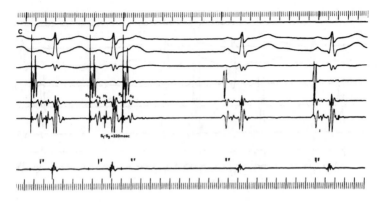

Figure 5.20 (*continued*)

His–Purkinje structures are usually "protected" by the conduction delays in the AV node. Thus, block in the His–Purkinje system is seldom seen during the extrastimulus technique in normal patients.

Figure 5.21 shows an abnormally prolonged AV nodal ERP. At a coupling interval of 480 msec, the S2 impulse is blocked in the AV node. The significance of this finding would depend largely on whether the patient showed evidence of symptomatic bradyarrhythmias. If so, and if the AV nodal dysfunction were intrinsic

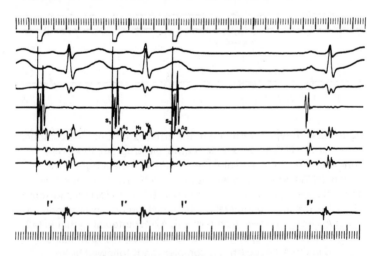

Figure 5.21 Abnormal AV nodal function brought out by the extrastimulus technique. The same leads are depicted as in Figure 5.20. With an S1–S2 coupling interval of 480 msec, block occurs in the AV node.

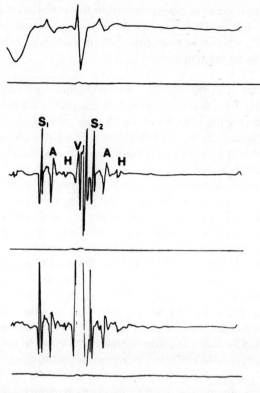

Figure 5.22 Abnormal His–Purkinje function brought out by the extrastimulus technique. With an S1–S2 coupling interval of 460 msec, block occurs below the His bundle (the H spike is not followed by a V complex). A surface ECG lead and two His-bundle electrograms are shown.

(i.e. not reversible), pacing might be considered. Note that in this example, it would be difficult to diagnose concomitant His–Purkinje disease because the long ERP (and thus the long FRP) of the AV node prevents us from evaluating the effect of early impulses on the more distal structures. To evaluate the His–Purkinje system in such a patient, it would be necessary to attempt to improve AV nodal function by administering atropine or isoproterenol.

An example of abnormal His–Purkinje function is shown in Figure 5.22. At an S1–S2 interval of 460 msec, the impulse is conducted normally to the His bundle through the AV node (we know this from the normal AH interval), but infranodal block is present because the impulse is not conducted to the ventricles (i.e. the H spike is not followed by a V spike). Block in the His–Purkinje system at an H1–H2 interval of greater than 400 msec indicates significant distal conducting system disease.

Incremental pacing   With this technique (illustrated in Figure 5.23), long sequences of right atrial pacing are introduced while observing the behavior of the AV node and the His–Purkinje system. A pacing rate slightly faster than the underlying sinus rate is used initially. The pacing rate is gradually increased with each subsequent pacing sequence.

The normal response to incremental pacing is shown in Figure 5.23. At progressively faster atrial pacing rates, the AH interval gradually increases until the refractory period of the AV node is reached, at which time second-degree AV block occurs, typically in a Mobitz I pattern. In this case, the AH interval gradually prolongs from 110 msec at a paced cycle length of 600 msec (Figure 5.23a) to 160 msec at a cycle length of 450 msec (Figure 5.23b). Finally, in Figure 5.23c, at a cycle length of 400 msec, Mobitz I second-degree AV block is seen (note the gradually increasing AH intervals prior to the dropped beat). The atrial pacing rate at which Mobitz type I block occurs is called the *Wenckebach cycle length*. Normally, the Wenckebach cycle length is less than or equal to 450 msec.

During incremental atrial pacing, the Wenckebach cycle length is normally encountered before any prolongation of the HV interval is seen. Lengthening of the HV interval, or block in the His bundle, occurring at a paced cycle length of greater than or equal to 400 msec indicates an abnormal distal conducting system. An example of distal block is shown in Figure 5.24. At a cycle length of 460 msec, intermittent second-degree AV block is seen. The His electrogram reveals a constant AH interval, with intermittent block occurring in the His–Purkinje system (in dropped beats, H spikes are not followed by V spikes). Once again, if distal conducting system disease is suspected but the AV nodal refractory periods are too long to allow the His–Purkinje system to be fully evaluated, autonomic maneuvers should be considered to reduce the refractoriness of the AV node and to permit further testing of the infranodal conducting system.

Bundle branch block

As we saw in Chapter 1, the His bundle divides into two main branches—the right and left bundle branches. Electrical impulses exiting the AV conduction system are rapidly transmitted through the right and left bundle branches, then through successive branches of Purkinje fibers, and finally to the right and left ventricular myocardium. The bundle branches and Purkinje system distribute the electrical impulse across the ventricular myocardium in such a way as to optimally coordinate the contraction of both ventricles.

The bundle branches and Purkinje fibers are subject to the same sorts of disorder as the rest of the cardiac conducting system. When there is a general slowing of conduction in or distal to the bundle branches, the distribution of the electrical impulse to the

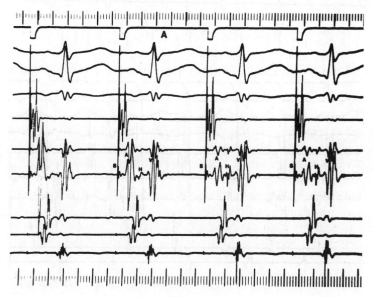

Figure 5.23 The normal response to incremental atrial pacing. Three surface ECG leads followed by one right atrial electrogram, two His-bundle electrograms, two coronary sinus electrograms, and one right ventricular electrogram are shown. (a) Incremental pacing from the high right atrium at a cycle length of 600 msec results in normal AV conduction (as shown in the labeled His-bundle electrogram). (b). At a faster incrementally paced cycle length (450 msec), prolongation in the AH interval (compared to (a)) is apparent. All atrial impulses, however, are conducted. (c). At a paced cycle length of 400 msec, Mobitz I conduction occurs. Note the progressive prolongation in the AH intervals in the beats preceding the nonconducted P wave. Thus, the Wenckebach cycle length is 400 msec (a normal value).

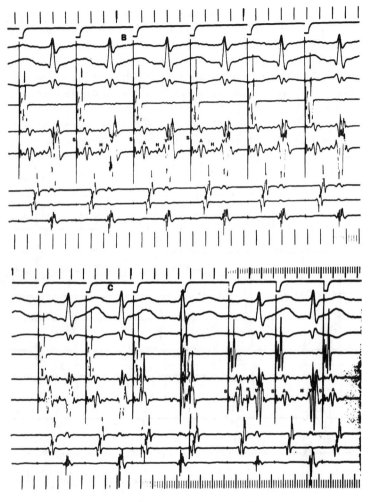

Figure 5.23 (*continued*)

ventricular myocardium is delayed, and an intraventricular conduction delay (IVCD) is said to be present. An IVCD is manifested on a surface ECG by a wide QRS complex.

Delayed or blocked conduction is commonly limited specifically to either the right or the left bundle branch, conditions referred to as right or left bundle branch block. Thus, right bundle branch block (RBBB) and left bundle branch block (LBBB) are specific varieties of IVCD.

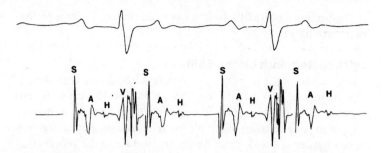

Figure 5.24 Distal AV block during incremental atrial pacing. In this figure, during incremental atrial pacing, 2 : 1 AV block occurs. The His-bundle electrogram shows that the block is in the distal conducting system—the AH interval is constant, and there is an H spike in the nonconducted beats.

Right bundle branch block (RBBB)

RBBB is a relatively common ECG finding that generally carries little prognostic significance. The incidence of RBBB gradually increases with age, from less than 1% in 50-year-olds to approximately 10% in octogenarians. Most younger patients with RBBB have no underlying heart disease.

The right bundle branch remains a relatively discrete structure for a few centimeters after splitting off from the His bundle, and for most of its course it is located just beneath the endocardial surface, where it is subject to stretch and trauma from conditions affecting the right ventricle. Thus, RBBB is common in conditions causing pulmonary hypertension or right ventricular hypertrophy, inflammation,'or infarction. RBBB can appear quite abruptly, with sudden elevations in right-sided cardiac pressures, as in pulmonary embolism. RBBB can also occur during right heart catheter insertions due to localized trauma to the right bundle branch—this latter form of RBBB, which is seen in roughly 5% of right heart catheterizations, is usually transient.

The prognosis of patients with RBBB is dictated not by the RBBB itself, but almost entirely by the type and severity of any underlying heart disease. If there is no underlying heart disease—that is, if RBBB is an isolated finding in an otherwise normal patient—the long-term prognosis appears virtually normal.

As long as the left bundle branch functions normally, patients with RBBB do not appear to suffer from clinically significant ventricular dyssynchrony; that is, left ventricular contractions remain coordinated and efficient.

The presence of RBBB alone is never an indication for a permanent pacemaker.

Left bundle branch block (LBBB)

LBBB, while not uncommon, is seen less frequently than RBBB. The incidence of LBBB is less than 0.5% in 50-year-olds, but increases to 5–6% by age 80 (the age-related increase in frequency seen with both varieties of bundle branch block suggests a degenerative disorder of the conducting system, similar to the process that causes SA nodal and AV conduction abnormalities in the same age group).

Younger patients with LBBB usually have no underlying heart disease, in which case the prognosis is thought to be excellent. In older patients, for whom the new onset of LBBB most often indicates the presence of progressive heart disease (most commonly coronary artery disease, cardiomyopathy, or valvular heart disease), LBBB is an independent predictor of mortality.

There are at least two reasons why LBBB may indicate a worse prognosis in patients with underlying heart disease. The first is related to the fact that the left bundle branch almost immediately divides into three major fascicles after splitting off from the His bundle, and thus quickly becomes a relatively diffuse system. For this reason, the presence of LBBB (in contrast to RBBB) both suggests a diffuse pathological process instead of a localized one and frequently indicates that advanced heart disease is present. The second reason is that the LBBB itself produces disordered left ventricular contraction and in patients with underlying systolic dysfunction can directly worsen cardiac performance (see Chapter 9, especially Figure 9.1, for an explanation of how LBBB produces ventricular dyssynchrony). In many cases, patients with LBBB and heart failure can be helped with cardiac resynchronization therapy (CRT)— specialized pacemakers that pace both ventricles simultaneously, thus recoordinating ventricular contraction (see Chapter 9 for a detailed discussion of CRT).

The presence of LBBB alone does not constitute an indication for a standard, anti-bradycardia permanent pacemaker. As noted, however, in some clinical circumstances patients will have an indication for CRT pacemakers by virtue of their LBBB. Further, when performing a right heart catheterization in patients with LBBB, provisions for immediate temporary pacing support should be available, since there is a 5% chance of causing transient RBBB (and thus complete heart block) during the procedure. In addition, some patients experiencing block in one of the fascicles of the left bundle branch in combination with RBBB (a condition known as bilateral fascicular block) and a myocardial infarction have an increased risk of complete heart block and should receive permanent pacemakers.

A brief overview of permanent pacemakers

Major indications for pacemakers

In the preceding discussion, we have touched upon the major indications for permanent pacemakers. The following list makes these indications more explicit:

1. Symptomatic sinus bradycardia:
   a. symptomatic sinus bradycardia at rest;
   b. inability to increase the sinus rate appropriately with exercise (i.e. chronotropic incompetence), thus limiting exercise capacity;
   c. syncope of unknown origin in patients who are shown to have significant SA nodal abnormalities on electrophysiologic testing.
2. AV conduction disease:
   a. acquired third-degree AV block;
   b. second-degree AV block below the AV node;
   c. second-degree AV nodal block if persistent and symptomatic;
   d. new bilateral fascicular block following an acute myocardial infarction;
   e. congenital complete heart block with severe bradycardia, significant symptoms, or wide-QRS escape rhythm;
   f. markedly prolonged HV interval (>100 msec) or split His.
3. Other indications for pacing:
   a. cardioneurogenic syncope (also known as vasodepressor syncope; see Chapter 10), in which there is a severe or persistent component of bradycardia, in patients in whom more conservative therapeutic attempts have failed;
   b. syncope of unknown origin in the presence of bilateral fascicular block, where no other cause of syncope can be identified;
   c. bradycardia-induced ventricular tachyarrhythmias;
   d. cardiac resynchronization therapy (CRT). CRT is indicated for many patients with significant LV dysfunction (ejection fraction less than 0.35) and wide QRS complex (QRS duration more than 120 msec). CRT is discussed in detail in Chapter 9.

Pacemaker nomenclature

While in practical terms most pacemakers can be separated into one of two categories—single-chambered or dual-chambered—any pacemaker can be programmed to a potentially bewildering array of "modes." If we view a pacemaker as a tiny computer enclosed within an implantable metal can, the pacing mode can be thought of as the set of instructions—or the software program—that tells the pacemaker how to function under various circumstances.

By convention, pacing modes are described by a *three-letter code*.

The first letter indicates the chamber or chambers that are paced. "A" indicates the atrium; "V" indicates the ventricle; and "D" (which stands for "dual chamber") indicates both atrium and ventricle.

The second letter indicates the chamber or chambers in which sensing occurs. Again, "A" indicates the atrium; "V" indicates the ventricle; "D" indicates both atrium and ventricle; and "O" means no sensing is occurring.

The third letter indicates how the pacemaker responds to a sensed event. "I" means that a sensed event causes inhibition of the pacing impulse (and resets the timing intervals). "T" means a sensed event triggers a pacing impulse. "D," which is only used in dual-chambered devices, means there is a "dual" (or two kinds of) response—a sensed event can either inhibit or trigger a pacing impulse, depending on circumstances. "O" means that a sensed event neither inhibits nor triggers a pacing impulse—it is "ignored."

In addition, *a fourth letter* is often employed to indicate that rate-responsive pacing is being used. Rate-responsive pacing incorporates a sensor into the pacing system that continually monitors the physiologic needs of the patient. The rate of pacing is thereby adjusted to the physiologic requirements of the patient from moment to moment. The sensors used most commonly in today's pacemakers monitor either activity or respiratory rate—the more active the patient or the more rapidly they are breathing, the higher the rate of pacing (within a programmed limit). The fourth letter "R" is added to the three-letter code if rate-responsive pacing is active.

Common modes of pacing

For practical purposes, only two modes are used with any frequency: the VVI (or AAI) mode for single-chambered pacemakers and the DDD mode for dual-chambered pacemakers.

VVI or AAI pacing

Single-chambered pacemakers function in the VVI mode when the pacing lead is positioned in the ventricle and in the AAI mode when the lead is in the atrium. These pacemakers simply maintain a minimum programmable heart rate. Each timing sequence is initiated by either a paced impulse or a sensed (i.e. intrinsic) impulse. If an intrinsic beat does not occur (i.e. is not sensed) by the end of this timing sequence, a paced impulse is delivered and a new timing sequence is begun (thus a VVI pacemaker paces in the ventricle (V) and senses intrinsic beats occurring in the ventricle (V), and a sensed event causes it to inhibit pacing and resets the timing sequence (I)). Essentially then, the doctor programs a minimum heart rate, and whenever the patient's intrinsic heart rate falls below that value, pacing occurs at the programmed rate; if the intrinsic heart rate is above the programmed rate, pacing is inhibited. An electrogram from a VVI pacemaker is illustrated in Figure 5.25.

AAI pacemakers work in exactly the same way, except that the pacing lead is located in the atrium instead of the ventricle. AAI pacing is used exclusively in patients with isolated SA nodal

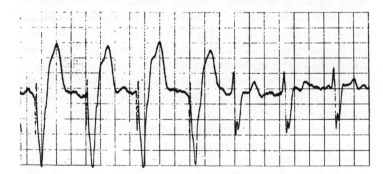

Figure 5.25 This surface ECG tracing is from a patient with a VVI pacemaker. A VVI pacemaker paces the ventricle at a fixed rate, unless intrinsic ventricular activity is sensed during the pacemaker escape interval (the length of time after a QRS complex during which the pacemaker waits for an intrinsic QRS complex before firing). The first four beats show ventricular pacing. After the fourth paced beat, an intrinsic QRS complex occurs during the pacemaker escape interval. This inhibits the pacemaker from firing and resets the pacemaker escape interval. Two more intrinsic QRS complexes occur, and the pacemaker remains appropriately inhibited.

dysfunction; that is, patients who show no evidence of AV conduction disease. For such patients, AAI pacing provides both rate support and AV synchrony and is an excellent choice. AAI pacing is not used commonly in the United States (apparently American doctors are afraid either of occult AV conduction disease or of American lawyers) but is employed quite frequently in many other countries.

VVI pacemakers offer perfectly acceptable protection from bradyarrhythmias but do not restore AV synchrony. In general, VVI pacemakers are used in patients who are felt to need only rare to occasional ventricular pacing support.

Practically speaking, almost all single-chambered pacemakers in use today are programmed to rate-responsive modes (i.e. either AAIR or VVIR pacing modes), so the rate of pacing is not fixed but adjusts from minute to minute according to the needs of the patient. Since AAI pacing is used exclusively in patients with SA nodal disease, and thus in patients who are likely to have a blunted heart-rate response to exercise, it is difficult to imagine a circumstance in which AAI pacing would be chosen over AAIR pacing. VVIR pacemakers are a good choice for patients with chronic atrial fibrillation.

Pacemaker syndrome The major clinical problem inherent in VVI/R pacing is *pacemaker syndrome*. Pacemaker syndrome arises when intrinsic atrial impulses occur during or just after ventricular pacing, thus causing the atria to contract against closed AV valves and producing reflux of atrial blood through the superior vena cava and pulmonary veins. Symptoms may include headache, dizziness, fatigue, lethargy, neck throbbing, cough, dyspnea, chest "fullness," and, occasionally, orthostatic hypotension or syncope. Pacemaker syndrome is especially prevalent in patients who have intact retrograde conduction, where retrograde impulses stimulate atrial contraction immediately after ventricular pacing. In some series, more than 20% of patients who require frequent VVI pacing display some degree of pacemaker syndrome. Pacemaker syndrome is resolved by changing over to a dual-chambered pacemaker. Patients with chronic atrial fibrillation are not subject to pacemaker syndrome.

DDD pacing

Modern dual-chambered pacemakers almost always function in the DDD mode. In DDD pacing, pacing occurs in both the right atrium and the right ventricle (D), sensing in both the atrium and the ventricle (D), and a sensed event can either trigger or inhibit a pacing output (D); see Figure 5.26.

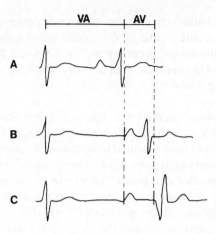

Figure 5.26 DDD pacing is designed to maintain AV coordination under most circumstances. DDD pacing can be described largely by considering two escape intervals: the VA interval and the AV interval (both of which are programmable with DDD pacemakers). When a QRS complex occurs (either intrinsic or paced), the VA interval is reset. If no intrinsic atrial or ventricular activity is sensed by the end of the VA interval, an atrial pacing spike is delivered. Once an atrial event occurs (either a paced or an intrinsic atrial event), the AV interval is initiated. If no intrinsic ventricular activity occurs during the AV interval, a ventricular pacing spike is delivered at the end of that interval. (a) An intrinsic P–QRS complex occurs during the VA interval, and all pacing is inhibited. (b) No atrial or ventricular activity is sensed during the VA interval, and atrial pacing occurs. During the ensuing AV interval, normal conduction occurs to the ventricle, so ventricular pacing is inhibited. (c) Same as in (b), except that this time conduction to the ventricles does not occur during the AV interval, so the ventricle is paced.

DDD pacemakers are designed to preserve the normal sequence of AV contraction under a wide range of circumstances and, if the SA node is functioning normally, to allow tracking of the intrinsic sinus rate. Atrial pacing occurs if the intrinsic atrial rate falls below the minimum programmed heart rate. After a paced or sensed atrial event, the pacemaker will wait a certain length of time (i.e. the programmed AV interval) for the ventricle to depolarize. If no intrinsic ventricular activity is detected during that interval, the ventricle is then paced.

Most dual-chambered pacemakers used today offer a rate-responsive mode (i.e. the DDDR mode) to allow higher heart rates in response to physiologic needs, even if the SA nodal dysfunction is present. DDDR pacing is ideal for patients with both SA nodal and AV conduction disorders.

Mode-switching   In the past, DDD pacing was often difficult to manage in patients with episodic atrial tachyarrhythmias, since the pacemaker would track the atrial tachycardia and pace the ventricle at inappropriately high rates. Most modern dual-chambered pacemakers now provide a *mode-switching* feature that largely eliminates this problem. Under mode-switching, when an atrial tachyarrhythmia occurs, the pacemaker automatically switches to a non-atrial-tracking mode, most commonly the VVI (or VVIR) mode. When the atrial arrhythmia terminates, the pacemaker switches back to the DDD (or DDDR) mode.

Pacemaker tachycardia   The most common clinical problem inherent to DDD pacemakers is *pacemaker tachycardia*, in which (a) a premature ventricular complex causes a retrograde impulse to be transmitted to the atrium; where (b) it is sensed by the atrial lead and interpreted by the pacemaker as an intrinsic atrial beat; so that (c) the pacemaker then triggers a ventricular paced beat; which again (d) transmits a retrograde impulse to the atrium–thus establishing a pacemaker-mediated "reentrant tachycardia" (Figure 5.27). In the typical case, pacemaker tachycardia occurs at the maximum programmed pacing rate.

A number of methods have been used to control pacemaker tachycardia:

- Lengthening the post-ventricular atrial refractory period (PVARP) can essentially "blind" the atrium for a time after a ventricular event, to reduce the odds that a retrograde P wave will be sensed. Unfortunately, increasing the PVARP also reduces the maximum tracking rate the pacemaker will allow.
- The sensitivity of the atrial lead can be reduced, so that SA nodal impulses can still be detected but retrograde P waves (which often have relatively small amplitudes) cannot.
- Many modern pacemakers incorporate a feature that automatically lengthens PVARP for one cycle following a premature ventricular complex, which can inhibit the initiation of pacemaker tachycardia.

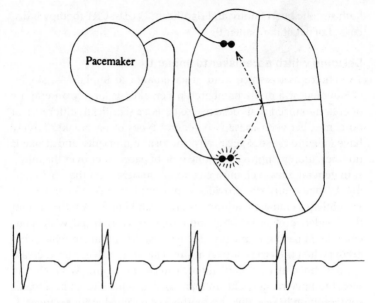

Figure 5.27 Pacemaker tachycardia. With DDD pacemakers, the potential for a reentrant tachycardia exists, the pacemaker itself serving as the antegrade limb of the reentrant circuit. Pacemaker tachycardia is most often initiated by a PVC, which conducts retrogradely to the atrium. The atrial electrode of the pacemaker senses the retrograde atrial impulse and initiates the AV escape interval (see Figure 5.26) of the DDD pacemaker. At the end of the AV interval, a ventricular pacing spike is delivered. If this paced ventricular impulse again conducts retrogradely to the atrium, an incessant tachycardia can result.

- Special algorithms, available in some pacemakers, can automatically withhold a single ventricular paced impulse after a certain number of beats, whenever the pacemaker is pacing at the maximum tracking rate. This single inhibited ventricular impulse will terminate pacemaker tachycardia.

In general, by using one or more of these strategies, pacemaker tachycardia can be managed adequately.

CRT pacing

Cardiac resynchronization therapy—also known as *biventricular pacing*—is done not to provide bradycardia support, but instead to improve left ventricular hemodynamic function in patients with both systolic heart failure and significant IVCDs. CRT therapy is discussed in detail in Chapter 9.

Deciding which pacemaker to implant

The choice as to which kind of pacemaker to implant—a single-chambered or a dual-chambered pacemaker–is largely an empiric one. Randomized trials designed to detect a significant difference in outcomes between these two general types of pacemaker largely have failed to do so. Specifically, the risk of mortality and stroke is not measurably improved for one type of pacemaker over the other.

In general, however, most electrophysiologists feel that maintaining AV synchrony still provides significant benefits. Avoiding overt or subtle pacemaker syndrome is one such benefit. Another is that the incidence of atrial fibrillation appears be reduced with dual-chambered pacing (quite possibly because the atrial stretching that occurs when the atria contract against closed AV valves may increase the likelihood of atrial fibrillation). Thus, maintaining AV synchrony seems to have real benefits in many patients and should be a major consideration in selecting the appropriate pacemaker for a patient.

The other major consideration is maintaining rate-responsiveness, since the ability to perform physical activity is strongly dependent on the ability to increase the heart rate appropriately with exercise.

Keeping these two major considerations in mind (i.e. maintaining both AV synchrony and rate-responsiveness), the appropriate pacemaker can usually be selected by answering two fairly simple questions (Figure 5.28). The first is: "Is there chronic atrial fibrillation?" If so, maintaining AV synchrony becomes

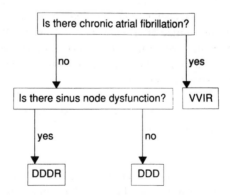

Figure 5.28 Decision tree for the selection of a pacemaker.

moot, and a single-chambered VVIR pacemaker should be used. In virtually all other cases, a dual-chambered pacemaker is preferable. The second question is: "Is there SA nodal dysfunction?" If the SA node is known to be normal then a simple DDD pacemaker can provide both AV coordination and rate-responsiveness. On the other hand, if the SA node is either known or suspected to be abnormal then a dual-chambered pacemaker capable of the DDDR mode should be used.

Is the electrophysiology study helpful in selecting the right pacemaker?

Generally, the electrophysiology study is *not* helpful in selecting the right pacemaker, but on occasion it can be. If one would like to use a DDD instead of a DDDR pacemaker in a patient with AV block, for instance, firm evidence of normal SA nodal activity would be helpful, and an electrophysiology study could provide that evidence. There is, however, little advantage at present in choosing a dual-chambered pacemaker that does not provide rate-responsive pacing, as the cost differential between DDD and DDDR pacemakers is now usually quite small. Indeed, almost all currently manufactured dual-chambered pacemakers offer rate-responsive pacing.

The other circumstance in which electrophysiologic testing may be helpful is when considering an AAIR pacemaker (in deference to American electrophysiologists, AAIR pacing is not included in Figure 5.28). In patients with pure SA nodal disease and normal AV conduction, an AAIR pacemaker will result in both AV synchrony and rate-responsiveness and would be a very reasonable choice. Unfortunately, at least one-third of patients with SA nodal disease have concomitant AV conduction disease. Thus, electrophysiologic testing should be considered prior to the use of AAI pacing, in order to rule out subtle conduction abnormalities. Indeed, one advantage of avoiding the AAI mode altogether is that doing so virtually eliminates the need to ever do electrophysiologic testing in deciding which pacemaker to implant.

6 The Electrophysiology Study in the Evaluation of Supraventricular Tachyarrhythmias

The electrophysiology study has revolutionized our understanding and treatment of supraventricular tachyarrhythmias. The ability to study these arrhythmias accurately has allowed us to classify them precisely according to mechanism, and this reclassification has helped greatly to direct appropriate therapy. Correlating findings from the electrophysiology laboratory with findings on the surface ECG has allowed clinicians to choose specific therapy in many patients, even without invasive testing. Further, the electrophysiology study has allowed us to identify effective therapy for patients with complex or difficult forms of supraventricular arrhythmia whose therapy would likely have been unsatisfactory in earlier days.

The study of supraventricular tachyarrhythmias is the most challenging and intellectually satisfying type of electrophysiology study. Unlike the studies performed for bradyarrhythmias (the novelty of which soon fades for the budding electrophysiologist), no two studies of supraventricular tachyarrhythmias are exactly alike. When investigating supraventricular tachycardia, unpredicted findings are commonplace. The electrophysiologist must therefore be alert for unexpected results and must be ready to alter the procedural plan to pursue fully those findings. As opposed to studies performed for ventricular tachyarrhythmias, there is no need to take it on faith during studies for supraventricular tachycardias that the arrhythmias being induced are reentrant. In many patients with supraventricular tachyarrhythmias, the anatomic pathways for the reentrant circuit can be defined with surprising accuracy. In fact,

Electrophysiologic Testing, Fifth Edition. Richard N. Fogoros.
© 2012 John Wiley & Sons, Ltd. Published 2012 by John Wiley & Sons, Ltd.

most electrophysiologists starting off in the profession do not truly believe in the reality of reentrant circuits until they perform a few electrophysiology studies in patients with supraventricular tachycardia.

In this chapter, we will review the various types of supraventricular tachyarrhythmia and describe how the electrophysiology study helps to elucidate the mechanisms and most appropriate therapy for them.

General classification of supraventricular tachyarrhythmias

As described in Chapter 2, most supraventricular tachyarrhythmias are caused by either abnormal automaticity or reentry.

Automatic supraventricular tachyarrhythmias

Automatic supraventricular tachyarrhythmias are relatively uncommon, except in acutely ill patients. When they do occur, they are usually associated with fairly obvious metabolic disturbances, the most common being myocardial ischemia, acute exacerbations of chronic lung disease, acute alcohol ingestion, and electrolyte disturbances. The arrhythmias usually arise from ectopic automatic foci located somewhere within the atrial myocardium. Characteristically, automatic atrial tachycardias display the typical warm-up phenomenon seen with automatic rhythms (i.e. the rate accelerates after its initiation). The peak rate is usually less than 200 beats/min. There is a discrete P wave before each QRS complex, and the P wave configuration generally differs from the sinus P wave (depending on the location of the automatic focus within the atria). Because the AV node is not necessary for the maintenance of the arrhythmia, AV block is commonly seen during automatic atrial tachycardia; interventions that affect AV conduction may produce block but do not affect the tachycardia itself.

Digitalis toxicity often presents as atrial tachycardia with AV block and, while the mechanism is felt to be triggered automaticity, this arrhythmia is clinically indistinguishable from standard automatic atrial tachycardia. Thus, any unexplained atrial tachycardia with block should prompt a search for digitalis toxicity.

Multifocal (or chaotic) atrial tachycardia (Figure 6.1) is a form of automatic atrial tachycardia characterized by multiple (usually at least three) P wave morphologies and irregular PP intervals. It is thought to be due to multiple atrial automatic foci that are firing at

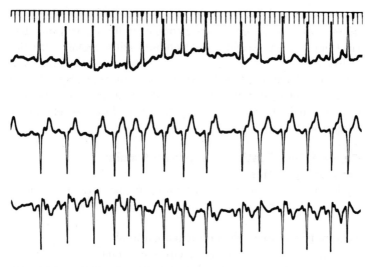

Figure 6.1 Multifocal atrial tachycardia. This is an irregularly irregular rhythm with multiple (but discrete) P wave morphologies. It is thought to be due to multiple atrial automatic foci.

differing rates. Multifocal atrial tachycardia is often seen with acute pulmonary disease and may be related to theophylline use.

Inappropriate sinus tachycardia (IST) is a unique type of automatic tachycardia originating in the sinus node. Consequently, except for the clinical setting, IST is identical to normal sinus tachycardia (IST is discussed in detail in Chapter 11 and is mentioned here mainly to point out how it differs from other, more typical forms of automatic tachycardia). IST occurs in young, otherwise healthy patients who do *not* have reversible metabolic abnormalities, drug toxicities, or any other transient conditions producing the arrhythmia. Instead, IST is a chronic or persistent condition that is probably related to an underlying autonomic imbalance, and which can become quite debilitating over time.

For all forms of automatic supraventricular tachycardia, the basic principle of therapy is to attempt to reverse the underlying cause. Digitalis toxicity should be suspected in any patient who has been taking this drug, and digitalis should be withheld until toxic levels are ruled out. If the ventricular response is rapid enough to produce hemodynamic instability, the ventricular rate can usually be slowed with digitalis (if toxicity has been ruled out), verapamil, or β-blockers. In addition, if rapid 1:1 conduction is occurring during an automatic atrial tachycardia, an immediate slowing of the ventricular response can sometimes be accomplished by pacing the atria even faster than the rate of the tachycardia—fast enough to produce 2 : 1 or 3 : 1 AV block. Because these arrhythmias are not reentrant, they cannot be pace-terminated and usually do not respond well to direct current (DC) cardioversion. Class Ia antiarrhythmic drugs can be used in an attempt to terminate the arrhythmias, but, unless the underlying cause is reversed, these drugs tend to be relatively ineffective. The electrophysiology study offers no benefit in patients with automatic supraventricular tachyarrhythmias.

Reentrant supraventricular tachyarrhythmias

The vast majority of supraventricular tachyarrhythmias seen in ambulatory patients are due to reentry. In contrast to automatic atrial tachycardias, reentrant supraventricular tachycardias are seen in patients who are not acutely ill. Further, in contrast to reentrant ventricular tachyarrhythmias (see Chapter 7), reentrant supraventricular tachycardias are usually seen in patients who are free of chronic heart disease. Although reentrant circuits in the ventricle generally do not appear unless disease of the ventricular myocardium is present, the reentrant substrate for supraventricular arrhythmias tends to be congenital. Overt heart disease is therefore not necessary in order for a patient to develop these arrhythmias. Thus, the typical patient with reentrant supraventricular tachycardia is young and healthy.

There are five general categories of reentrant supraventricular tachyarrhythmia: AV nodal reentry, bypass tract-mediated macro-reentry, intraatrial reentry, SA nodal reentry, and atrial flutter/atrial fibrillation. Many clinicians still tend to lump these reentrant arrhythmias (except for atrial flutter and atrial fibrillation) together into one large group called PAT (paroxysmal atrial tachycardia—generally, any regular, narrow-complex tachycardia with sudden onset and sudden termination). The term PAT, however, is a vestige from the days when the mechanisms for supraventricular arrhythmias were poorly understood. The electrophysiology study has now made it clear that PAT is almost always due to one of the categories of reentrant supraventricular tachyarrhythmia just listed. In many cases, the knowledgeable clinician can tell which type of supraventricular tachyarrhythmia he or she is dealing with (and therefore what type of therapy to use) merely by keeping these categories in mind while examining a 12-lead ECG of the arrhythmia.

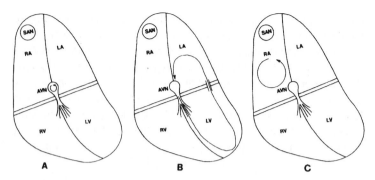

Figure 6.2 The three most common reentrant supraventricular tachycardias. (a) AV nodal reentrant tachycardia. In this arrhythmia, the reentrant circuit is small and is thought to be localized entirely within the AV node. (b) Bypass tract-mediated macroreentrant tachycardia. An AV bypass tract serves as one pathway (usually the retrograde) and the normal AV conduction system serves as the other of this large (hence, macroreentrant) reentrant circuit. (c) Atrial reentrant tachycardia. In this arrhythmia, the reentrant circuit is contained within the atrial myocardium.

AV Nodal Reentrant Tachycardia

AV nodal reentrant tachycardia is the most common type of reentrant supraventricular tachycardia and is the operative mechanism in up to 60% of patients presenting with PAT. In AV nodal reentry, the reentrant circuit is usually said to be enclosed within the AV node (Figure 6.2a). In patients with AV nodal reentry, the AV node is functionally divided into two longitudinal pathways (dual AV nodal pathways). These dual pathways form the reentrant circuit. Because, for all practical purposes, the reentrant circuit in AV nodal reentry involves the AV node exclusively, this arrhythmia responds well to autonomic maneuvers and drugs that affect the AV node (digitalis, calcium blockers, and β-blockers).

Bypass tract-mediated macroreentrant tachycardia

Bypass tract-mediated macroreentrant tachycardia is the next most common type of arrhythmia presenting as PAT (30%). In macroreentrant tachycardia, an AV bypass tract is present. (The majority of patients presenting with macroreentrant tachycardia do not have overt Wolff–Parkinson–White syndrome. Instead, they have concealed bypass tracts—bypass tracts that are incapable of conducting in the antegrade direction and therefore generate no delta waves.)

In these patients, the bypass tract acts as one pathway (almost always the retrograde pathway), and the normal AV conducting system acts as the other (the antegrade pathway), of the reentrant circuit (Figure 6.2b). Because this reentrant circuit is a large circuit involving the AV node, the His–Purkinje system, and the ventricular and atrial myocardia as well as the bypass tract, it is termed a macroreentrant circuit. Also, because the circuit consists of several types of cardiac tissue, it can be attacked on many levels by many types of drug.

Intraatrial reentry

Intraatrial reentry accounts for only a small percentage of patients presenting with PAT. In intraatrial reentry, the reentrant circuit is entirely within the atrial myocardium and does not involve the AV conducting system (Figure 6.2c). It resembles automatic atrial tachycardia in that discrete P waves, which usually differ from normal sinus P waves, precede each QRS complex, and AV block can occur without affecting the arrhythmia itself. It differs from automatic arrhythmias through its paroxysmal onset and offset and the fact that it can be induced and terminated by pacing. Class Ia drugs are often effective. Because the AV node is not part of the reentrant circuit, attacking the AV node does not affect this arrhythmia.

SA Nodal Reentry

SA nodal reentry is a fairly uncommon arrhythmia in which the reentrant circuit is thought to be enclosed within the SA node. Discrete P waves identical to sinus P waves precede each QRS complex. SA nodal reentrant tachycardia is distinguishable from both normal sinus tachycardia and IST by its onset, which is paroxysmal and does not display warm-up, by its equally sudden termination, and by the fact that it is inducible and terminable with pacing. Because the reentrant circuit is enclosed within the SA node, autonomic maneuvers and drugs such as digitalis, calcium blockers, and β-blockers tend to ameliorate this arrhythmia.

Atrial flutter and atrial fibrillation

Finally, *atrial flutter and atrial fibrillation* are forms of reentrant atrial tachycardia. These arrhythmias are generally distinctive enough not to be considered to be PAT by clinicians who still use this terminology. In atrial flutter, the atrial rate is regular and in excess of 220 beats/min, and usually displays a typical sawtooth pattern (Figure 6.3). Atrial flutter can usually be terminated by pacing.

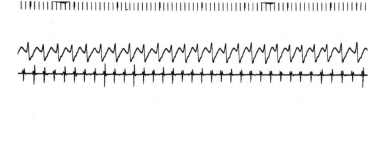

Figure 6.3 Atrial flutter. One surface ECG lead and the right atrial electrogram are shown. Note the rapid, regular atrial rate (cycle length approximately 200 msec) and the 3 : 2 atrioventricular conduction.

Atrial flutter is virtually always accompanied by AV block, usually in a 2 : 1 pattern. In atrial fibrillation, the atrial activity is continuous and chaotic, and definite P waves cannot be distinguished (Figure 6.4). The ventricular response is irregular, reflecting the chaotic atrial activity. Both atrial flutter and atrial fibrillation are similar to intraatrial reentry (and to automatic atrial tachycardia) in that attacking the AV node does not directly affect these arrhythmias. In general, therapy is aimed at either converting the patient to normal sinus rhythm (with class I or class III drugs or cardioversion, or both) or simply controlling the ventricular response with AV nodal blocking agents.

In summary, reentrant supraventricular tachyarrhythmias include several types of arrhythmia, which have different therapies, depending on the location and characteristics of the respective

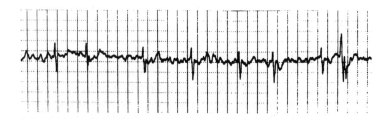

Figure 6.4 Atrial fibrillation. Note the chaotic atrial activity, absence of discrete P waves, and irregularly irregular ventricular response.

reentrant circuits. Most of these arrhythmias are commonly lumped together as PAT, a practice that is counterproductive to appropriate therapy. Once these arrhythmias are understood, the proper diagnosis can often be made (and proper therapy initiated) without resorting to invasive testing. The electrophysiology study, however, can be vital in managing patients with reentrant supraventricular tachyarrhythmias, especially because the majority of these arrhythmias can now be cured with transcatheter ablation techniques (see Chapter 8).

General outline of the electrophysiology study in reentrant supraventricular tachyarrhythmias

The key to studying supraventricular tachyarrhythmias in the electrophysiology laboratory is the capability of inducing these arrhythmias with programmed pacing techniques, while at the same time recording intracardiac electrograms from various key locations within the heart. As noted in Chapter 2, inducing any reentrant rhythm requires the existence of an appropriate anatomic substrate to form a reentrant circuit. In supraventricular tachyarrhythmias, the reentrant circuits can incorporate SA or AV nodal tissue, bypass tracts, and atrial and ventricular myocardial tissue. By recording strategically placed intracardiac electrograms and studying the patterns of activation, by examining the mode of initiation and termination of arrhythmias, and by studying the response to programmed pacing, most supraventricular tachyarrhythmias can be fully characterized in the electrophysiology laboratory. Specifically, the electrophysiology study seeks to determine the anatomic location and electrophysiologic characteristics of the reentrant circuit, the propensity of the circuit to sustain arrhythmias, the characteristics of those arrhythmias, and the response of the reentrant arrhythmias to various therapies.

Positioning the catheters

To localize the reentrant circuits in supraventricular tachyarrhythmias, it is important to record electrograms from all four major cardiac chambers, as well as from the His-bundle region. These recordings can generally be obtained by positioning four electrode catheters: one in the right atrium, one in the right ventricle, one in the His position, and one in the coronary sinus (to record both left atrial and left ventricular deflections; Figure 6.5). With catheters in these four positions, one can record electrograms from the most critical locations and introduce paced impulses from the right

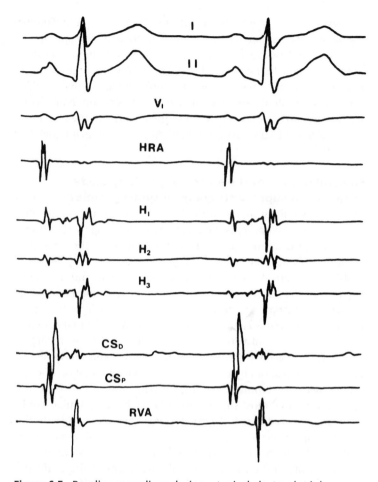

Figure 6.5 Baseline recordings during a typical electrophysiology study for supraventricular tachycardia. Surface leads I, II, and V_1 allow estimation of the QRS axis. The high right atrial (HRA) electrogram records activity near the SA node. The His-bundle electrogram is recorded from several electrode pairs on the His catheter (three in this example). Two recordings are made from the coronary sinus (both of which record left atrial and left ventricular activity)—coronary sinus distal (CS_D) is recorded from the distal electrode pair on the coronary sinus catheter and coronary sinus proximal (CS_P) is recorded from the proximal pair of electrodes. Finally, a recording is made from the right ventricular apex (RVA). With this combination of recordings, the electrophysiologist can keep track of events in all four cardiac chambers, as well as in the normal AV conducting system.

ventricle and from both atria (pacing from the coronary sinus catheter generally produces capture in the left atrium alone).

Evaluation of supraventricular tachyarrhythmias

Once the catheters are positioned, the characteristics of the arrhythmia can be deduced by answering four general questions. First, what is the mode of initiation and termination of the tachycardia? Second, what are the patterns of antegrade and retrograde activation during sinus rhythm and during tachycardia? Third, what is the evidence that atrial or ventricular myocardium is necessary to the reentrant circuit? Fourth, what are the effects of autonomic maneuvers and drugs on the tachycardia? These questions must be addressed for each type of supraventricular tachycardia that is induced during the study.

What is the mode of initiation and termination of the tachycardia?

In assessing the mode of initiation of tachycardia, the electrophysiologist addresses several points.

First, is the tachycardia more readily inducible from one location than another? As noted in Chapter 4, inducing a reentrant arrhythmia requires the delivery of a premature impulse to the reentrant circuit at just the right moment. A major element influencing the inducibility of reentrant arrhythmias, then, is the distance between the pacing catheter and the reentrant circuit—the closer the catheter is to the circuit, the more likely it is that a paced premature beat will arrive at the circuit early enough to induce reentry. Thus, for instance, if a reentrant rhythm is significantly easier to induce with left atrial pacing (i.e. pacing from the coronary sinus) than it is with right atrial pacing, then the reentrant circuit may be expected to involve a left-sided bypass tract.

It is important to observe whether supraventricular tachycardia is readily inducible with ventricular pacing. Inducing tachycardia with ventricular pacing is readily accomplished in macroreentrant tachycardias, is relatively difficult in AV nodal reentry, and is rare with intraatrial reentry (in intraatrial reentry, the arrhythmia can be induced by ventricular stimulation only indirectly and infrequently, by means of retrograde stimulation of the atrium).

Another point relating to the mode of initiation of the tachycardia is the site of the conduction delay that typically occurs with the onset of reentrant supraventricular tachyarrhythmias. The reason for this conduction delay can be seen by reviewing the mechanism for inducing reentrant arrhythmias (see Figure 2.6). As described in Chapter 2, a reentrant circuit requires two roughly parallel pathways (labeled pathways A and B) connecting proximally and distally to common conducting tissues, forming an anatomic circuit. Pathway B has a longer refractory period than pathway A, and pathway A conducts impulses slower than pathway B. The initiation of reentry occurs when a premature impulse enters the circuit at a time when pathway B is still refractory from the previous normal impulse but pathway A has already recovered.

Note that, since pathway B conducts faster than pathway A, a normal (i.e. not premature) impulse will conduct via pathway B rather than pathway A (Figure 6.6a). When an early impulse initiates reentry, this impulse is blocked in pathway B (the fast pathway) and instead conducts via pathway A (the slow pathway). Thus, a beat that initiates reentry is commonly accompanied by conduction delay (Figure 6.6b). The electrophysiologist must pay

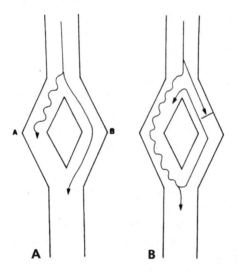

Figure 6.6 Why reentry is accompanied by a conduction delay. (a) In this generic reentrant circuit, a normal impulse travels from top to bottom by the fastest available pathway (pathway B). No conduction delay is seen. (b) When a premature impulse blocks in pathway B and initiates reentry, that impulse must travel from top to bottom via the slow pathway (pathway A). Thus, an observer watching the exit of the impulse from the circuit will see a conduction delay whenever reentry is initiated.

SUPRAVENTRICULAR TACHYARRHYTHMIAS

particular attention to the occurrence of conduction delay in association with the onset of tachycardia. The site of this delay virtually always points to one of the pathways within the reentrant circuit.

An additional issue relating to the mode of initiation is the tachycardia (or echo) zone. The tachycardia zone is the range of coupling intervals of premature beats that will initiate reentrant tachycardia. As one introduces a series of premature impulses with progressively shorter coupling intervals, one impulse will eventually encounter the reentrant circuit during the effective refractory period (ERP) of pathway B (i.e. the impulse blocks in pathway B). At this point, reentry is often initiated. The latest premature impulse that blocks in pathway B (if it were any later, the impulse would not encounter refractory tissue) usually defines the beginning of the tachycardia zone. If one now continues to introduce premature impulses with progressively shorter coupling intervals, reentry will typically be induced with each succeeding premature beat until the ERP of pathway A is finally encountered. At this point, the premature impulse blocks in both pathways of the reentrant circuit and no further reentry occurs. The ERP of pathway A thus defines the end of the tachycardia zone. Note that the width of the tachycardia zone is related to the difference between the refractory periods of the two pathways constituting the reentrant circuit. The wider the tachycardia zone, the more likely a premature impulse will fall within that zone and induce reentry. During the electrophysiology study for supraventricular tachycardia, one thus tries to identify the refractory periods (and thus the tachycardia zone) of the various pathways involved in the reentrant circuit. By doing so, one can attempt to tailor therapy to reduce the width of the tachycardia zone.

The mode of termination of the arrhythmia is somewhat less helpful than the mode of initiation in localizing the bypass tract. Nonetheless, careful observation of the precise mechanism of termination of reentry can offer clues as to the type of reentrant rhythm. This point will be discussed in detail later.

What are the patterns of antegrade and retrograde activation during sinus rhythm and during supraventricular tachycardia?
Abnormalities in the pattern of activation of impulses traveling from the atria to the ventricles and from the ventricles to the atria can help to localize portions of the reentrant circuit.

We have already discussed normal antegrade activation patterns (see Chapter 1). Impulses arising in the SA node traverse the atria

113

in a radial fashion until they encounter the fibrous skeleton of the heart at the AV groove. There, the impulses are abolished, except in the AV conducting system (the AV node and His–Purkinje structures). Because of its electrophysiologic properties, impulses conduct relatively slowly through the AV node. Further, premature impulses conduct even more slowly (manifested in the His electrogram as a prolonged AH interval). Typically, if one introduces single atrial extrastimuli with progressively shorter coupling intervals, the delay in AV nodal conduction (and the AH interval) increases gradually. Eventually, the ERP of the AV node is reached and the early impulse is blocked.

This normal pattern of gradually increasing AH intervals with progressively premature atrial impulses is shown graphically in Figure 6.7. This AV nodal conduction curve shows the normal smooth and continuous prolongation in AH intervals with progressively premature beats. This normal pattern can be disrupted by two

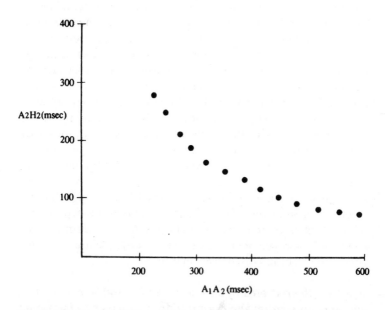

Figure 6.7 A normal AV conduction curve. With progressively shorter coupling intervals, premature atrial beats display a progressive conduction delay in the AV node. In this graph, the conduction intervals (A_1A_2) are shown on the x axis, and the resulting AH intervals (A2H2) are shown on the y axis. The normal AV conduction curve is smooth and continuous, as shown.

general conditions that produce supraventricular tachycardias: dual AV nodal pathways and AV bypass tracts. These two conditions will be discussed in detail later.

When an impulse is conducted from the atria to the ventricles via the normal AV conducting system, ventricular activation follows a typical pattern. First, the intraventricular septum is depolarized, then the apices of the right and left ventricles, then the ventricular free walls, and finally the basilar portions of the ventricles. The area of the ventricles that is depolarized last is the left ventricular poster-obasilar area. This normal pattern of ventricular activation is altered if there is a bypass tract that preexcites the ventricle. Studying the ventricular activation pattern in the electrophysiology laboratory can help to localize the ventricular insertion of a bypass tract.

The characteristics of normal retrograde conduction (i.e. the conduction of impulses from the ventricles to the atria that occurs during ventricular pacing) are important in evaluating supraventricular tachycardias. Normally, retrograde conduction occurs over the normal AV conducting system—the impulse travels from the ventricular myocardium to the Purkinje fibers, then to the His bundle, to the AV node, and finally to the atria, where it spreads in a radial fashion (i.e. from the atrial septum to the right and left atria). Although some retrograde conduction can be seen in most individuals, in most cases retrograde conduction is not as efficient as antegrade conduction. Thus, in most individuals, retrograde block occurs at longer coupling intervals than antegrade block (this is not always the case, however—e.g. a substantial minority of patients with complete AV block have intact retrograde conduction).

In normal individuals, if one introduces progressively earlier extrastimuli from the ventricle and measures the retrograde conduction intervals, one will see a progressive prolongation of the VA interval (Figure 6.8), similar to the gradual prolongation in the AH interval that one sees with antegrade conduction. Normally, block will occur first in the His–Purkinje system. In practical terms, however, one is only rarely able to discern the H spike in the His electrogram during retrograde conduction, as it is usually hidden in the large V complex.

In studies of supraventricular tachyarrhythmias, the pattern of retrograde atrial activation is important. With normal retrograde conduction, the earliest atrial activation is seen in the His electrogram because that electrogram records the atrial activity near the AV node (i.e. the point of entry of the impulse into the atrial myocardium during normal retrograde conduction). The retrograde

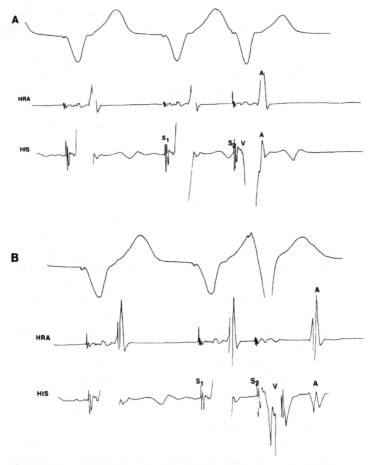

Figure 6.8 Normal VA conduction during right ventricular pacing. A surface ECG lead, a high right atrial (HRA) electrogram, and a His bundle electrogram are shown. (a) With a relatively long S1–S2 coupling interval, retrograde conduction to the atrium is rapid (the VA interval following the S2 is short). Note that the retrograde atrial impulse is recorded in the His electrogram (near the AV node) before it reaches the high right atrium. This suggests retrograde conduction via the normal AV conducting tissues. (b) With a shorter coupling interval, retrograde conduction still occurs, but it is slower (the VA interval following the S2 is longer than in the previous figure). This retrograde conduction delay with shorter coupling intervals is normal when retrograde conduction occurs via the normal AV conducting tissues.

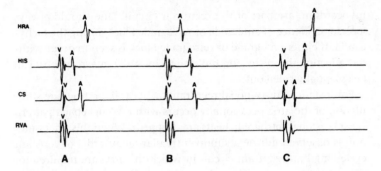

Figure 6.9 Patterns of retrograde atrial activation are important for localizing AV bypass tracts. This figure shows electrograms from the high right atrium (HRA), the His bundle, the coronary sinus (CS), and the right ventricular apex (RVA) during pacing from the RVA. (a) The normal pattern of retrograde atrial activation. This pattern is seen when retrograde conduction occurs via the normal AV conducting system or with septal bypass tracts. The atrial septum is activated first (His electrogram), followed by left atrial (CS electrogram) and right atrial activation. (b) Retrograde activation pattern with a right-sided bypass tract. The right atrium is activated first because retrograde conduction occurs via a right-sided bypass tract. The septal atrium and the left atrium are then activated. (c) Retrograde activation pattern with a left-sided bypass tract. The left atrium is activated first (CS electrogram) because retrograde conduction occurs via a left-sided bypass tract. The atrial septum and the right atrium are then activated.

impulse then spreads radially across the atria, and the right atrial electrogram and left atrial electrogram are inscribed more or less at the same time (Figure 6.9a). This normal pattern of retrograde activation can be disrupted if an AV bypass tract is present. In this case, eccentric retrograde activation of the atria can occur. With a right-sided bypass tract, for instance, the right atrial electrogram will be inscribed earliest (Figure 6.9b); with a left-sided bypass tract, the left atrial electrogram will be inscribed earliest (Figure 6.9c). Mapping of retrograde atrial activation is one of the most useful methods for localizing AV bypass tracts.

What is the evidence that atrial or ventricular myocardium is necessary to the reentrant circuit?

Once a reentrant tachycardia has been induced, it can be helpful to attempt to deduce whether the atrial myocardium and ventricular myocardium are part of the reentrant circuit. One should always look for evidence of antegrade or retrograde block during the tachycardia. If either antegrade or retrograde block is seen to occur without affecting the cycle length of the tachycardia, macroreentry can be essentially ruled out.

For instance, in AV nodal reentrant tachycardia, retrograde stimulation of the atria occasionally occurs with a Wenckebach pattern (i.e. occasional retrograde beats are dropped). When this phenomenon is observed during a supraventricular tachycardia of constant cycle length, a reentrant circuit in which the atria are required for the maintenance of tachycardia can be ruled out.

The effect of bundle branch block on the cycle length of the tachycardia can also be instructive. In AV nodal reentry, bundle branch block does not change the reentrant circuit because the circuit does not involve the bundle branches. In macroreentry, however, the sudden occurrence of bundle branch block on the same side as the AV bypass tract (such as left bundle branch block (LBBB) occurring during a macroreentrant tachycardia involving a left-sided bypass tract) will increase the cycle length of the tachycardia (Figure 6.10).

What are the effects of autonomic maneuvers and drugs on the tachycardia?

When attempting to define the anatomic substrate of, and effective therapy for, reentrant supraventricular tachyarrhythmias, it is often helpful to take advantage of the differential effects of autonomic maneuvers and drugs on various cardiac structures. As noted in previous chapters, the AV node has rich autonomic innervation and is exquisitely sensitive to changes in both sympathetic and parasympathetic tone. In contrast, atrial and ventricular myocardial tissue responds moderately to changes in sympathetic tone but only minimally to changes in parasympathetic tone. Thus, vagal maneuvers, by increasing the refractory period and decreasing the conduction velocity of the AV node, can terminate reentrant arrhythmias in which the AV node is part of the reentrant circuit (such as AV nodal reentry and macroreentry). If the AV node is excluded from the reentrant circuit (as in intraatrial reentry), vagal maneuvers may increase heart block but will not directly alter the reentrant impulse.

Likewise, drugs that have a specific effect on the AV node (such as digitalis, calcium blockers, and β-blockers) can be effective in terminating or preventing reentrant arrhythmias that include the AV node as part of the circuit. In contrast, class Ia drugs have relatively little effect on the AV node but increase the refractory periods and

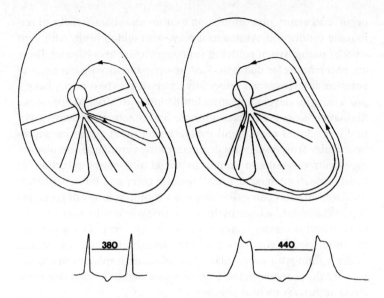

Figure 6.10 Effect of bundle branch block on macroreentrant tachycardia. In this figure, macroreentrant tachycardia involving a left-sided bypass tract is present. Initially, no bundle branch block is present, and the tachycardia cycle length is 380 msec. If LBBB occurs, it will now take longer for the reentrant impulse to reach the left-sided bypass tract, and the tachycardia cycle length will be prolonged to 440 msec.

slow conduction velocity in atrial and ventricular myocardium and in bypass tracts. Thus, reentrant circuits that involve these structures can be altered by class Ia drugs. Class Ib drugs affect the ventricular myocardium (and bypass tracts) but not atrial myocardium or the AV node. Because some supraventricular tachycardias (i.e. macroreentry) involve ventricular myocardium, the class Ib drugs may be useful in some cases. The class Ic drugs slow conduction in all cardiac tissues, including the AV node. Although offering relatively little help in identifying the anatomic substrate, class Ic drugs can be helpful in treating many forms of supraventricular tachyarrhythmia.

General procedure for performing the electrophysiology study in patients with supraventricular tachyarrhythmias

When studying patients with supraventricular tachyarrhythmias, once the electrode catheters are in position most electrophysiologists begin with ventricular stimulation to study the characteristics of retrograde conduction. Although it may seem odd to begin with ventricular pacing when studying supraventricular arrhythmias, there are two reasons for doing so. First, many patients who have supraventricular tachycardias (especially those with bypass tracts) have a propensity for developing atrial fibrillation with atrial pacing. Atrial fibrillation, since it entails continuous and chaotic atrial activity, virtually precludes meaningful evaluation of other reentrant supraventricular arrhythmias. By first performing ventricular stimulation, the electrophysiologist hopes to avoid the early induction of atrial fibrillation. Second, for AV nodal reentry and for bypass tract-mediated macroreentry (the two most common forms of reentrant supraventricular tachyarrhythmia), retrograde conduction is a prominent and necessary component of reentry. Thus, the characteristics of retrograde conduction and the retrograde activation pattern of the atrium with ventricular stimulation are important in characterizing these arrhythmias. It is therefore logical to evaluate these characteristics as early as possible.

Generally, retrograde conduction is evaluated using the extrastimulus and incremental pacing techniques. Single ventricular extrastimuli are introduced (either in sinus rhythm or following a train of paced beats) with gradually decreasing coupling intervals until the extrastimulus fails to capture the ventricle. With each extrastimulus, the electrophysiologist notes the presence or absence of retrograde stimulation of the atrium, the pattern of atrial activation, and the conduction time of the retrograde impulse (the VA interval; see Figure 6.8). The coupling interval at which retrograde conduction is blocked (the retrograde ERP) is also noted. Next, incremental trains are introduced with progressively shorter cycle lengths. Note is taken of the cycle length at which 1 : 1 retrograde conduction no longer occurs.

After ventricular stimulation is completed, pacing is performed from the high right atrium. The procedure here is similar to that described in Chapter 5—atrial extrastimuli and incremental atrial pacing are used to assess the characteristics of AV conduction and of SA nodal function.

Next, similar stimulation is performed using left atrial pacing (i.e. with the coronary sinus catheter). This is done to look for evidence of a left-sided AV bypass tract.

When a bypass tract is suspected, pacing from multiple atrial sites is often performed (by moving the right atrial and/or coronary sinus catheters to various positions) to try to localize the bypass tract—the closer to the bypass tract one paces, the more preexcitation will occur.

For the vast majority of patients with reentrant supraventricular tachyarrhythmias, the reentrant arrhythmia will be induced during one or more of these pacing maneuvers. Whenever reentrant tachycardia is induced, the protocol is interrupted so that the characteristics of the arrhythmia can be studied. Specifically, the mechanism of the tachycardia is noted, the cycle length is recorded, an assessment of the patient's hemodynamic stability and level of symptoms is made, and atrial or ventricular stimulation is carried out to examine the effect of such stimulation on the arrhythmia.

If reentrant supraventricular tachycardia is not induced with standard pacing techniques, multiple extrastimuli are used and drug administration (such as an isoproterenol infusion) is implemented to try to bring out the arrhythmia.

If a bypass tract is known or suspected to occur, the final step during the baseline (drug-free) study is to induce atrial fibrillation. This is done to assess the ability of the bypass tract to conduct rapidly enough during atrial fibrillation to pose a lethal risk to the patient.

Finally, at the end of the baseline study, after the reentrant circuits have been localized and the mechanism of tachycardia has been deduced, drug studies may be carried out in an attempt to devise effective therapy for the patient. Drug studies for supraventricular tachycardias, however, are becoming ever more rare now that most of these arrhythmias are routinely treated with ablation procedures.

Although this general outline of the electrophysiology study for supraventricular tachyarrhythmias is fairly representative, no two electrophysiologists follow precisely the same protocol. In fact, no single electrophysiologist follows precisely the same protocol in every patient. Even within the same general category of arrhythmias, supraventricular arrhythmias show tremendous variability from patient to patient. Thus, every electrophysiology study has to be individualized. Electrophysiologists usually approach these patients with a general outline of a protocol, tailoring the study as they go, depending on the findings.

With this introduction, we will now review the electrophysiologic evaluation of specific types of supraventricular tachyarrhythmia.

The electrophysiology study in AV nodal reentrant tachycardia

As we have noted, AV nodal reentrant tachycardia is the most common type of arrhythmia presenting as PAT, probably accounting for 60% of all such arrhythmias. AV nodal reentry is seen in all age groups and occurs in both sexes equally. The incidence of underlying heart disease in patients with this arrhythmia is no greater than in the normal population.

Mechanism of AV nodal reentry

One can think of the AV node in patients with AV nodal reentrant tachycardia as being shaped like a doughnut (Figure 6.11). The AV node in these patients behaves functionally as if there were two separate pathways through the node. The two pathways (the alpha and the beta pathways) are differentiated by their characteristic

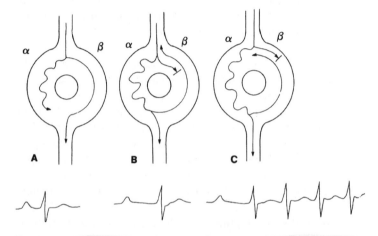

Figure 6.11 AV nodal reentrant tachycardia. (a) In AV nodal reentry, the AV node is functionally divided into two pathways (alpha and beta). The alpha pathway conducts more slowly than the beta, and the beta pathway has a longer refractory period than the alpha. A normal atrial impulse reaches the ventricles via the beta pathway. (b) A premature atrial impulse can find the beta pathway refractory at a time when the alpha pathway is not. In this case, the premature impulse conducts via the alpha pathway. Because conduction down the alpha pathway is slow, the resultant PR interval is prolonged. (c) If conditions are right, a premature impulse can block in the beta pathway and travel down the alpha pathway (as in (b)), then travel retrograde up the beta pathway and reenter the alpha pathway in the antegrade direction. A circuitous impulse is thus established within the AV node, and AV nodal reentrant tachycardia results. Note the prolonged PR interval in the beat that starts AV nodal reentry (caused by jumping from the beta to the alpha pathway). This conduction delay is typically seen in reentrant supraventricular arrhythmias.

electrophysiologic properties. The alpha pathway (or the slow pathway) usually has a relatively short ERP and conducts slowly. The beta pathway (or the fast pathway) usually has a relatively long ERP and conducts more rapidly. Patients whose AV nodes are arranged in such a fashion are said to have dual AV nodal pathways (see Chapter 8 for a more detailed discussion of the anatomy and physiology of dual AV nodal pathways).

In patients with dual AV nodal pathways, a normally timed sinus impulse will conduct through the AV node via the beta pathway, since the beta conducts more rapidly than the alpha pathway (Figure 6.11a). However, a premature atrial impulse can arrive at the AV node at such a time that the beta pathway (with a relatively long ERP) is still refractory from the previous normal beat but the alpha pathway (with a relatively short ERP) is no longer refractory. This early impulse will then traverse the alpha pathway, reaching the His bundle after a prolonged conduction time through the AV node (since the alpha pathway conducts slowly (Figure 6.11b)). This AV nodal conduction delay is manifested by a prolonged PR interval on the surface ECG. If the beta pathway recovers by the time the impulse reaches the distal portion of the alpha pathway, the impulse may conduct retrogradely up the beta pathway (producing an atrial echo beat). If this retrograde impulse is then able to reenter the alpha pathway, a continuously circulating impulse can be established within the AV node. This is AV nodal reentrant tachycardia (Figure 6.11c).

Thus, in AV nodal reentrant tachycardia, the reentrant circuit is located within the AV node. In most cases, both the atria and the ventricles are stimulated by impulses exiting from the circuit during each lap. Neither the atria nor the ventricles, however, are necessary for the maintenance of that reentrant circuit. It is thus possible to have block in the His bundle, preventing the ventricles from being stimulated, without affecting the reentrant circuit itself. It is also possible to have retrograde block, preventing the atria from being stimulated, but without affecting the arrhythmia.

There is evidence that in some patients the beta pathway may not be typical AV nodal tissue. In such patients, the beta pathway does not respond to AV nodal drugs (digitalis, calcium blockers, β-blockers) so well as the alpha pathway. In these patients, the beta pathway may be more affected by class Ia drugs than is typical for AV nodal tissue.

Mode of initiation and termination of AV nodal reentry

Most often, AV nodal reentrant tachycardia is induced with atrial extrastimuli. If one introduces progressively earlier atrial premature impulses, impulses with relatively longer coupling intervals will conduct down the beta (fast) pathway, just as sinus beats do (Figure 6.12a). When the coupling interval of a premature impulse becomes shorter than the ERP of the beta pathway, however, that impulse blocks in the beta pathway and jumps to the alpha (slow) pathway (thus producing the typical conduction delay in the AV node). It is at this point that AV nodal reentry is usually first seen (Figure 6.12b). Premature impulses that are yet earlier will also induce AV nodal reentry, until the ERP of the alpha pathway is reached (at which point the premature impulse is blocked entirely). The tachycardia zone in AV nodal reentry is from the ERP of the beta pathway to the ERP of the alpha pathway. In this arrhythmia, the tachycardia zone tends to be quite reproducible (that is, successive measurements will yield the same result).

Atrioventricular nodal reentry is also commonly induced with incremental atrial pacing at the Wenckebach cycle length. At this cycle length, progressive prolongation in AV nodal conduction is seen until block occurs in the beta pathway and conduction is instead down the alpha pathway—at this point, AV nodal reentry is usually seen.

Atrioventricular nodal reentry is less often, and less reproducibly, induced with ventricular pacing. Normally in patients with dual AV nodal pathways, ventricular pacing produces retrograde impulses that enter the AV node and begin traveling up both the beta and the alpha pathways (Figure 6.13a). Because conduction in the beta pathway is faster, the retrograde impulse reaches the atria via the beta pathway. Reentry is not induced, however—the impulse is not able to turn around and travel back down the alpha pathway because the alpha pathway has just been stimulated itself by the retrograde impulse and is still refractory. Relatively rarely, AV nodal reentry is induced by ventricular pacing if a ventricular extrastimulus can be interpolated between two sinus beats. In this case, the beta pathway can be rendered refractory by the retrograde impulse, so that the next sinus impulse blocks in the beta pathway and conducts down the alpha pathway, thus producing reentry (Figure 6.13b).

Termination of AV nodal reentrant tachycardia follows the typical pattern described in Chapter 4 (see Figure 4.11). Relatively late premature impulses can encounter refractory tissue and be

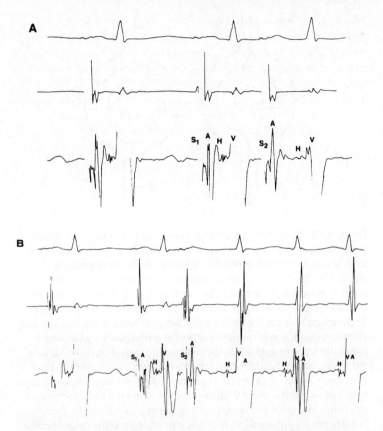

Figure 6.12 Initiation of AV nodal reentry with atrial extrastimuli. One surface ECG lead, one high right atrial electrogram, and one His bundle electrogram are shown. (a) An S2 impulse conducts through the normal AV conducting system with a moderate prolongation in the AH interval. This response is normal and is similar to the normal conduction pattern shown in Figure 5.2. (b) With a slightly shorter S1–S2 coupling interval, a large jump in the resultant AH interval occurs (compared to the previous figure), and AV nodal reentry is initiated. The sudden increment in AH intervals represents a shift in conduction from the beta to the alpha pathway in this patient with dual AV nodal pathways. Note (in the last two beats in this figure) that during AV nodal reentry, the retrograde A spike (which is labeled on the His electrogram) occurs very soon after the V spike. This is because retrograde conduction occurs via the rapidly conducting beta pathway. On the surface ECG, the retrograde P wave is usually buried in the QRS complex (as in this figure) during AV nodal reentrant tachycardia.

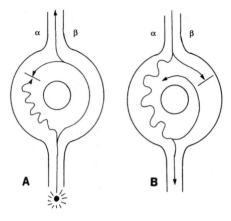

Figure 6.13 Initiation of AV nodal reentry with a ventricular paced beat. Because the reentrant circuit in AV nodal reentry is exposed to both the atria and the ventricles, it is possible that a premature ventricular beat (as well as a premature atrial beat) can initiate reentry. However, in practice this event is rare. (a) A ventricular paced impulse begins traveling up both the beta and the alpha pathways. The impulse reaches the atria via the beta pathway (since this pathway conducts rapidly) and cannot reenter the alpha pathway because it encounters the retrograde impulse traveling slowly up it. This is why AV nodal reentry is difficult to initiate with ventricular pacing. (b) If the events shown in (a) occur at just the right time, the following sinus beat can encounter the AV node at a time when the beta pathway is still refractory from the recent retrograde impulse. Thus, AV nodal reentry can be initiated indirectly by a premature ventricular impulse.

prevented from entering the circuit (see Figure 4.11a). Early impulses may enter the circuit via the alpha pathway, resulting in a resetting of the tachycardia (see Figure 4.11b). Still earlier impulses can terminate the tachycardia (see Figure 4.11c). The ability to cause a premature impulse to reach the AV node early enough to terminate AV nodal reentry depends on the distance of the pacing catheter from the AV node and on the refractory and conduction characteristics (i.e. the functional refractory period (FRP)—see Chapter 4) of the intervening tissue. If terminating the tachycardia with single atrial or ventricular extrastimuli is not possible, one can improve the chances of terminating the arrhythmia by repositioning the catheter or, more commonly, by introducing multiple extrastimuli. This latter maneuver has the effect of reducing the FRP of intervening myocardial tissue.

Patterns of activation with AV nodal reentry

Dual AV nodal pathways are the rule in patients with AV nodal reentrant tachycardia. Because there are two pathways of conduction through the AV node, the AV nodal conduction curve can be expected to be abnormal. Figure 6.14 shows a typical AV nodal conduction curve in a patient with dual AV nodal pathways. With extrastimuli having relatively long coupling intervals, conduction through the AV node occurs via the beta pathway. As atrial extrastimuli are introduced with progressively shorter coupling intervals, the AH interval increases gradually at first, as it would in a normal AV node. At the point at which the ERP of the beta pathway is

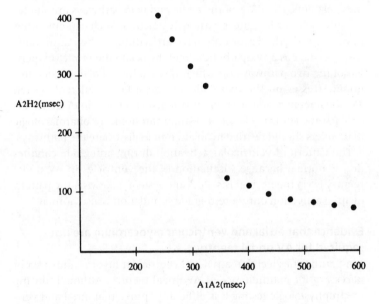

Figure 6.14 A typical AV conduction curve from a patient with AV nodal reentrant tachycardia. Compare this curve to the normal curve in Figure 6.7. In AV nodal reentry, dual AV nodal pathways are present. Premature atrial impulses with longer coupling intervals conduct down the beta pathway. With earlier premature atrial impulses, the refractory period of the beta pathway is reached, and conduction jumps to the slower alpha pathway. It is at this point that AV nodal reentry may occur. On the AV conduction curve, this jump from faster to slower conduction is manifested by a sudden discontinuity in the curve. The sudden lengthening of the AH interval when conduction shifts from the beta to the alpha pathway is also seen in Figure 6.12.

reached, however, conduction suddenly shifts to the alpha pathway, at which time there is a sudden increment in the AV nodal conduction time. This increment is manifested by a sudden jump in the AH interval. The AV nodal conduction curves in patients with dual AV nodal pathways show a discontinuity—the discontinuity represents the point at which conduction shifts from the beta to the alpha pathway.

Occasionally, patients with dual AV nodal pathways will manifest their two pathways during normal sinus rhythm—these patients can be seen to have two distinct PR intervals during sinus rhythm. In other patients with dual AV nodal pathways, evidence for dual pathways is not seen during baseline electrophysiologic testing. In these patients, the ERPs of the alpha and beta pathways are similar (i.e. the tachycardia zone is extremely narrow). Such patients either have few arrhythmias or only have arrhythmias when autonomic stresses (such as a sympathetic surge) dissociate the refractory periods of the two pathways (in which case a differential effect of autonomic stresses on the two pathways must be postulated). When AV nodal reentry is suspected in patients who have no evidence for dual pathways during baseline testing, autonomic or pharmacologic maneuvers should be tried in an attempt to dissociate the pathways.

The pattern of ventricular activation during antegrade conduction is normal because stimulation of the ventricles in AV nodal reentry is via the normal His–Purkinje system. Likewise, the pattern of atrial activation during retrograde stimulation is also normal.

Evidence that atrial and ventricular myocardium are not required for AV nodal reentry

Most authorities feel that atrial and ventricular myocardium are not necessary for maintenance of AV nodal reentry. Although during electrophysiologic testing it is difficult to prove that atrial and ventricular tissues are not required to maintain AV nodal reentry, evidence is sometimes present spontaneously during AV nodal reentrant tachycardia. One should always be alert for the phenomenon of retrograde Wenckebach conduction during tachycardia. If the tachycardia cycle length is constant at the same time that the relationship of the retrograde P waves to the QRS complex is changing, or especially if occasional retrograde P waves are dropped, that is strong evidence that the atria are not required for the maintenance of the tachycardia. Likewise, if occasional antegrade block occurs without a change in the tachycardia cycle length, the ventricles are thus not required for maintenance of tachycardia.

Finally, because the activation pattern of the ventricular myocardium has no bearing on the cycle length of the reentrant circuit, if bundle branch block should develop during AV nodal reentry, no change in the rate of the tachycardia should occur.

If these spontaneous events are not seen, extrastimuli from the atria and the ventricles can help to show that the atria and ventricles are not required. Capture of the atria near the AV node or capture of the His bundle without changing the tachycardia suggests that the reentrant circuit is localized to the AV node. In practice, it is difficult and impractical to prove that the atria and the ventricles are not necessary by using extrastimuli. Fortunately, it is also usually unnecessary because the diagnosis of AV nodal reentry rarely hinges on rigorous documentation that the atria and ventricles are not required.

Other observations in AV nodal reentry

Relationship of P waves to QRS complexes during AV nodal reentry

One of the most useful observations made in the electrophysiology laboratory in patients with AV nodal reentry is the relationship between retrograde P waves and the QRS complexes on the surface ECG during the tachycardia. During AV nodal reentry, the atrium is stimulated in the retrograde direction by impulses exiting to the atria via the beta pathway. Because the beta pathway tends to conduct rapidly, retrograde atrial activation tends to occur during or just after ventricular depolarization. On the surface ECG, P waves thus tend either to be buried within the QRS complex or to occur just at the end of the QRS. In patients presenting with regular, narrow-complex tachycardia in which P waves cannot be discerned at all in a good-quality 12-lead ECG, one can make the diagnosis of AV nodal reentry with some confidence.

Atypical AV nodal reentry

In patients with atypical AV nodal reentry, the ERP of the alpha pathway is longer than that of the beta pathway. In these individuals, reentry occurs in the opposite direction (i.e. up the alpha pathway and down the beta pathway), and the P to QRS relationship is not typical of AV nodal reentry (because retrograde conduction occurs through the slow pathway). Patients with this unusual form of AV nodal reentry tend to have incessant tachycardia.

Treatment of AV nodal reentry

Because both pathways in AV nodal reentry involve AV nodal tissue, drugs and maneuvers that increase the refractory period and slow the conduction velocity of AV nodal tissue are very effective at terminating the arrhythmia. In addition to maneuvers that increase vagal tone (the Valsalva maneuver, carotid sinus massage, and ice-water immersion), the digitalis agents, calcium blockers, and β-blockers tend to be effective. In most instances, these agents work by producing Wenckebach conduction in the slow pathway. They thus cause termination of reentrant tachycardia after a few cycles, when an impulse that has conducted retrogradely through the beta pathway fails to reenter the alpha pathway.

Because occasionally the alpha and beta pathways respond differently to various agents, it is sometimes possible to potentiate tachycardia with drugs. For instance, in some patients, the beta pathway is relatively unaffected by drugs that normally depress AV nodal function. Thus, a drug might slow conduction in the alpha pathway without prolonging refractoriness in the fast pathway. In this case, any premature impulse traveling down the alpha pathway would tend to be so delayed that the beta pathway would be much more likely to have recovered by the time the impulse reached it. Reentry, then, would tend to be easier to start and more difficult to stop.

Patients in whom standard AV nodal drugs seem to be ineffective may respond to class Ia or class Ic drugs. The beta pathway in such patients seems to behave less like AV nodal tissue and more like atrial or ventricular myocardial tissue.

During the last 15 years, techniques for performing transcatheter ablation of the slow (alpha) pathway in patients with AV nodal tachycardia have become quite advanced (see Chapter 8). Transcatheter ablation of AV nodal reentry can now be performed successfully in well over 95% of patients who undergo this procedure. Ablation should be strongly considered in any patient with AV nodal reentry who has frequent or disabling episodes.

Bypass tract-mediated supraventricular tachyarrhythmias

As described in Chapter 1, there is normally only one way for electrical impulses to travel from the atria to the ventricles—that is, by the normal AV conduction system. Of every thousand individuals, however, several are born with a second electrical connection between the atria and the ventricles. These extra connections are called bypass tracts (or accessory pathways), because they offer a potential route for electrical impulses to bypass all or part of the normal AV conduction system. Bypass tracts consist of tiny bands of myocardial tissue that most commonly insert in atrial muscle on one end and in ventricular muscle on the other. They tend to occur sporadically, although patients with Ebstein's anomaly and mitral valve prolapse have a somewhat higher incidence than the general population.

The electrophysiologic characteristics of these bypass tracts vary, but they generally behave much more like myocardial tissue than AV nodal tissue. Thus, they do not display slowing of conduction with premature impulses as the AV node does. Also, when stimulated rapidly, bypass tracts develop block in the manner of His–Purkinje tissue rather than AV nodal tissue. That is, the block is sudden (of the Mobitz II variety) instead of gradual (i.e. Wenckebach conduction does not occur).

Bypass tracts are generally invisible to the naked eye (significantly, surgeons cannot see them when attempting surgical disruption) and therefore must be located by their electrophysiologic effects alone. Bypass tracts can occur virtually anywhere along the AV groove (except in the space between the aortic valve and the mitral valve) and can also occur more or less parallel to the AV conducting system in the septal area. There are four general types of bypass tract (Figure 6.15): AV bypass tracts (the "typical" bypass tracts, in which the tract is located along the AV groove and

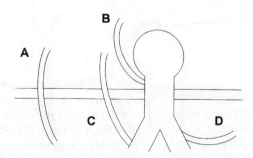

Figure 6.15 Four types of bypass tract. Tract A is an AV bypass tract, connecting atrial myocardium to ventricular myocardium. Tract B is an AV nodal bypass tract, connecting atrial myocardium to the His–Purkinje system. Tract C is a "Mahaim" tract, connecting the distal atrium (near the AV node) to the right bundle branch. Tract D connects the distal conducting system to the ventricular myocardium.

connects atrial and ventricular muscle; tract A in Figure 6.15); AV nodal bypass tracts (which connect the low atrial myocardium to the His–Purkinje system; tract B); bypass tracts that connect the distal atrial myocardium (near the AV node) to the right bundle branch (so-called "Mahaim" tracts; tract C); and bypass tracts that connect the His or Purkinje fibers to ventricular myocardium (tract D). AV bypass tracts are by far the most common variety.

Bypass tracts may or may not conduct in the antegrade direction. When they do (in which case the patient is said to have Wolff–Parkinson–White syndrome), the surface ECG often shows preexcitation of the QRS complex (Figures 6.16 and 6.17). Preexcitation

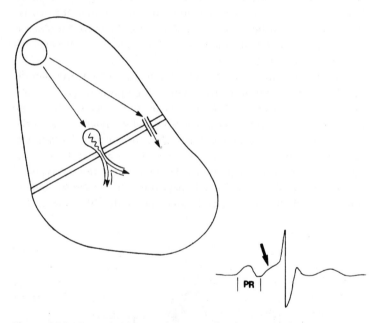

Figure 6.16 Preexcitation. In this example, there is a left-sided AV bypass tract. An impulse arising from the SA node stimulates the ventricles via both the normal conducting system and the bypass tract. Thus, the resulting QRS complex represents a fusion beat between normal and eccentric activation. Because conduction through the bypass tract does not display the normal conduction delay seen in the AV node, earliest ventricular activation classically occurs via the bypass tract. Hence, the PR interval is shorter than normal, and the QRS complex has a slurred onset known as a delta wave (*thick arrow*). Patients whose bypass tracts conduct antegradely, as shown, are said to have Wolff–Parkinson–White syndrome.

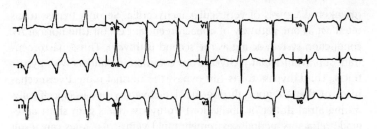

Figure 6.17 A typical 12-lead ECG from a patient with an AV bypass tract. Note the short PR interval and the delta wave visible on most leads.

refers to antegrade conduction over a bypass tract that stimulates the ventricle prematurely. This ventricular stimulation is premature because the bypass tract conducts rapidly, like most myocardial tissue. Thus, an impulse traveling over the bypass tract does not display the delay seen when an impulse encounters the AV node. Preexcitation is usually manifested by a short PR interval and a slurring of the onset of the QRS complex (which is termed a "delta wave"). In patients whose bypass tracts are capable of antegrade conduction, most QRS complexes are actually fusion beats between ventricular stimulation via the normal AV conduction system and ventricular stimulation via the bypass tract. The degree of preexcitation then depends on several factors, including the AV nodal conduction time (the slower AV nodal conduction, the larger the delta wave), the conduction velocity and the refractory period of the bypass tract itself (more preexcitation occurs in tracts with rapid conduction velocity and shorter refractory periods), and the proximity of the bypass tract to the SA node (the atrial impulse reaches a right-sided bypass tract earlier than it reaches a left-sided bypass tract, and thus right-sided bypass tracts tend to preexcite more).

In many patients who present with supraventricular tachycardia mediated by bypass tracts, the bypass tracts are incapable of antegrade conduction. Instead, they conduct in the retrograde direction only. Such bypass tracts are called concealed bypass tracts, because they never manifest delta waves or short PR intervals and are totally unapparent on the ECG when the patient is in normal sinus rhythm.

Bypass tracts are clinically significant for three reasons. First, they can confuse the clinician. Delta waves can masquerade as Q waves and lead to the false diagnosis of myocardial infarction. Marked preexcitation that occurs during an atrial tachycardia can lead to the mistaken diagnosis of ventricular tachycardia. Second, bypass tracts often act as one pathway of a macroreentrant circuit (the normal AV conduction system acting as the second pathway). Thus, macroreentrant supraventricular tachycardia is common in patients with bypass tracts. Third, bypass tracts can bypass the normal protective mechanism of the AV node during atrial tachyarrhythmias (specifically, during atrial flutter or fibrillation). In bypass tracts with short antegrade refractory periods, extremely rapid ventricular rates can result during atrial tachyarrhythmias. This problem is life-threatening.

The electrophysiology study can play a major role in characterizing the significance of bypass tracts and developing appropriate therapy. The electrophysiology study can be used to determine the characteristics of the pathways of a macroreentrant circuit and can help to select effective therapy for macroreentrant arrhythmias. In addition, the electrophysiology study can help to determine the potential of the bypass tract to mediate lethal arrhythmias (the potential for lethal arrhythmias is not an issue in patients with concealed bypass tracts, since it depends on efficient antegrade conduction). Finally, and most importantly, the electrophysiology study can be used to precisely localize and ablate the bypass tract (see Chapter 8). Indeed, rare is the electrophysiologist today who identifies a bypass tract without ablating it.

The electrophysiology study in bypass tract-mediated macroreentry

The mechanism of macroreentrant supraventricular tachycardia

Macroreentrant "supraventricular" tachycardia is actually a misnomer because the reentrant circuit involves ventricular as well as supraventricular structures. The mechanism of this arrhythmia is illustrated in Figure 6.18. A bypass tract acts as one of the pathways of the reentrant circuit. Like pathway B in our model of reentry, the bypass tract conducts rapidly, and often has a relatively long refractory period. The pathway A of the reentrant circuit is formed by the normal AV conduction system, which displays the characteristics of slow conduction and a relatively short ERP. In short, in a heart containing a bypass tract, the characteristics of an ideal reentrant circuit are often present (Figure 6.18a). A macroreentrant rhythm can then often be started simply by introducing an atrial premature impulse at a time when the bypass tract is still refractory from the previous impulse but when the AV node has recovered

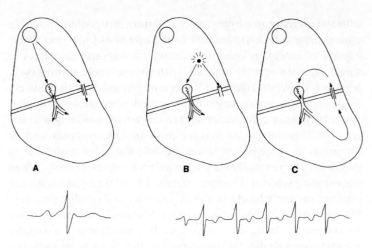

Figure 6.18 Bypass tract-mediated macroreentry. In this illustration, a left-sided AV bypass tract is present. (a) A normal impulse arising in the SA node stimulates the ventricle via both the normal conducting system and the bypass tract, as in Figure 6.16. The resulting ECG shows the typical short PR interval and delta wave. (b) A premature atrial complex occurs during the refractory period of the bypass tract (which typically has a longer refractory period than the AV node). The impulse thus blocks in the bypass tract and reaches the ventricle solely via the normal conducting pathway, and with a normal PR interval (depending on the site of origin of the premature atrial contraction (PAC)) and a normal (i.e. no delta wave) QRS complex. (c) Because the PAC has blocked antegradely in the bypass tract, the bypass tract may no longer be refractory by the time the impulse reaches the ventricles by way of the normal conducting system. In this case, the bypass tract may be able to conduct the impulse retrogradely back to the atrium. Thus, a reentrant impulse is established, which travels antegradely down the normal conducting system and retrogradely up the bypass tract. This form of macroreentry is extremely common in patients with AV bypass tracts.

(Figure 6.18b and c). The macroreentrant tachycardia has a normal QRS complex because antegrade conduction is via the normal AV conduction system.

Mode of initiation and termination of macroreentry
Bypass tract-mediated macroreentrant supraventricular tachyarrhythmias can usually be both initiated and terminated with either atrial or ventricular pacing.

In the presence of a bypass tract, macroreentry is often inducible with a single atrial extrastimulus. In the case of a bypass tract that is capable of antegrade conduction, a typical response to a series of single premature atrial impulses with progressively shorter cycle lengths is shown in Figure 6.19. Premature impulses with relatively long coupling intervals may show only moderate preexcitation (Figure 6.19a). As coupling intervals are shortened, conduction in the AV node is prolonged, so that the resultant QRS complexes show progressively more preexcitation (i.e. impulses have more time to depolarize the ventricles via the bypass tract (Figure 6.19b)). When the coupling interval is shorter than the ERP of the bypass tract, the impulse suddenly blocks in the bypass tract and conducts entirely via the normal AV conduction system. The resultant QRS complex shows no preexcitation (Figure 6.19c). If conduction of this impulse through the normal AV conduction system is slow enough, the bypass tract may have enough time to recover so that the impulse can conduct retrogradely back to the atria, thus initiating macroreentry. The conduction delay seen with the onset of macroreentrant tachycardia represents the shift in AV conduction from the bypass tract to the AV node. The beginning of the tachycardia zone in macroreentry is thus related to the ERP of the bypass tract. In general, with even earlier premature atrial stimuli, macroreentry will be reproducibly inducible until the ERP of the AV conduction system is reached (the end of the tachycardia zone).

In the case of concealed bypass tracts (which are not capable of antegrade conduction), the initiation of macroreentry is somewhat more difficult to visualize. If there were truly no antegrade conduction down the bypass tract, one would expect every normally conducted sinus beat to conduct retrogradely back up the bypass tract and thus to initiate reentry. Because this is not the case, sinus beats must partially penetrate the bypass tract in the antegrade direction, rendering it refractory to subsequent retrograde conduction (Figure 6.20). (This phenomenon of conduction into a structure that cannot be directly observed but that one can deduce because of its effect on subsequent refractoriness is called *concealed conduction*.) To initiate macroreentry with atrial extrastimuli in patients with a concealed bypass tract, the extrastimulus must occur early enough that concealed conduction into the bypass tract is blocked (i.e. the extrastimulus must occur during the antegrade ERP of the concealed bypass tract (Figure 6.20)). In addition, the extrastimulus must occur early enough to cause sufficient delay in AV conduction so that the bypass tract has time to recover from

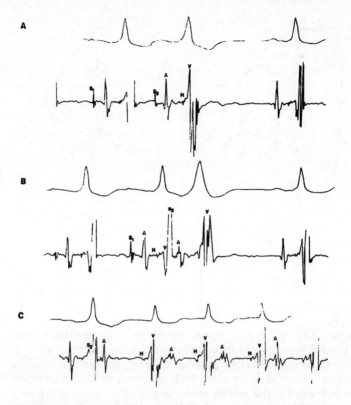

Figure 6.19 Induction of macroreentry with a single extrastimulus from the right atrium (i.e. by the mechanism illustrated in Figure 6.18). A surface ECG lead and the His bundle electrogram are depicted. (a) At a relatively long S1–S2 coupling interval, the premature atrial impulse conducts down both the normal conducting system and the bypass tract. The resultant QRS complex resembles the QRS complex in sinus rhythm (the last complex in (a)). (b) A premature atrial impulse with a shorter coupling interval encounters more delay in the AV node than was present in (a). Thus, the resultant QRS complex shows more preexcitation (more of the ventricle is depolarized via the bypass tract, while the impulse slowly wends its way through the AV node). The H spike is not visible during the premature beat in (b) because the His bundle is not stimulated until well into ventricular depolarization. (c) An even earlier atrial premature beat now encounters the refractory period of the bypass tract. Thus, the premature impulse reaches the ventricles entirely through the normal conducting system. Note the relatively long AH interval following the S2 impulse, and the narrow (nonpreexcited) QRS complex. The impulse then returns to the atria retrogradely via the bypass tract, and macroreentrant tachycardia is established.

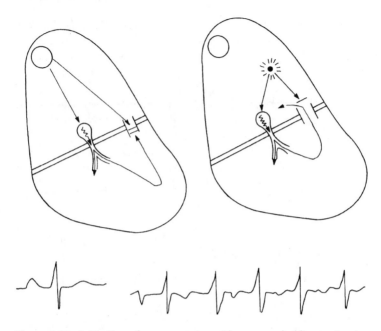

Figure 6.20 Initiation of macroreentry with a concealed bypass tract. No atrial impulses are capable of reaching the ventricles via a concealed bypass tract. However, some antegrade penetration of the bypass tract must be occurring, otherwise every atrial impulse would initiate reentry. This hidden conduction into the concealed bypass tract (called concealed penetration) is depicted in the first panel. Concealed antegrade penetration renders the bypass tract refractory to retrograde conduction and prevents reentry. Note that with a concealed bypass tract, the PR interval is normal and there is no delta wave. In the second panel, a premature atrial impulse occurs during the refractory period of the bypass tract, preventing concealed penetration from occurring. Because the bypass tract is not stimulated in the antegrade direction, the impulse may now conduct retrogradely back up the bypass tract and thus initiate reentry.

concealed conduction. Induction of macroreentry in patients with concealed bypass tracts is facilitated by pacing near the bypass tract. Concealed conduction into the bypass tract then occurs early, and the bypass tract has more time to recover for subsequent retrograde conduction.

With either typical or concealed bypass tracts, macroreentry can also be induced with incremental atrial pacing, as long as pacing is rapid enough to cause complete or intermittent antegrade block in the bypass tract.

As opposed to AV nodal reentry, bypass tract-mediated macro-reentry is often easy to induce with ventricular pacing. This is because retrograde conduction via the normal AV conduction system is often inefficient and therefore quick to block. Ventricular impulses that block retrogradely in the His bundle but conduct up the bypass tract will often induce reentry.

Termination of macroreentrant tachycardia can be accomplished with either atrial or ventricular extrastimuli. Atrial premature beats generally terminate macroreentry when they occur early enough to block antegradely in the AV node. Likewise, ventricular premature beats terminate macroreentry most commonly by preexciting the atrium (retrogradely via the bypass tract) early enough to produce antegrade block in the AV node.

Patterns of atrial and ventricular activation in bypass tract-mediated reentry

In bypass tracts that are capable of antegrade conduction, the ventricular activation patterns in sinus rhythm or with premature atrial complexes will be abnormal to the extent that preexcitation occurs. If one could record intracardiac electrograms along the ventricular side of the AV groove, the earliest ventricular activation would be seen at the ventricular insertion of the bypass tract. Because bypass tracts usually conduct rapidly and with constant conduction times until block occurs, the AV interval (or the PR interval) remains relatively constant with progressively premature atrial impulses until the ERP of the bypass tract is reached. The AV conduction curve is thus flat until block in the bypass tract occurs and AV conduction shifts to the AV node (Figure 6.21).

In patients with concealed bypass tracts, no preexcitation is seen. In these patients, the AV conduction curve is normal, unless there are concomitant and unrelated dual AV nodal pathways.

Retrograde activation of the atrium is abnormal in patients who have left-sided or right-sided bypass tracts (see Figure 6.9). Often, with ventricular paced beats that have relatively long coupling intervals, atrial fusion occurs between normally conducted retrograde impulses and impulses that conduct up the bypass tract. With shorter coupling intervals, conduction up the normal pathways is delayed or blocked and retrograde activation patterns are frankly abnormal.

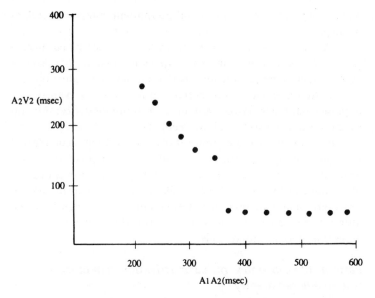

Figure 6.21 A typical AV conduction curve in a patient with an AV bypass tract. At longer coupling intervals, premature atrial impulses are conducted to the ventricles via the bypass tract. Because the bypass tract does not typically display slowing in conduction with premature beats, this portion of the curve is flat. When the refractory period of the bypass tract is reached, AV conduction shifts to the normal AV conducting system. Thus, the curve is discontinuous. At the point where the curve shifts, the delta wave disappears from the resulting QRS complex. Also at this point, macroreentry is likely to occur. Intracardiac electrograms displaying this phenomenon are shown in Figure 6.19.

In patients who have anterior septal bypass tracts, the retrograde activation pattern of the atrium appears normal because the atrial insertion of these tracts is near the AV node. In these patients, however, progressively earlier ventricular paced beats do not result in a progressive delay in retrograde conduction time, as one would expect to see in retrograde conduction via the normal AV conduction system. The normal delay in retrograde atrial activation with progressively earlier ventricular stimulation is shown in Figure 6.8.

Requirement of the atria and ventricles in macroreentry
The reentrant circuit in macroreentrant tachycardia includes atrial and ventricular myocardium. Any instance of antegrade or

retrograde block occurring during the tachycardia, without producing a change in the tachycardia, rules out macroreentry, because a single blocked impulse in either direction should immediately terminate the arrhythmia. During tachycardia, premature atrial or ventricular extrastimuli can readily reset the tachycardia—this phenomenon can be used as evidence that the atria and ventricles are part of the circuit. An appropriately timed premature ventricular stimulus during tachycardia can often be shown to preexcite the atrium, which is strong evidence that retrograde stimulation via a bypass tract is operational (Figure 6.22). During macroreentry, the development of bundle branch block on the same side of the heart as the bypass tract will increase the cycle length of the tachycardia, strongly suggesting that the ventricles are part of the circuit (see Figure 6.10).

Relationship of P to QRS during macroreentrant tachycardia

Unlike AV nodal reentry, in which the atria and ventricles are depolarized nearly simultaneously, in macroreentry the atria and the ventricles are depolarized sequentially. Thus, distinct P waves are virtually always seen. P waves tend to be less than halfway between successive QRS complexes (the RP interval is shorter than the PR interval) because retrograde conduction via the bypass tract tends to be faster than antegrade conduction via the normal AV conducting system (Figure 6.23). Because atrial stimulation is in the retrograde direction, the P wave axis is superior—the P waves will be negative in the inferior leads (II, III, and AVF).

Treatment of macroreentrant supraventricular tachycardia

The main goal of pharmacologic therapy in macroreentry is to reduce the width of the tachycardia zone. Drugs that increase the refractory period of the AV node (digitalis, calcium blockers, and β-blockers) can decrease the width of the tachycardia zone. In practice, however, the best results are often obtained not so much by narrowing the tachycardia zone as by increasing AV nodal block, thus resulting in Wenckebach conduction whenever tachycardia begins. This is effective therapy because a single blocked beat immediately terminates the tachycardia.

Another approach is to attempt to increase the retrograde refractory period of the bypass tract with class Ia drugs. Unfortunately, class Ia drugs also usually increase the antegrade refractory period of the bypass tract, which has the effect of increasing the tachycardia zone. Thus, class Ia drugs tend to be beneficial only when they have

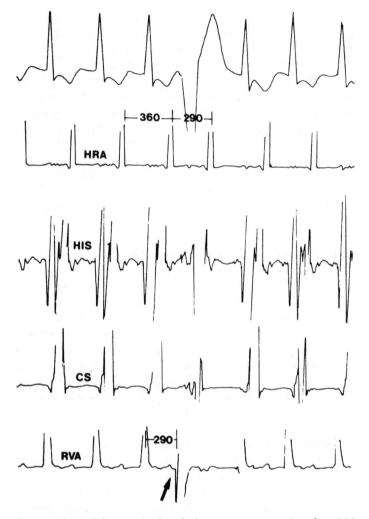

Figure 6.22 Atrial preexcitation during macroreentry. A surface ECG lead and intracardiac electrograms from the high right atrium (HRA), His bundle, coronary sinus (CS), and right ventricular apex (RVA) are shown. Macroreentrant tachycardia is present, with a cycle length of 360 msec. During the tachycardia, a single extrastimulus is delivered to the RVA at a coupling interval of 290 msec (*arrow*). This ventricular stimulation results in a premature retrograde atrial impulse at the same coupling interval (290 msec), best seen in the HRA electrogram. Preexcitation of the atrium with ventricular pacing during supraventricular tachycardia is strong evidence that an AV bypass tract is present.

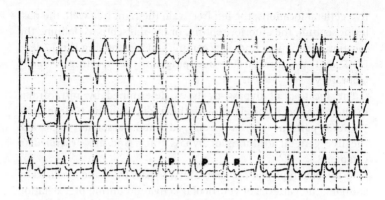

Figure 6.23 Macroreentrant tachycardia. Three surface EGG leads are shown, but P waves are best seen on the bottom tracing. The PR interval is typically longer than the RP interval.

an extreme effect on the bypass tract, achieving "pharmacological ablation." If the effect of the drug is only moderate, macroreentry is often potentiated.

In general, the best results with drug therapy are obtained by using drugs that affect AV nodal conduction and refractoriness, either alone or in combination with class Ia drugs. Class Ic drugs such as flecainide and propafenone are often effective in treating macroreentrant tachycardia. Amiodarone is likewise effective, but most electrophysiologists consider it potentially too toxic to use in patients with nonlethal arrhythmias.

Antitachycardia pacemakers have been used successfully in patients with macroreentrant tachycardias because these arrhythmias are almost always terminable by programmed pacing.

Today, however, all of these alternatives are considered suboptimal, since most bypass tracts can be ablated in the electrophysiology laboratory with a high degree of success.

Localization of bypass tracts

Defining the location of bypass tracts is important if transcatheter ablation of the tract is contemplated. As noted, bypass tracts can occur anywhere along the AV groove (except in the space between the aortic and mitral valves). The classification of bypass tracts as type A (positive QRS in lead V_1) or type B (negative QRS in lead V_1) is outmoded and of little use for localizing bypass tracts. Currently, AV bypass tracts are thought of as occurring in one of five general locations: the left free wall, the right free wall, the posterior septum, the anterior septum, or the midseptum. Defining the location of a bypass tract is accomplished by studying the 12-lead ECG and by intracardiac mapping in the electrophysiology laboratory.

The location of bypass tracts as determined by intracardiac mapping has been correlated with the findings on the 12-lead ECG. The ECG patterns that have emerged match reasonably well with the five general locations of bypass tracts and are described in Chapter 8.

In the electrophysiology laboratory, bypass tracts are localized by studying the patterns of ventricular activation during preexcitation and of atrial activation during retrograde conduction. Left-sided and posterior septal tracts are the easiest to localize. The coronary sinus catheter lies in the AV groove between the left atrium and the left ventricle, and the os of the coronary sinus lies in the posterior septal region. By recording electrograms from multiple electrode pairs from an electrode catheter in the coronary sinus, early activation of the left atrium during retrograde conduction (and of the left ventricle during preexcitation) can be precisely localized. Right free-wall and anterior septal tracts are more difficult to localize precisely because there is no structure analogous to the coronary sinus that allows mapping of the right AV groove. Nonetheless, in the past few years electrophysiologists have become quite adept at precisely localizing bypass tracts. See Chapter 8 for details.

Atrial flutter/fibrillation in patients with bypass tracts

For reasons that are not well understood, patients with bypass tracts seem more predisposed to developing atrial flutter and fibrillation than is the general population. Because some bypass tracts have the propensity for rapid conduction, an exceedingly rapid ventricular response can be seen in the presence of these arrhythmias (obviously, this is not a problem in patients with concealed bypass tracts). Patients who have rapidly conducting bypass tracts with short antegrade refractory periods are capable of conducting in excess of 300 beats/min (Figure 6.24). Thus, when performing electrophysiologic testing in patients with bypass tracts, it is important to assess the antegrade refractory period and the conduction velocity of the bypass tract during atrial fibrillation.

During the electrophysiology study, the refractory periods of the bypass tract are measured in sinus rhythm and with atrial pacing. It is important to keep in mind, however, that bypass tracts respond to

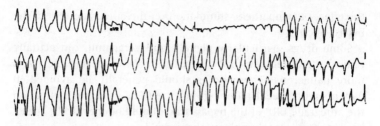

Figure 6.24 Atrial fibrillation in a patient with an AV bypass tract. Some patients with AV bypass tracts may experience extremely rapid conduction down the bypass tract during atrial tachyarrhythmias. The resulting QRS complexes are wide because ventricular stimulation is almost entirely via the bypass tract. This is a life-threatening arrhythmia.

rapid stimulation like atrial or ventricular myocardium and not like AV nodal tissue—the faster the tract is stimulated, the shorter its refractory periods and the faster its conduction. Thus, the only way to know for sure how fast the tract can conduct during atrial fibrillation or atrial flutter is to attempt to induce these arrhythmias during the study. Further, because bypass tracts tend to respond somewhat to sympathetic stimulation, it is best to test the effect of atrial fibrillation on the bypass tract during an isoproterenol infusion. In general, bypass tracts are considered to be benign when the shortest preexcited RR interval during atrial fibrillation is greater than 270 msec. If the RR intervals are shorter than this, most electrophysiologists feel compelled to administer therapy.

In the past, the most common treatment for potentially lethal bypass tracts was to administer drugs to increase the antegrade refractory period of the bypass tract, such as drugs in class Ia, Ic, or III. After administration of these drugs, their effect must be tested by reinducing atrial fibrillation/flutter. Quite commonly, such pharmacologic therapy appears effective until isoproterenol is again infused, at which time the benefit of the antiarrhythmic drug is often counteracted. In these instances, the addition of a β-blocker is often helpful.

In patients who have potentially lethal bypass tracts, the addition of a class Ia drug, by increasing the antegrade ERP of the bypass tract and thus widening the tachycardia zone, can make macroreentry much more likely to occur. In these patients, the addition of a drug that affects the AV node can often be of benefit (using a β-blocker in this instance can both reduce macroreentry and counter

145

the effect of sympathetic stimulation on the antegrade ERP of the bypass tract).

Some drugs, particularly digitalis and verapamil, can actually reduce the antegrade ERP of bypass tracts, rendering the tracts more dangerous. These drugs should generally be avoided in patients with preexcitation. If they are to be used, their effect on the antegrade ERP of the bypass tract should be specifically measured in the electrophysiology laboratory.

Given all the drawbacks to using chronic antiarrhythmic drug therapy in patients with potentially malignant bypass tracts, the treatment of choice for most of these patients is radiofrequency ablation of the bypass tract. Not only does ablation eliminate the bypass tract, it also eliminates the necessity of taking chronic daily antiarrhythmic drug therapy. This factor is especially important considering that the majority of patients presenting with bypass tracts are relatively young.

Uncommon varieties of bypass tract

AV Nodal Bypass Tracts

AV nodal bypass tracts (tract B in Figure 6.15) are relatively rare bypass tracts that connect the low septal atrium to the distal conducting system (usually to the His bundle), thus bypassing the AV node. On the surface ECG, patients with AV nodal bypass tracts display short PR intervals and normal QRS complexes. The His electrogram in patients with such bypass tracts reveals a short AH interval.

These bypass tracts display the same electrophysiologic characteristics as the bypass tracts we have been discussing; that is, they behave like myocardial tissue rather than AV nodal tissue. Although patients with AV nodal bypass tracts can occasionally have reentrant arrhythmias that use the bypass tract as the retrograde pathway and the normal AV node as the antegrade pathway, the major clinical problem with these tracts is their propensity to conduct impulses to the ventricle extremely rapidly during atrial fibrillation. Drug therapy to prevent rapid conduction during atrial tachyarrhythmias consists of class Ia or Ic drugs because these tracts do not respond to the usual AV nodal blocking agents, but, again, ablation of these tracts is generally the treatment of choice.

Mahaim bypass tracts

Mahaim bypass tracts (tract C in Figure 6.15) form connections between atrial muscle and the right bundle branch (atriofascicular tracts) or between atrial muscle and ventricular muscle (atrio-ventricular fibers). These tracts, which are discussed in more detail in Chapter 8, do not have typical bypass tract electrophysiology but instead display the kind of decremental conduction seen in AV nodal tissue. Reentrant tachycardia, when it occurs with Mahaim tracts, uses the tract in the antegrade direction and the normal conducting system in the retrograde direction. Since right bundle branch preexcitation occurs in tachycardia mediated by these tracts, the tachycardia display an LBBB configuration.

Fasiculoventricular bypass tracts
Fasiculoventricular bypass tracts (tract D in Figure 6.15) connect the His bundle or the Purkinje fibers to ventricular myocardium. They are extremely rare and, because they almost never mediate reentrant arrhythmias, they have little clinical significance. Their only manifestation is a short HV interval.

Multiple bypass tracts
Approximately 10% of patients with bypass tracts have more than one. Multiple bypass tracts, when present, can be difficult to diagnose in the electrophysiology laboratory, because one bypass tract almost always predominates and prevents other tracts from manifesting themselves. Additional tracts become clinically significant most often following ablation of a bypass tract—successful ablation of the target bypass tract allows the hidden tract to become apparent. Multiple bypass tracts are more likely to be present if the 12-lead ECG shows atypical delta waves (including delta waves that appear to shift axis over time) or preexcited tachycardias. Multiple tracts are also likely if either multiple routes of atrial activation or mismatch of antegrade and retrograde activation during macroreentrant tachycardia are seen during electrophysiologic testing.

Surgical treatment of bypass tracts
During the mid to late 1980s, surgical disruption of bypass tracts became an attractive therapeutic option for patients whose arrhythmias could not be controlled with pharmacologic regimens. Although surgery to ablate bypass tracts has been almost entirely supplanted by transcatheter ablation techniques, such surgery is still rarely required when catheter techniques have failed. Surgical disruption of bypass tracts is usually performed while the patient is on cardiopulmonary bypass. Generally, a blunt dissection of the portion of the AV groove that contains the bypass tract is performed via an

atriotomy. Before surgery, careful electrophysiologic testing is performed to characterize and localize the bypass tract as fully as possible, and mapping is repeated in the operating room before the patient is placed on cardiopulmonary bypass.

The electrophysiology study in intraatrial reentry

Intraatrial reentry is the mechanism of arrhythmia in less than 5% of patients presenting with supraventricular tachycardias. In intraatrial reentry, the reentrant circuit is entirely contained within the atrial myocardium. Superficially, intraatrial reentry resembles automatic atrial tachycardia because distinct P waves precede each QRS complex, P wave morphology almost always differs from normal sinus P waves, and AV block can occur without affecting the arrhythmic mechanism. Unlike automatic atrial reentry, however, intraatrial reentry is inducible and terminable with pacing.

Induction of intraatrial reentry is accomplished with atrial pacing. Invariably, whether the arrhythmia is induced with a single extrastimulus or with incremental atrial extrastimuli, induction occurs only when a premature impulse is early enough to produce intraatrial conduction delay (i.e. during the RRP of the atrium). The requirement for intraatrial conduction delay is further evidence that the arrhythmia being induced is reentrant in mechanism and that the atrial myocardium forms at least part of the reentrant circuit.

During intraatrial reentry, the atrial activation pattern differs from the normal atrial activation pattern because the atria are usually activated from a different location than during sinus rhythm. If the site of intraatrial reentry is near the SA node, however, the activation pattern can be indistinguishable from normal. In these cases, intraatrial reentry can often be distinguished from SA nodal reentry by the necessity of intraatrial conduction delay for initiation of the arrhythmia.

Because intraatrial reentrant circuits are contained entirely in atrial tissue, AV nodal block or block in the more distal conducting system can often be observed to occur without affecting the reentrant mechanism, thus demonstrating that the arrhythmia does not require the ventricular myocardium.

The pharmacologic treatment of intraatrial reentry requires drugs that affect the atrial myocardium; namely, antiarrhythmic drugs in classes Ia, Ic, and III. Drugs that affect primarily the AV node do not affect this arrhythmia (except perhaps to induce heart block). Antitachycardia pacemakers have occasionally been used to terminate intraatrial reentry. Transcatheter ablation of intraatrial reentry,

using radiofrequency energy, has also been performed. This procedure, however, tends to be more difficult than the transcatheter
ablation of slow AV nodal pathways or of bypass tracts.

The electrophysiology study in SA nodal reentry

SA nodal reentry is a rare form of reentrant supraventricular tachycardia in which the reentrant circuit is enclosed entirely within the
SA node. Because SA nodal tissue is electrophysiologically similar to
AV nodal tissue, the mechanism of SA nodal reentry is felt to be the
same as that of AV nodal reentry. Most likely, there are dual tracts
within the SA node that form a potential reentrant circuit. The
P wave morphology on the surface ECG and the atrial activation
pattern during SA nodal reentry are normal. SA nodal reentry is
distinguished from standard sinus tachycardia by its paroxysmal
onset and termination and by the ability to induce and terminate
the arrhythmia by pacing.

Inducing and terminating SA nodal reentry is possible with atrial
pacing, using either single extrastimuli or incremental pacing.
Unlike in intraatrial reentry, conduction delay within the atrial
myocardium is not necessary for the induction of SA nodal reentry.
It is likely that the conduction delay necessary for the initiation of
reentry occurs in a reentrant circuit enclosed within the SA node,
where it cannot be demonstrated.

Treatment of SA nodal reentry is similar to the treatment of AV
nodal reentry. This arrhythmia responds to vagal maneuvers and to
drugs that decrease conduction and increase refractoriness in the
SA and AV nodes (digitalis, calcium blockers, and β-blockers). SA
nodal ablation can also be performed, but a permanent pacemaker
may be required as a consequence.

The electrophysiology study in atrial flutter and atrial fibrillation

Atrial flutter and atrial fibrillation are felt to be reentrant supraventricular tachyarrhythmias in which the reentrant circuits are
located entirely within the atrial myocardium. Both are inducible
with single atrial extrastimuli or incremental atrial pacing during
the atrial relative refractory period (RRP; i.e. during pacing with
coupling intervals short enough to produce intraatrial conduction
delay). In atrial flutter, distinct P waves are seen, classically in a
sawtooth pattern. In atrial fibrillation, atrial activity is continuous
and chaotic, hence distinct P waves are not seen. In both arrhythmias, second-degree AV block is the rule.

Atrial flutter

Patients who have paroxysms of atrial flutter often have normal hearts, whereas patients with chronic atrial flutter usually have underlying heart disease that causes atrial distention or dilation. Most often, chronic atrial flutter eventually converts to chronic atrial fibrillation.

Patients in whom atrial flutter is inducible during electrophysiologic testing tend to have demonstrable intraatrial conduction abnormalities. In these patients, atrial flutter is usually induced with atrial pacing at cycle lengths that are short enough to produce intraatrial conduction delays.

As already noted, these same characteristics are also typical for intraatrial reentrant tachycardias. It is probably legitimate to think of intraatrial reentry, atrial flutter, and atrial fibrillation as forming a spectrum of arrhythmias that have the same essential mechanism— that is, intraatrial reentry. Atrial flutter is distinguished from intraatrial reentrant tachycardia by its rate (flutter occurs from 220 to 350 beats/min, whereas intraatrial reentrant tachycardia occurs from 120 to 220 beats/min) and by its mode of termination. Whereas intraatrial reentrant tachycardia can often be terminated with single programmed atrial premature impulses, atrial flutter cannot. Atrial flutter generally requires rapid atrial pacing for several seconds at rates from 20 to 50% faster than the flutter rate to terminate the arrhythmia.

The intraatrial electrogram recorded during atrial flutter normally shows rapid regular deflections with uniform cycle lengths and amplitude; the deflections correlate with the P waves on the surface ECG (Figure 6.25a). If this typical pattern is seen, the atrial flutter can almost always be terminated with rapid atrial pacing. In some cases of flutter, however, the intraatrial electrogram shows variability in the cycle length and amplitude of the atrial deflections. This second type of flutter is probably actually a form of atrial fibrillation (Figure 6.25b). When this pattern is seen on the intraatrial electrogram, termination of the arrhythmia with rapid atrial pacing is usually not possible. On the surface ECG, this intermediate form of flutter is often called atrial fib-flutter because the atrial activity appears flutter-like but somewhat irregular, and the ventricular response is often irregular.

When vigorous attempts to pace-terminate the typical form of atrial flutter are made, two basic responses are commonly seen. The rhythm may be converted to sinus rhythm or to atrial fibrillation. Generally, atrial fibrillation is more likely to result when faster

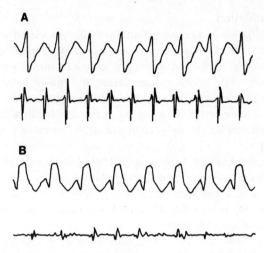

Figure 6.25 Two types of atrial flutter. A surface ECG lead and a right atrial electrogram are shown in both panels. (a) Typical atrial flutter displays a constant amplitude and cycle length on the intracardiac electrogram. This type of flutter is relatively easy to terminate with pacing. (b) Atypical flutter shows a somewhat variable cycle length and amplitude on the intracardiac electrogram. This type of flutter may be intermediate between atrial flutter and atrial fibrillation and is relatively difficult to terminate with pacing.

pacing rates are used (paced cycle lengths approaching 150% of the atrial flutter cycle length). When atrial fibrillation is the result of pace-termination of atrial flutter, the fibrillation usually spontaneously converts to sinus rhythm within 24 hours.

Treatment of atrial flutter

In general, the treatment of atrial flutter consists of restoring and maintaining sinus rhythm. Restoring sinus rhythm is most readily accomplished either by pace-termination of the flutter or by DC cardioversion. If atrial flutter recurs, chronic therapy to prevent atrial flutter should be considered. In the past, such chronic suppressive therapy was limited to antiarrhythmic drugs (class Ia, Ic, or III drugs). During the past few years, however, effective transcatheter ablation techniques have been developed for the prevention of atrial flutter. Transcatheter ablation of this arrhythmia (described in Chapter 8) should be considered for any patient in whom chronic antiarrhythmic drug therapy is being contemplated.

Atrial fibrillation

Atrial fibrillation can be paroxysmal (usually associated with normal hearts) or chronic (usually associated with heart disease). Although atrial fibrillation is thought to be a reentrant arrhythmia of the atrial myocardium, its continuous and chaotic atrial activity precludes both meaningful analysis by recording intraatrial electrograms and pace-termination of the arrhythmia. Thus, although atrial fibrillation can be induced by pacing, it cannot be terminated by pacing.

During standard electrophysiologic testing of the SA node and AV conduction, a few seconds of atrial fibrillation are induced in 5% of normal patients. The induced atrial fibrillation is likely to terminate spontaneously within seconds, unless the patient has a history of spontaneous atrial fibrillation.

Patients with a history of atrial fibrillation have a high incidence of intraatrial conduction defects on electrophysiologic testing, like patients who have atrial flutter and intraatrial reentrant tachycardia. In patients with atrial fibrillation, however, the conduction defects tend to be more generalized, often involving the SA node and AV conduction system as well.

Treatment of atrial fibrillation

Atrial fibrillation is one of the most common cardiac arrhythmias seen in medical practice, so it is unfortunate that it is also one of the most difficult to treat. The difficulty stems from the fact that there are no widely applicable, reliable, and safe methods for restoring and maintaining sinus rhythm in patients with atrial fibrillation. So, in many instances, the most expedient path is to allow the arrhythmia to persist, while controlling the ventricular rate and anticoagulating. In any case, the fundamental decision that must be made when treating atrial fibrillation is whether to aim for rhythm control or for rate control.

Rhythm control

Opting for rhythm control commits the physician to first restoring then trying to maintain sinus rhythm.

Restoring sinus rhythm is usually straightforward—the main issue involves the timing of cardioversion, so as to reduce the risk of systemic embolization. If atrial fibrillation is known or suspected to have been present for more than 48 hours, one should assume that atrial thrombi exist and delay the cardioversion until 3–4 weeks of anticoagulation can be given. If immediate cardioversion is required and the duration of atrial fibrillation is longer than 48 hours (or is unknown), the safety of cardioversion is improved if no atrial thrombi are seen during transesophageal echocardiography.

There are two standard methods for restoring sinus rhythm: DC cardioversion and drug therapy. Electrical cardioversion has the advantage of being highly efficacious as well as nonproarrhythmic. If the patient is stable, however, several drugs are available that can be effective in restoring sinus rhythm, including dofetilide, flecainide, ibutilide, and propafenone. The efficacy of these drugs is generally reported to be 30–60%; because all of them can cause proarrhythmia, patients need to be monitored for at least several hours after the drugs are administered.

When restoring sinus rhythm, one should consider the possibility that the patient has diffuse electrical system disease (as many elderly patients with atrial fibrillation do). Especially if the ventricular response is relatively slow in the absence of AV blocking drugs, precautions should be taken to make sure that immediate pacing support is available after cardioversion, if needed.

Only 20–30% of patients restored to sinus rhythm will remain free of atrial fibrillation for 1 year without antiarrhythmic drug therapy. This success rate can be increased to around 50% with class Ia, Ic, or III drugs, though evidence exists that amiodarone may be able to increase this 1-year success rate to 60–70%.

Some implantable defibrillators offer atrial defibrillation in addition to standard ventricular therapies. These atrial defibrillators sometimes can be helpful in supporting a rapid-cardioversion maintenance strategy in patients with occasional episodes of atrial fibrillation. These devices can be programmed to deliver a DC shock either automatically or only in response to a "triggering" signal from either the patient or his or her doctor. The shocks delivered by these devices are quite painful and are not substantially more convenient than an external DC cardioversion, unless the doctor is willing to activate the automatic or patient-triggered modes—an uncommon scenario. Perhaps not surprisingly, implanted atrial defibrillators have not gained much traction in clinical practice.

Because antiarrhythmic drugs are only modestly effective in maintaining sinus rhythm and can be quite toxic, a major focus of electrophysiologists over the past 20 years has been on trying to figure out how to "cure" atrial fibrillation, using ablation techniques. While significant progress has been made, the ablation of atrial fibrillation is still tedious, not completely effective, and a relatively risky procedure, and should be offered only to carefully selected patients by experienced electrophysiologists. The ablation of atrial fibrillation will be discussed in Chapter 8.

Rate control

If maintaining sinus rhythm in patients with atrial fibrillation was easy and safe, nobody would opt for rate control. The fact that rate control is nevertheless the standard of therapy speaks volumes about the difficulty and risks of rhythm control.

Controlling the ventricular rate in atrial fibrillation can usually be accomplished by administering drugs that affect AV nodal conduction and refractoriness (digitalis, calcium blockers, and β-blockers). Often, all three types of drug need to be used in combination to achieve adequate rate control.

If rate control cannot be achieved by pharmacologic means, there is a more drastic (though effective and relatively safe) method for doing so—ablating the AV conduction system to produce complete heart block, and then inserting a permanent rate-responsive pacemaker. This option virtually guarantees excellent rate control, and in patients whose symptoms are related to persistently high heart rates, it often creates a dramatic improvement in quality of life. This method is discussed in detail in Chapter 8.

Rhythm control versus rate control

For decades it has been a point of controversy whether patients with atrial fibrillation are best managed with rhythm control or with rate control.

Two large randomized clinical trials—the AFFIRM trial (Wyse DG et al., N Engl J Med 2002 Dec 5; 347:1825) and the RACE trial (VanGelder IC et al., N Engl J Med 2002 Dec 5; 347:1834)—showed no benefit to patients with atrial fibrillation assigned to rhythm control (using antiarrhythmic drugs) when compared to patients assigned to rate control. Indeed, in both trials there was a tendency toward better clinical outcomes in the rate-control groups; this latter finding is generally interpreted as yet more evidence of the toxicity of antiarrhythmic drugs. Furthermore, systemic embolization was *not* reduced in the rhythm-control group, so once a patient has had chronic or persistent atrial fibrillation, chronic anticoagulation apparently remains necessary, even if sinus rhythm is successfully restored and maintained. The bottom line: for now, in general, rate control is the generally accepted standard of treatment for patients with chronic or persistent atrial fibrillation.

AFFIRM and RACE do not, however, tell the whole story. Consider the following:

- Some patients have significant symptoms when they are in atrial fibrillation, even if their heart rates are controlled. Usually, these patients have relatively "stiff," noncompliant ventricles (i.e. diastolic dysfunction). Such patients rely heavily on effective atrial contractions, which allow them to maintain the high left ventricular end-diastolic pressures they require while at the same time maintaining relatively normal mean left atrial pressures. With the onset of atrial fibrillation, the only way to maintain these high left ventricular end-diastolic pressures is to immediately and dramatically elevate the mean left atrial pressures, leading to symptoms related to pulmonary congestion. In individuals like this, no matter what the randomized trials might say, maintaining sinus rhythm is imperative.
- Patients with normal hearts and occasional episodes of atrial fibrillation almost always feel much better in sinus rhythm. Maintaining sinus rhythm in these patients is often the favorable approach. These patients were underrepresented in both AFFIRM and RACE.
- A substudy from the AFFIRM trial suggests that patients who actually achieved chronic sinus rhythm (as opposed to patients merely randomized to rhythm control) had improved clinical outcomes (Corley SD *et al.*, Circulation 2004; 109:1509).

These considerations emphasize once again that rate control is the standard of therapy not because it is a perfectly adequate treatment, but because the alternatives are so unappealing. The lack of benefit from rhythm control seen in randomized trials seems most likely to be an artifact of our current ineffective and risky methods for maintaining sinus rhythm. With the further refinement and generalized ability of techniques for ablating atrial fibrillation, this equation is likely to change eventually. Nonetheless, in general, rate control now ought to be the predominant treatment strategy used in patients with chronic or persistent atrial fibrillation.

For patients with paroxysmal or recent-onset atrial fibrillation—in other words, patients who do not have chronic or persistent atrial fibrillation—virtually all experts agree that restoring sinus rhythm is still the best course of action, though not many are enthusiastic about using antiarrhythmic drugs to maintain sinus rhythm even in these patients. Patients with frequent episodes of paroxysmal atrial fibrillation—whose arrhythmias are now thought often to be triggered by ectopic foci located in the pulmonary veins—are probably those who stand to benefit the most from ablation techniques centered around the electrical isolation of the pulmonary veins (see Chapter 8).

Evaluation of patients with supraventricular tachyarrhythmias—when is electrophysiologic testing necessary?

Although the study of supraventricular tachyarrhythmias is probably the most intellectually stimulating and satisfying type of electrophysiology study one can perform, the fact is that many patients with supraventricular tachycardias can be managed adequately without invasive testing. Electrophysiology studies are often not necessary for two reasons. First, if one understands the mechanisms of supraventricular tachyarrhythmias, the astute clinician can often diagnose and treat an arrhythmia based on examination of the surface ECG and on the response to vagal maneuvers. Second, in most cases, supraventricular tachyarrhythmias are not life-threatening. Therefore, if one guesses incorrectly on therapy, the patient will survive, and one will have an opportunity to change the recommended treatment (the major exception to this rule is in patients with bypass tracts that have very short antegrade refractory periods).

The examination of the surface ECG can help immensely in diagnosing the mechanism of supraventricular tachycardia. Atrial flutter and atrial fibrillation can be diagnosed almost immediately from the ECG and do not present a diagnostic problem. In the other types of supraventricular tachycardia, the relationship of P waves to QRS complexes and the morphology of P waves during tachycardia can be most helpful. Figure 6.26 shows the essential characteristics of the P waves in the four types of reentry that are commonly lumped under the heading "PAT."

In the majority of patients with AV nodal reentry (the most common form of PAT), the retrograde P waves occur during the QRS complex and are therefore invisible on the 12-lead ECG. In every other kind of PAT, P waves can usually be identified on careful inspection of the ECG. Therefore, if there are no P waves, AV nodal reentry is the likely diagnosis.

In bypass tract-mediated macroreentry (the next most common type of PAT—approximately 90% of patients presenting with PAT have either this or AV nodal reentry), P waves virtually always can

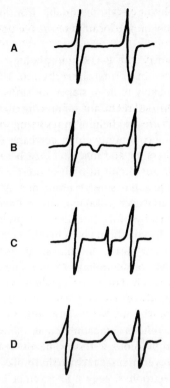

Figure 6.26 Typical P wave relationships in four types of supraventricular tachycardia. Surface ECG lead II is depicted. (a) In AV nodal reentrant tachycardia, the P wave is usually buried within the QRS complex and is not discernible. (b) In bypass tract-mediated macroreentry, the inferior leads usually show a negative P wave, with the RP interval shorter than the PR interval. (c) In intraatrial reentry, discrete P waves are almost always seen. The P wave morphology can have any configuration, and the PR interval is normal or short. (d) In SA nodal reentry, P waves and the PR interval appear normal.

be seen. Because the P waves are generated retrogradely during this tachycardia, they are always negative in the inferior leads. Generally, the RP interval is less than the PR interval. Because the RP interval is relatively short, the retrograde P wave is often mistaken for a bump on the T wave by the unwary observer.

In intraatrial reentry, P waves are invariably seen on the 12-lead ECG. The PR interval is usually shorter than the RP interval and therefore the P waves are more obvious than in macroreentry.

The P wave morphology is quite variable from patient to patient and depends entirely on the location of the reentrant circuit within the atrium.

In SA nodal reentry, the P–QRS morphology is almost exactly identical to that seen in normal sinus rhythm. Thus, this arrhythmia is much more likely to be mistaken for sinus tachycardia than any of the other forms of reentrant supraventricular tachycardia.

Vagal maneuvers are also helpful in resolving these arrhythmias. Increased vagal tone commonly either decreases the rate of or terminates AV nodal reentry and macroreentry, because the AV node is part of the reentrant circuit in both of these arrhythmias. Likewise, vagal maneuvers may slow or terminate SA nodal reentry. In intraatrial reentry, however, vagal maneuvers have no effect on the cycle length of the tachycardia, but they may prolong the PR interval or produce AV block without changing the tachycardia.

Most of the time, the correct mechanism of PAT can be deduced by these noninvasive considerations. Appropriate therapy can then be instituted immediately. For instance, when one recognizes that a patient has intraatrial reentry, one can correctly predict that the patient is one of the famous 5–10% presenting with PAT who will *not* respond to intravenous verapamil or adenosine.

Normally, electrophysiologic testing needs to be performed in patients with supraventricular tachyarrhythmias in three general situations. First, electrophysiology studies can be helpful in patients whose arrhythmias appear refractory to treatment. In such patients, the arrhythmias usually have not responded to therapy, either because the mechanism of the arrhythmia is unknown or misunderstood, or because the reentrant circuit has unusual characteristics and does not respond to treatment in the usual way. Invasive studies can help immeasurably by identifying the exact mechanism of the arrhythmias and by fully characterizing the various portions of the reentrant circuit. Pharmacologic or nonpharmacologic therapy can then be chosen based on that information.

Second, electrophysiology studies are indicated in patients with bypass tracts that are suspected to be capable of mediating life-threatening arrhythmias. Certainly such patients would include those who have already demonstrated the propensity of the bypass tract to conduct dangerously rapidly during atrial fibrillation or flutter. Many electrophysiologists advocate invasive studies in any patient with a bypass tract who has had symptomatic arrhythmias of any type. Some even recommend studying any patient who is seen to have preexcitation on an ECG, on the premise that any bypass tract that conducts antegradely may have lethal potential until proven otherwise.

Third, electrophysiology studies are done for the purpose of performing transcatheter ablation. With the remarkable success of transcatheter ablation using radiofrequency energy over the past few years for most varieties of supraventricular tachycardia, it is now advisable to refer any patient for electrophysiologic testing who would otherwise be subjected to daily long-term pharmacologic therapy.

7 The Electrophysiology Study in the Evaluation and Treatment of Ventricular Arrhythmias

Ventricular tachyarrhythmias and sudden death

Sudden death (death that is instantaneous and completely unexpected) may well be the major public health problem in the United States today. If this statement seems surprising, consider that each year, approximately 400 000 Americans die suddenly, and that sudden death is the most common form of death in the United States. Although most Americans are touched by sudden death, few realize that the majority of these deaths are due to electrical disturbances of the heart and are therefore, at least in theory, preventable.

Consider a typical sudden cardiac death: a 59-year-old man who has suffered a myocardial infarction within the past 12 months has recovered, is now feeling well, and is leading a happy and productive life. He has followed his physician's advice and has altered his lifestyle in an exemplary fashion—he has stopped smoking, is on a low-fat and low-cholesterol diet, and has joined an exercise program. He is back at work, and his new sense of mortality has resulted in a broader and more tolerant perspective on everyday job-related stresses. In many ways, he feels better than he has in years.

Then one day, while watching television with his wife, he gasps softly and slumps over. An ambulance is called, but within minutes he is dead. The grieving widow is told by the emergency room physician (who has never seen the victim before) that her husband has died of a heart attack. Later, the victim's personal physician is only too quick (often through the honest desire to allay any feelings of

Electrophysiologic Testing, Fifth Edition. Richard N. Fogoros.
© 2012 John Wiley & Sons, Ltd. Published 2012 by John Wiley & Sons, Ltd.

guilt among surviving family members) to corroborate the "inevitability" of the event.

This scene takes place, on average, almost once every minute in the United States. The tragedy is compounded by a lack of understanding by both the lay public and the medical profession as to the reason for these sudden deaths. Most often, sudden death is not caused by acute myocardial infarction or bradycardia, as is commonly claimed. Instead, the vast majority of the 400 000 sudden deaths that occur each year in the United States are due to ventricular tachycardia or ventricular fibrillation. To the extent that ventricular tachyarrhythmias can be adequately treated, most of these sudden cardiac deaths can be prevented.

During the past 2 or 3 decades, remarkable advances have been made in treating ventricular tachycardia and fibrillation, largely thanks to what has been learned in the electrophysiology laboratory. It was the recognition that the great majority of lethal arrhythmias are due to the mechanism of reentry, and that they therefore lend themselves nicely to study in the electrophysiology laboratory, that catalyzed the rapid expansion of electrophysiology centers during the 1980s. The original "Holy Grail" for electrophysiologists was to solve the problem of sudden cardiac death.

This goal was pursued for years through the careful study of ventricular tachyarrhythmias in the electrophysiology laboratory. For almost 20 years, electrophysiologists spent much of their time inducing and terminating ventricular arrhythmias, and most especially, trying to identify effective therapy for those arrhythmias by the serial testing of antiarrhythmic drugs.

Thankfully, serial drug testing for ventricular arrhythmias now has virtually disappeared from the electrophysiologist's repertoire. So, in contrast to early editions of this book, where much space in this chapter was devoted to the technique of, and rationale for, serial drug testing, the author now offers instead a chilling speculation on how future historians of medicine might view these recent times:

> The reader no doubt will be disturbed to learn that, during the last decades of the 20th century, doctors calling themselves "electrophysiologists" submitted thousands of patients to multiple inductions of cardiac arrest, followed by resuscitations, over periods of days to weeks; and further, that this practice was not only legal, but was represented as being therapeutic, and was accepted—and in some instances honored and admired—by

their medical colleagues. It is not recorded what these "electrophysiologists" did to sublimate their proclivities once this "serial drug testing" was no longer considered a legitimate medical practice.

In this chapter, we will review the current management of ventricular tachyarrhythmias—and the role that electrophysiologic testing plays in their evaluation and treatment. This role is clearly very different today than it was in the recent past. Nonetheless, the electrophysiology study can still be helpful in managing patients with ventricular tachyarrhythmias, both in diagnosing their problem and in devising optimal treatment. And, despite the smug superiority that (the author fears) may color future historians' view of the matter, it is what we have learned in the electrophysiology laboratory that enables our treatment of these arrhythmias today and (if we allow ourselves to follow the science) opens a path to substantially reducing the millions of sudden deaths that threaten to occur in the future.

The evaluation of ventricular tachyarrhythmias

The mechanisms of ventricular arrhythmias

The appropriate evaluation and treatment of ventricular arrhythmias largely depends on the mechanism of those arrhythmias. Table 7.1 lists the most common ventricular arrhythmias according to their mechanisms. Whatever the mechanism, however, ventricular arrhythmias have similar appearances on the ECG: premature ventricular complexes (PVCs), ventricular tachycardia, or ventricular fibrillation. Figuring out which mechanism is responsible when faced with any of these arrhythmias depends to a great extent on the clinical setting in which the arrhythmia occurs—and sometimes on its characteristics in the electrophysiology laboratory.

We will discuss these arrhythmias in the order of their clinical frequency, beginning with reentrant ventricular arrhythmias.

Reentrant ventricular arrhythmias

Reentry accounts for the majority of ventricular arrhythmias. Reentrant ventricular arrhythmias are most often associated with chronic underlying heart disease. Reentrant circuits within the ventricles usually do not appear until patients develop some form of heart disease which causes scarring in the ventricular myocardium. Such scarring mainly occurs with ischemic heart disease and the

Table 7.1 Mechanisms of ventricular arrhythmias

Automatic ventricular arrhythmias
- Premature ventricular complexes
- Ventricular tachycardia and fibrillation associated with acute medical conditions:
  - ° Acute myocardial infarction or ischemia
  - ° Electrolyte and acid–base disturbances, hypoxemia
  - ° Increased sympathetic tone

Reentrant ventricular arrhythmias
- Premature ventricular complexes
- Ventricular tachycardia and fibrillation associated with chronic heart disease:
  - ° Previous myocardial infarction
- Cardiomyopathy (including bundle branch reentry and ventricular arrhythmias associated with arrhythmogenic right ventricular dysplasia)

Triggered activity
- Pause-dependent triggered activity
- Catechol-dependent triggered activity

Miscellaneous ventricular arrhythmias
- Idiopathic left ventricular tachycardia
- Outflow tract ventricular tachycardia (repetitive monomorphic ventricular tachycardia)
- Brugada syndrome
- Catecholaminergic polymorphic ventricular tachycardia

various cardiomyopathies. In ischemic heart disease, reentrant circuits arise during the healing and ventricular remodeling that follow an acute myocardial infarction—usually, the reentrant circuits form in the border zone between the scar tissue and the normal myocardium. In contrast to automatic arrhythmias, in which the typical substrate (such as acute ischemia) is temporary in nature and most often reversible, in the case of reentrant arrhythmias the substrate (i.e. the reentrant circuit) is not temporary but fixed. Once a reentrant circuit is formed, it is always present and can generate a reentrant ventricular tachyarrhythmia at any time and without warning. Thus, the "late" sudden deaths that occur in patients with myocardial infarction (i.e. sudden death occurring at a time between roughly 24 hours and months or even years after the acute infarction) are usually due to reentrant arrhythmias. Reentrant arrhythmias, then, are commonly seen in patients who have a history of cardiac disease but are not acutely ill at the time of the arrhythmia. The vast majority of sudden cardiac deaths in the United States are due to reentrant ventricular tachyarrhythmias.

Risk factors for reentrant ventricular arrhythmias

It is relatively straightforward to predict which patients are at risk for reentrant ventricular tachyarrhythmias (and, therefore, at risk for sudden cardiac death), as long as one has an understanding of the pathophysiology of reentrant arrhythmias. A reentrant arrhythmia requires both an anatomic circuit with electrophysiologic properties appropriate for sustaining a reentrant impulse and an appropriately timed premature impulse to trigger the reentrant arrhythmia.

Because reentrant circuits are common only in the setting of myocardial disease, the major risk factor for ventricular reentry is the presence of underlying cardiac disease. As noted, myocardial infarctions and cardiomyopathic diseases are the most common disorders associated with reentrant ventricular arrhythmias. Nonetheless, any cardiac condition that causes even a small amount of ventricular fibrosis can give rise to reentrant circuits. Such conditions include myocardial trauma, a myocardial infarction that has been "aborted" by thrombolytic therapy, subclinical infarctions associated with bypass surgery, and subclinical viral myocarditis.

In general, the more extensive the myocardial fibrosis, the higher the likelihood of developing a reentrant circuit. With disease states that cause large fibrotic patches (such as a myocardial infarction), reentrant circuits are reasonably likely to develop. In disease states that cause only microscopic fibrosis, however, the likelihood of reentrant arrhythmias is proportional to the degree of myocardial involvement in the underlying disease process.

Once an anatomic circuit exists whose electrophysiologic properties are appropriate for sustaining reentry, an appropriately timed premature impulse is required to trigger the reentrant arrhythmia. Thus, another risk factor for developing reentrant ventricular arrhythmias is ventricular ectopy. Complex ventricular ectopy is generally considered to be present if, on 24-hour Holter monitoring, there are more than 10 PVC complexes per hour, or repetitive forms such as couplets, triplets, or runs of nonsustained ventricular tachycardia. Patients with underlying cardiac disease who have complex ventricular ectopy have a higher risk of sudden death than patients who have the same underlying disease without complex ectopy. Frequent ectopic beats are not, however, a requirement for developing reentrant arrhythmias, since a single PVC (or even a premature atrial complex (PAC)) has the potential to trigger a reentrant ventricular tachyarrhythmia, given the right reentrant circuit. Indeed, a substantial proportion of patients resuscitated from lethal arrhythmias have only negligible ventricular ectopy. It should also be noted that complex ventricular ectopy in patients with normal heart muscles (who are therefore extremely unlikely to have a reentrant circuit within their ventricles) has never not been shown to increase the risk of sudden death.

An individual's risk for sudden cardiac death from a reentrant tachycardia, therefore, is most directly dependent on the presence or absence of underlying myocardial disease and on the extent of that disease. In general, since lower ejection fractions imply more extensive scarring and therefore indicate a higher likelihood that a reentrant circuit is present, the lower the ejection fraction, the higher the probability of sudden death. Most fatal arrhythmias occur in patients who have left ventricular ejection fractions of less than 40%. As we have noted, some degree of ectopy must also be present to trigger the reentrant arrhythmia, but that ectopy does not necessarily have to be very frequent for an arrhythmia to occur. The probability that a reentrant circuit will generate an arrhythmia is much more dependent on the characteristics of the circuit itself (e.g. the tachycardia zone of the circuit) than on the frequency of ectopic beats.

Many studies have been done to attempt to quantify an individual's risk of sudden death, and most have focused on three risk factors: the presence of a prior myocardial infarction, the presence of a depressed left ventricular ejection fraction (arbitrarily, less than 40%), and the presence of complex ventricular ectopy. At the risk of greatly oversimplifying the vast body of literature examining this issue, let us make the following generalizations. First, the presence of underlying heart disease is more important in determining risk than the presence of complex ectopy, because underlying heart disease alone increases one's risk for sudden death, whereas complex ectopy alone does not. Second, having one of these risk factors alone (except for complex ectopy) yields a 1-year risk of sudden death that can be grossly estimated at approximately 5%. Third, the risk entailed by the presence of more than one of these risk factors appears to be roughly additive (Table 7.2). Thus, the presence of either a previous myocardial infarction or a depressed ejection fraction gives a 1-year risk of about 5%. The presence of any two risk factors gives a risk of about 10%, and the presence of all three factors gives a risk of about 15%. Obviously, these values represent

Table 7.2 Risk factors and probabilities of sudden cardiac death

Moderate-risk group	
Risk factors	*1-year risk of sudden death*
Previous MI or LV EF < 40%	50%
Previous MI + LV EF < 40% or previous MI + complex ectopy or LV EF < 40% + complex ectopy	10%
Previous MI + LV EF < 40% + complex ectopy	15%
High-risk group	
Risk factors	*1-year risk of sudden death*
Sudden-death survivor	30–50%
VT with syncope	30–50%
VT with minimal symptoms	20–30%

Values on this table are loosely derived from data reported by the Multicenter Post-infarction Research Group (Bigger JT *et al.*, Circulation 1984; 69:250) and the Multicenter Investigation of the Limitation of Infarction Size (Mukharji J *et al.*, Am J Cardiol 1984; 54:31). MI, myocardial infarction; LV EF, left ventricular ejection fraction; VT, ventricular tachycardia.

only a gross estimate derived from the available literature. The severity of each risk factor is also important. For instance, a large myocardial infarction yields a higher risk than a small infarction, an ejection fraction of 15% yields a higher risk than an ejection fraction of 35%, and the presence of nonsustained ventricular tachycardia yields a higher risk than a single PVC. Thus, a patient with a previous large myocardial infarction with severely depressed ventricular function and long runs of nonsustained ventricular tachycardia will have a 1-year risk substantially higher than 15%.

Another indicator that is sometimes used to estimate risk of reentrant ventricular arrhythmias is the signal-averaged surface ECG. The signal-averaging process digitizes and processes a series of QRS complexes (usually several hundred) recorded from the body surface. The result is a clean, high-fidelity average QRS complex in which small (low-amplitude) details can be seen which are not visible on a normal ECG. In many patients at risk for lethal arrhythmias, low-amplitude afterpotentials can be seen immediately following the QRS complex (Figure 7.1). In theory, these afterpotentials may represent electrical activity caused by localized slow conduction in one or more reentrant circuits. If so, the signal-averaged ECG may be a method of detecting the presence of

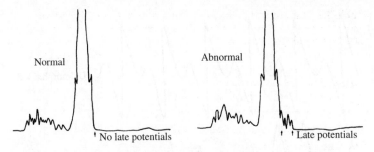

Figure 7.1 Signal-averaged ECG. The first panel shows a normal signal-averaged ECG, in which no late potentials are present. The second panel shows an abnormal signal-averaged ECG. The late potentials may indicate areas of slow conduction within the ventricular myocardium, suggesting the presence of a reentrant circuit.

reentrant circuits in patients who have underlying cardiac disease known to predispose to reentry. When considered with other risk factors, as listed in Table 7.2, the prognostic value of the signal-averaged ECG appears to be roughly additive. Thus, for instance, a patient with a depressed ejection fraction, a prior myocardial infarction, complex ectopy, and a positive signal-averaged study would have a 1-year risk of sudden death of 20–30%. The signal-averaged ECG should always be interpreted along with these other risk factors.

In summary, patients who have survived a myocardial infarction or who have a depressed left ventricular ejection fraction from any cause are at increased risk for sudden death from reentrant ventricular tachyarrhythmias. The risk increases when the underlying cardiac disease is accompanied by complex ventricular ectopy or a positive signal-averaged ECG. Considering only the fact that each year between 500 000 and 1 000 000 people suffer myocardial infarctions, the pool of patients at risk for sudden cardiac death is seen to be huge. It is from this very large pool of individuals that most of the 400 000 sudden-death victims each year are drawn.

Clinical characteristics of reentrant ventricular tachyarrhythmias

The reentrant ventricular tachyarrhythmias take two major forms—ventricular tachycardia and ventricular fibrillation—and result in three major symptom complexes: sudden cardiac death, syncope, or minimal symptoms such as dizziness and palpitations.

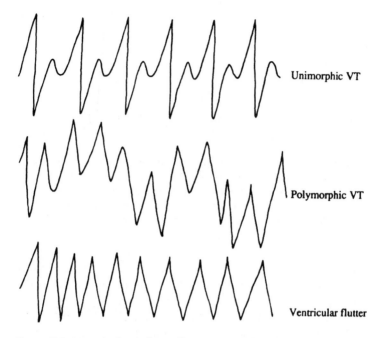

Figure 7.2 Ventricular tachycardia. In unimorphic (or monomorphic) ventricular tachycardia, all QRS complexes are similar in morphology. In polymorphic ventricular tachycardia, the QRS complexes have constantly changing morphologies. In ventricular flutter, the ventricular rate is so rapid that the QRS complexes cannot be readily distinguished from T waves.

Ventricular tachycardia (Figure 7.2) is a relatively organized tachyarrhythmia with discrete QRS complexes. It can be either sustained or nonsustained and can be monomorphic or polymorphic—polymorphic ventricular tachycardias tend to be faster and less stable than monomorphic tachycardias. The rate of ventricular tachycardia can be from 100 to more than 300 beats/min. At slower rates, ventricular tachycardia often does not cause significant hemodynamic compromise and may be relatively asymptomatic. The symptoms produced by ventricular tachycardia also depend on the morphology of the tachycardia, the severity of the underlying heart disease, the vascular tone, the geometry of ventricular contraction during the tachycardia, and whether the patient is upright or supine. At faster rates (usually 220 beats/min or faster), the tachycardia is so rapid that it may be impossible to distinguish the QRS

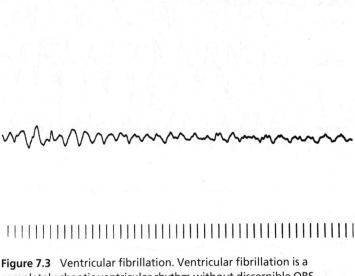

Figure 7.3 Ventricular fibrillation. Ventricular fibrillation is a completely chaotic ventricular rhythm without discernible QRS complexes.

complex from the T waves. This type of ventricular tachycardia is often referred to as ventricular flutter.

Ventricular fibrillation (Figure 7.3) is a completely disorganized tachyarrhythmia without discrete QRS complexes. This arrhythmia causes instant hemodynamic collapse and rapid loss of consciousness, because the heart immediately ceases to contract meaningfully. When ventricular fibrillation begins, it is associated with a coarse electrical pattern. As the heart becomes less viable (over a period of a few minutes), the amplitude of fibrillation waves seen on the ECG becomes finer and finer. Finally, all electrical activity ceases (flatline).

Recordings from patients who wore Holter monitors at the time of sudden cardiac death have often displayed the following progression of arrhythmias (Figure 7.4): an acute increase in ventricular ectopy is followed within a few seconds to minutes by ventricular tachycardia, which in turn degenerates (again in seconds to minutes) to coarse and then fine ventricular fibrillation. After another 5–7 minutes, there is no electrical activity. Patients who are successfully resuscitated during such an episode (electrophysiologists have called them, oxymoronically, "sudden-death survivors") are often

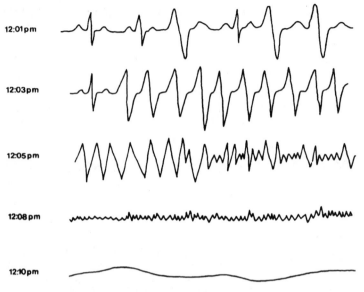

Figure 7.4 A typical sequence of events in sudden death. This figure shows tracings from a Holter recording made in a patient who experienced sudden death. At 12:01 pm the patient is in sinus rhythm with PVCs. At 12:03 pm ventricular tachycardia occurs, which degenerates to ventricular fibrillation at 12:05 pm. By 12:08 pm, fine ventricular fibrillation is present. All electrical activity has ceased by 12:10 pm.

labeled as having had primary ventricular fibrillation, because that is the rhythm commonly seen by the time rescuers arrive. If the rescuers are a little too late, they see the flatline pattern of the dead heart. This has led to the popular misconception that sudden bradycardia is responsible for a large proportion of sudden deaths. The 1-year risk of arrhythmia recurrence for sudden death survivors is between 30 and 50%. Most recurrences are fatal.

When syncope occurs in a patient who has a history of previous myocardial infarction or cardiomyopathy (especially if complex ventricular ectopy is present), a spontaneously terminating ventricular tachyarrhythmia must be high on the list of differential diagnoses. Such patients have up to a 50% chance of having inducible ventricular tachycardia during electrophysiologic testing, and those who have inducible arrhythmias subsequently have a high risk of sudden death (nearly as high as in sudden-death survivors). It is unlikely that a patient will survive multiple episodes of hemodynamically unstable (i.e. syncope-producing) ventricular arrhythmias. Indeed, patients with underlying heart disease who present with a single syncopal episode actually have a worse prognosis than patients who present with multiple syncopal episodes (in these latter patients, there is likely to be some other cause for the syncope).

Despite the fact that reentrant ventricular tachyarrhythmias are responsible for hundreds of thousands of sudden deaths each year in the United States, it is not unusual for sustained reentrant ventricular tachycardia to present with relatively minimal symptoms (minimal symptoms being palpitations, dizziness, lightheadedness, and other minor symptoms that are less severe than loss of consciousness). Sustained ventricular tachycardia that produces only minimal symptoms almost invariably presents as a monomorphic wide-complex tachycardia whose rate is less than 200 beats/min. Patients who present with these minimally symptomatic arrhythmias have a lower risk of sudden death than patients who have lost consciousness with their presenting arrhythmias—but their risk is still far higher than normal.

Owing to the lack of severe symptoms, a major problem that occurs with these patients is that physicians often mistake their relatively well-tolerated ventricular tachycardia for supraventricular tachycardia with aberrancy. At some time in their careers, all physicians memorize a list of clues that helps them to distinguish ventricular tachycardia from supraventricular tachycardia with aberrancy in patients presenting with wide-complex tachycardia. Such a list of clues is presented in Table 7.3.

Unfortunately, within 15 minutes of taking the examination for which they memorized those clues, most physicians forget all of them. Instead, they often substitute the following simple rule (because it is easy to remember): "Ventricular tachycardia always causes loss of consciousness." This tenet is patently false and often leads to mistaking sustained ventricular tachycardia for paroxysmal atrial tachycardia (PAT) with aberrancy. Patients thus misdiagnosed are then sent out of the emergency room without appropriate treatment. Because their reentrant ventricular tachycardia is not recognized, the opportunity to intervene to reduce their long-term risk of sudden death is missed.

Intravenous adenosine has come into common usage for termination of supraventricular tachycardias and thus is often administered to patients with wide-QRS-complex tachycardia. When adenosine is administered, useful clues can often be seen that can

Table 7.3 Clues for distinguishing ventricular tachycardia from supraventricular tachycardia with aberrancy

	Ventricular tachycardia	Supraventricular tachycardia with aberrancy
AV dissociation present	50%	Never
QRS duration	Often >0.14 seconds	Often <0.14 seconds
Precordial concordance	Often present	Usually not present
If RBBB configuration:		
lead V$_1$	Initial R taller (Rsr)	Second R taller (rsR)
lead V$_6$	Monophasic QRS common	Triphasic QRS common
	Axis commonly <−30°	Axis usually >−30°
If LBBB configuration:		
lead V$_1$	Wide R wave, >0.04 seconds	Narrow R wave

Concordance, either all QRS complexes are positive or all are negative.
RBBB, right bundle branch block; LBBB, left bundle branch block.

lead one to a diagnosis of ventricular tachycardia. When supraventricular tachycardia of any type is treated with adenosine, careful observation usually reveals *some* transient change in the rhythm, even if the supraventricular tachycardia is not terminated. For instance, patients with atrial flutter or atrial tachycardia most commonly will have transient second- or third-degree AV block following IV adenosine, thus revealing the underlying mechanism of the arrhythmia. In contrast (unless the patient has one of the rare forms of ventricular tachycardia that responds to verapamil and adenosine), when adenosine is administered to a patient with ventricular tachycardia, *nothing happens*. Thus, when a patient with wide-complex tachycardia has no response at all to adenosine, ventricular tachycardia should immediately become the leading diagnosis.

Because the clues listed in Table 7.3 are difficult to remember, the author proposes an alternative simple rule:

When patients with previous myocardial infarction or cardiomyopathy present with wide-complex tachycardia, it is ALWAYS ventricular tachycardia, regardless of symptoms.

This rule will lead to the correct diagnosis in more than 95% of patients with underlying cardiac disease who present with wide-complex tachycardia. If such patients are referred for a more aggressive evaluation, the few who do have supraventricular arrhythmias will be diagnosed during electrophysiologic testing.

The electrophysiologic study in the evaluation of reentrant ventricular tachyarrhythmias

The electrophysiology study has revolutionized our understanding and management of lethal ventricular arrhythmias. Through the electrophysiology study, we have come to learn that most patients with ventricular tachyarrhythmias have reentrant foci as the source of their arrhythmias, that the arrhythmias can be reproduced safely in the laboratory, that some reentrant circuits can be successfully ablated using transcatheter techniques, and that no matter how thorough and aggressive one may be in testing antiarrhythmic drugs, these drugs cannot be fully relied upon to protect against recurrent ventricular arrhythmias.

The reasons for performing electrophysiology studies in patients known or suspected to have sustained ventricular tachyarrhythmias are: (1) to diagnose the presence of a reentrant circuit that can cause a ventricular tachyarrhythmia; (2) to test the effect of antiarrhythmic drugs on the inducible arrhythmias; (3) to assess the feasibility of mapping and ablating a reentrant circuit; and (4) to optimize the programming of an antitachycardia device.

Inducing ventricular arrhythmias   In considering the techniques used for inducing ventricular arrhythmias, we should begin by reviewing the prerequisites for reentry. First, an appropriate anatomic circuit should be present (see Figure 2.6). Second, the electrophysiologic characteristics of the circuit should be such that an appropriately timed premature impulse can block down one pathway (pathway B) and conduct down the other (pathway A) to establish a continuously circulating impulse. Third, the initiating premature impulse must reach the circuit at a critical instant in time (i.e. when pathway B is refractory and pathway A has recovered).

The successful induction of ventricular tachycardia in the electrophysiology laboratory depends on the first two prerequisites being in place: an anatomic circuit with appropriate electrophysiologic characteristics must be present. The only prerequisite for reentry supplied by the electrophysiologist is the critically timed premature impulse. By programmed stimulation, the electrophysiologist attempts to deliver a premature impulse to the reentrant circuit at just the right moment to induce ventricular tachycardia.

Delivering a premature impulse to a reentrant circuit at just the right moment is sometimes not easy. As noted in Chapter 4, the distance between the pacing electrode and the reentrant circuit, as well as the refractory characteristics and conduction velocity (i.e. the functional refractory period (FRP)) of the intervening tissue, determine whether it is possible for a paced impulse to reach the reentrant circuit early enough to initiate an arrhythmia. Unfortunately, the precise location of the suspected reentrant circuit is almost always unknown, and the FRP of the tissue between the pacing electrode and the reentrant circuit cannot be measured. Thus, the measures used to optimize conditions to allow premature paced impulses to arrive at the reentrant circuit early enough to initiate reentry are necessarily empiric.

As we have seen, pacing at faster rates (i.e. at shorter cycle lengths) decreases the refractory periods and increases the conduction velocity in ventricular myocardium, thus decreasing the FRP. Shorter FRPs will allow premature impulses to arrive at the reentrant circuit earlier and will increase the chances of initiating reentry. Stimulation protocols use two basic techniques to minimize the FRP of the ventricular myocardium: coupling multiple premature impulses together (typically up to three programmed extrastimuli) and pacing incrementally at rapid rates.

In addition, most stimulation protocols call for pacing from more than one catheter location, on the simple premise that one location may be closer to a reentrant circuit than another. Typically, pacing is performed initially from the right ventricular apex, and if no arrhythmias are induced, the electrode catheter is moved to the right ventricular outflow tract and pacing is repeated. Some electrophysiologists will also pace from the left ventricle. The experience of most, however, is that left ventricular stimulation is unlikely to induce an arrhythmia if no arrhythmias have been inducible from two right ventricular sites.

Finally, the inducibility of a reentrant ventricular arrhythmia can occasionally be improved by infusing isoproterenol. Presumably, in some patients, catecholamines act on potentially reentrant circuits to optimize the electrophysiologic characteristics for reentry.

Programmed stimulation protocols vary somewhat from institution to institution. The basic organization of stimulation protocols is to use progressively more aggressive pacing techniques, until either

Table 7.4 A typical stimulation protocol

End points for the electrophysiology study
- >10 beats of reproducibly inducible ventricular tachycardia (positive study)[a]
- Completing protocol without inducing ventricular tachycardia (negative study)

The following pacing sequences are introduced from the right ventricular apex
- Step 1: single extrastimulus brought in to ventricular refractoriness at three drive cycle lengths
- Step 2: double extrastimuli brought in to ventricular refractoriness at three drive cycle lengths
- Step 3: triple extrastimuli brought in to ventricular refractoriness at three drive cycle lengths
- Step 4: 8–12 incrementally paced beats brought in to ventricular refractoriness

If ventricular tachycardia is not induced, these steps are repeated from the right ventricular outflow tract.

If ventricular tachycardia is still not induced, isoproterenol is infused and pacing is repeated.

[a]Many authorities requires 30 seconds of induced ventricular tachycardia to consider a test positive.

the desired arrhythmia is induced or the protocol is finished (in which case the patient is declared to be noninducible).

A typical stimulation protocol is outlined in Table 7.4. The electrode catheter is initially positioned in the right ventricular apex. Following a drive train of eight incrementally paced beats (S1 beats) at a cycle length of 600 msec, a single programmed extrastimulus (S2) is introduced at a coupling interval of 500 msec (Figure 7.5a). If no arrhythmia is induced, the pacing sequence is repeated. With each pacing sequence, the coupling interval between the last S1 stimulus and the S2 stimulus is decreased by 10–20 msec, until the S2 no longer captures (i.e. the effective refractory period (ERP) for the S2 is reached). This procedure is then repeated, with S1 drive-train cycle lengths of 500 then 400 msec. If no ventricular tachycardia is induced with single extrastimuli at any of the three drive cycle lengths, the S2 stimulus is "parked" at a coupling interval approximately 20 msec longer than its ERP and a second extrastimulus (an S3) is added (Figure 7.5b). At drive cycle lengths of 600, 500, and 400 msec, the S1–S2–S3 coupling intervals are brought in as closely as possible. If double extrastimuli also fail

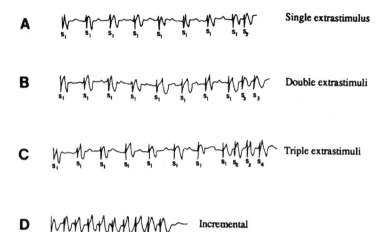

Figure 7.5 Typical stimulation protocol for inducing ventricular tachycardia. Right ventricular pacing is illustrated. (a) Pacing begins with the introduction of a single extrastimulus (S2) following drive trains of incrementally paced beats (S1). (b) If ventricular tachycardia is not induced, two extrastimuli are used (S3). (c) If ventricular tachycardia is not induced with two extrastimuli, three extrastimuli are used (S4). (d) If ventricular tachycardia is still not induced, incremental bursts are used.

to induce the arrhythmia, a third extra stimulus is added (S4; Figure 7.5c). At drive trains of 600, 500, and 400 msec, the S1–S2–S3–S4 intervals are brought in as tightly as possible. If no ventricular tachycardia is induced with single, double, or triple extrastimuli at any of the three drive cycle lengths, incremental pacing is performed. Incremental trains consisting of 8–12 stimuli are introduced with progressively shorter cycle lengths, beginning at a cycle length of 350 msec and decreasing to ventricular refractoriness (Figure 7.5d). If no ventricular tachycardia is induced from the right ventricular apex, the electrode catheter is repositioned to the right ventricular outflow tract, and the entire stimulation sequence is repeated. If ventricular tachycardia is not induced, an isoproterenol infusion is begun (to produce sinus tachycardia of 110–140 beats/min), and the entire stimulation sequence is repeated. If no ventricular tachycardia has been induced with any of these measures, the patient is deemed to be "noninducible."

We touch here on the endearing notion that the electrophysiology study defines the patient definitively as being in one of two states: inducible or noninducible. While this conceptualization is fundamentally flawed (as will be discussed later), it is still clinically useful in many cases.

For instance, the electrophysiology study is often performed for diagnostic purposes. The whole point of doing the study here is to see whether an arrhythmia is inducible or not. If it is, the patient is presumed to have a high probability of developing spontaneous ventricular tachyarrhythmias; if it is not, that probability is presumed to be low. Perhaps the best example of such a diagnostic study is the use of electrophysiologic testing for syncope of unknown origin. (The evaluation of syncope will be covered in Chapter 10.) Obviously, in such diagnostic tests, one wants the stimulation protocol to have a very high chance of inducing arrhythmias that are clinically relevant, but a very low chance of inducing arrhythmias that are never likely to become clinically manifest.

No two electrophysiologists completely agree on the "best" stimulation protocol or on the correct definition of "inducibility." Although ideally one wishes to minimize both false positives and false negatives, in reality, when the electrophysiologist selects a stimulation protocol and a definition of inducibility, he or she is deciding whether to err on the side of producing more false positives (inducing nonclinical arrhythmias, which can lead to inappropriately aggressive therapy) or more false negatives (failing to induce truly clinical arrhythmias, leading to undertreatment). The aggressive stimulation protocol outlined in Table 7.4 errs on the side of producing more false positives.

Studies in ostensibly normal patients suggest that in a substantial minority (20–30%), more than 10 beats of polymorphic ventricular tachycardia can be induced when triple extrastimuli are used, but that virtually none have inducible arrhythmias when only double extrastimuli are used. Thus, stimulation protocols using triple extrastimuli are likely to produce some false-positive studies. On the other hand, many patients who have had documented sustained ventricular tachyarrhythmias require triple extrastimuli to induce the clinical arrhythmias. Thus, stimulation protocols using less than three extrastimuli will tend to eliminate false positives but will miss some of the true positives.

Any definition chosen for "inducibility" necessarily takes into account the morphology and the duration of the induced arrhythmia. The morphology of the induced arrhythmia is an issue because the studies in "normals" mentioned earlier suggest that when a false-positive ventricular tachycardia is induced, the arrhythmia is almost always polymorphic. Thus, an induced arrhythmia that is polymorphic tends to be nonspecific. Some institutions accordingly attempt to limit their false-positive studies by stipulating that for a study to be considered positive, inducible ventricular tachycardia must be monomorphic. However, although induced polymorphic tachycardia is nonspecific, patients do, in fact, develop spontaneous polymorphic ventricular tachycardias. Insisting on a monomorphic arrhythmia will thus cause one to ignore some true-positive studies.

Regarding the duration of the induced tachycardia, most electrophysiologists recognize that in a substantial minority of patients presenting with sustained arrhythmias, only a nonsustained tachycardia will be inducible in the electrophysiology laboratory. Therefore, most laboratories will accept nonsustained tachycardia (if it is of sufficient duration) as a positive study. The determination of how many beats in duration that nonsustained tachycardia should be is completely empiric. In many laboratories, an inducible arrhythmia is defined by the ability to reproducibly induce at least 10 beats of ventricular tachycardia (Figure 7.6). The number 10 is chosen

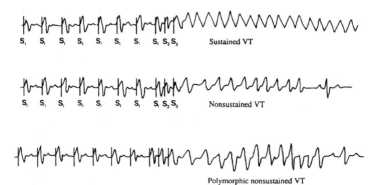

Figure 7.6 Types of inducible ventricular tachycardia. When inducing ventricular tachycardia in the electrophysiology laboratory, the goal is to induce sustained monomorphic ventricular tachycardia (*shown in the top panel*). This response is considered to be specific. The middle and bottom panels display two induced arrhythmias (nonsustained monomorphic ventricular tachycardia and polymorphic ventricular tachycardia) whose interpretation is controversial.

arbitrarily. Some electrophysiologists consider anywhere from 3 to 15 beats of induced tachycardia to represent a positive study. Others require at least 30 seconds of ventricular tachycardia before an arrhythmia is considered inducible.

One must be mindful of Baye's theorem when deciding on an appropriate stimulation protocol and definition of inducibility. Baye's theorem states that the specificity of any test is determined largely by the true incidence of the condition for which the test is being performed in the population being tested. In electrophysiology studies in patients who present with spontaneous sustained ventricular tachyarrhythmias, it is appropriate to use a more aggressive stimulation protocol and a more liberal definition of "inducibility." In such patients, positive tests are statistically less likely to be falsely positive than in the general population, and are more likely to be truly positive. If programmed stimulation is to be used in patients who are in lower-risk groups (such as patients with syncope of unknown origin), it might be reasonable to use a less-aggressive pacing protocol and a stricter definition of "inducibility," because the odds of a positive study being falsely positive are higher in such patients.

Electrophysiologists have perhaps done too much hand-wringing because they cannot agree on standardized pacing protocols and definitions of "inducibility." They worry that the many differences between centers render the electrophysiologic literature impossible to interpret. The author's opinion is that, on the contrary, the different approaches being used are not particularly harmful and may, in fact, be beneficial. An appraisal of the literature suggests that results with electrophysiologic testing in patients who present with sustained ventricular arrhythmias are actually quite similar among different centers. This suggests that in high-yield patient populations the variations in methodology have not been significant. Further, as noted previously, different approaches will probably be of benefit when the electrophysiology study is applied to different patient populations. It may be harmful to be locked into a standardized protocol that errs too much on the side of either false-positive or false-negative studies when studying new populations. Table 7.5 summarizes the factors that must be considered when estimating the specificity of the electrophysiology study.

Terminating ventricular arrhythmias Termination of induced ventricular tachyarrhythmias is accomplished by one of two methods: programmed stimulation (possible only with ventricular

Table 7.5 Estimating the specificity of a positive electrophysiology study

---

Factors increasing specificity of a positive study
- Induced arrhythmia is monomorphic ventricular tachycardia
- Induced ventricular tachycardia is sustained
- Tachycardia is induced with single or double extrastimuli
- Patient studied is in a high-risk group

Factors decreasing specificity of a positive study
- Induced arrhythmia is polymorphic ventricular tachycardia or ventricular fibrillation
- Induced arrhythmia is nonsustained
- Arrhythmia is induced with triple extrastimuli or incremental pacing
- Patient studied is not in a high-risk group

---

tachycardia, not with ventricular fibrillation) or direct current (DC) cardioversion/defibrillation.

Terminating a reentrant arrhythmia with programmed stimulation requires that a premature impulse encounters the reentrant circuit at a critical time. In this way, initiating and terminating reentry are similar, and the considerations for inducing arrhythmias discussed earlier (i.e. the distance between the electrode catheter and the reentrant circuit on one hand, and the FRP of the intervening tissue on the other) also pertain to termination of the tachycardia. Thus, techniques for pace-termination of ventricular tachycardia are similar to techniques for pace-induction.

Several methods for pace-termination of ventricular tachycardia have been proposed, but they essentially boil down to the incremental and extrastimulus techniques that we have seen before (Figure 7.7). The incremental method is used most commonly. Generally, incremental pacing to terminate ventricular tachycardia begins with 8–12 beats at a cycle length 10–20 msec faster than the cycle length of the tachycardia. If this is unsuccessful, pacing is repeated at faster rates. When the extrastimulus technique is used to terminate ventricular tachycardia, the extrastimuli are generally coupled to the intrinsic tachycardia beats rather than to a train of incrementally paced beats.

Whichever pacing method is used to terminate ventricular tachycardia, there is a real risk of accelerating the tachycardia or causing it to degenerate to ventricular fibrillation (Figure 7.8). This poor result tends to occur more frequently with more aggressive pace-

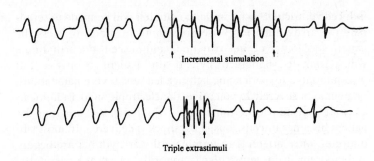

Incremental stimulation

Triple extrastimuli

Figure 7.7 Pace-termination of ventricular tachycardia. The top panel shows termination of ventricular tachycardia using a six-beat burst of incremental stimuli. The bottom panel shows termination of ventricular tachycardia using three programmed extrastimuli.

termination measures (such as rapid incremental pacing or triple extrastimuli), but these more aggressive pacing measures are also the most efficacious at terminating the tachycardia. If degeneration of the rhythm results from efforts at pace-termination, the patient usually needs to be rescued with a DC shock.

Successful pace-termination of ventricular tachycardia is easier to accomplish with arrhythmias that are relatively slow and mono-morphic. The faster and less organized the arrhythmia, the harder it is to pace-terminate.

The choice of the timing and method of terminating the induced arrhythmia depends on several factors, including the rate and mor-phology of the induced arrhythmia, the duration of the arrhythmia, the blood pressure, and the patient's symptoms and level of con-sciousness. In most laboratories, if the patient is tolerating the

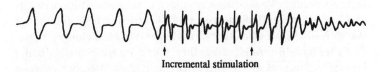

Incremental stimulation

Figure 7.8 Degeneration of ventricular tachycardia with pacing. This figure shows one of the inherent hazards in attempting to pace-terminate ventricular tachycardia. In this example, a six-beat burst of incremental stimuli degenerates the ventricular tachycardia into ventricular fibrillation.

induced ventricular tachycardia, no attempt will be made to terminate the arrhythmia for 30 seconds (both in order to assess the patient's tolerance of the arrhythmia and to see if the arrhythmia will terminate spontaneously). If the patient is awake but uncomfortable (experiencing lightheadedness, severe palpitations, or angina) or severely hypotensive, the electrophysiologist immediately attempts to pace-terminate the arrhythmia. If at any time the patient becomes unconscious, a DC shock is delivered. In most laboratories, once attempts to terminate the arrhythmia are begun, patients remain in ventricular tachycardia for an average of 10–15 seconds. Deaths from inducing ventricular arrhythmias in the electrophysiology laboratory are extremely rare (<0.01%), and even the need for full cardiopulmonary resuscitation is very uncommon (<0.10%).

Testing the effect of drugs on the reentrant circuit From the early 1980s until the mid 1990s, serial drug testing was the major reason for studying patients with reentrant ventricular tachyarrhythmias. This practice has largely fallen away for two reasons. First, large studies showed that pharmacologic therapy based on serial drug testing was not nearly as effective as had previously been thought. Second, results obtained with the implantable cardioverter–defibrillator (ICD) were far better than those obtained with serial drug testing—or with any other treatment. Today, serial drug testing is done only rarely, and is generally limited to patients who refuse therapy with the ICD, or for whom the intention is to reduce the frequency of recurrent arrhythmias in the presence of an ICD.

The principle behind drug testing for ventricular tachyarrhythmias is simple. As discussed in Chapter 3, antiarrhythmic drugs work by changing the shape of the cardiac action potential, thus altering the conduction velocity or refractoriness of cardiac tissue. By so doing, these drugs are capable of altering the electrophysiologic properties of a reentrant circuit to make a reentrant arrhythmia less (or more) likely to occur. If a ventricular arrhythmia that was inducible during baseline (drug-free) testing is no longer inducible after administering a drug, then that drug has probably had a favorable effect on the reentrant circuit (Figure 7.9). For years, it was thought that treatment with a drug that rendered a previously inducible arrhythmia noninducible would protect against recurrent arrhythmias. As it turns out, a drug defined as being "successful" during serial drug testing probably delays the onset of an arrhythmia, but may not substantially reduce the long-term risk.

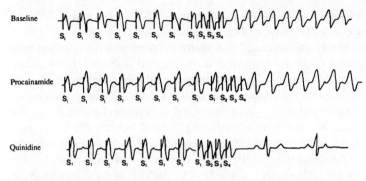

Figure 7.9 Successful serial drug testing for ventricular tachycardia. At baseline (*top*) and after administration of procainamide (*middle*), sustained ventricular tachycardia is inducible. After administration of quinidine (*bottom*), however, no ventricular tachycardia is inducible. Quinidine would appear to have a favorable effect on the reentrant circuit in this patient.

In the era of widespread serial drug testing, most centers averaged approximately three drug trials per patient and found successful drugs in 30–40% of patients tested. In some centers, no more than one or two drug studies were performed before moving directly to nonpharmacologic therapies. In other centers, exhaustive drug trials were carried out, including studies with multiple drug combinations. Despite differences in stimulation protocols, definitions of inducibility, and the number of drug studies performed, the long-term outcomes for patients who responded to drug testing and for patients who did not respond to drug testing were similar from center to center. Drug responders appeared to have a lower rate of recurrent arrhythmias than nonresponders (approximately 5–10% per year versus 30–50% per year). Unfortunately, since most recurrences were fatal, the proportion of surviving patients at the end of five years was similar in both groups.

The meaning of "inducibility" and "noninducibility"   The fact that serial drug testing is no longer commonly performed has significantly limited the use of the electrophysiology study in patients with ventricular arrhythmias. One remaining use, however, is diagnostic—that is, the assessment of patients who are thought, but not known beyond doubt, to have ventricular arrhythmias (the best example is patients with syncope of unknown origin, discussed in

Chapter 10). Especially in such cases, it is important to understand what "inducibility" and "noninducibility" really mean.

Earlier, we suggested that many electrophysiologists believe that the electrophysiology study sorts patients into one of two states: inducible or noninducible. If they are inducible, they have a potentially lethal reentrant circuit. If they are noninducible, then either they do not have such a circuit, or something that the doctor did (such as administer an antiarrhythmic drug) has effectively rendered their reentrant circuit nonfunctional. In other words, the "inducibility state" of the patient is thought of as a binary and deterministic feature, which is defined by the electrophysiology study.

Several years ago, the author conducted a study to test this proposition. In this study, patients with inducible ventricular tachycardia which was made noninducible during serial drug testing were immediately subjected to five additional, complete stimulation protocols over the next 24 hours, while being given the drug that had suppressed their inducible tachycardia. It turned out that the probability of inducing ventricular tachycardia during any one of the five subsequent drug trials remained constant—roughly 15–20%. In other words, the odds of failing trial number two (after having passed only one previous trial) were the same as the odds of failing trial number six (after having passed five previous trials). Such results strongly suggest that the inducibility of reentrant arrhythmias does *not* define a clear-cut binary state—that patients are *not* either inducible or noninducible—and that inducibility is best regarded as a probability function, not as a deterministic state.

This finding makes perfect sense when one considers that virtually all complex, multifactorial, physiologic events follow a probabilistic "dose-response" curve, in which a given "dose" of a stimulus yields a measurable probability that an event will occur. Figure 7.10 postulates such a probability curve for the induction of ventricular tachycardia. In this model, a successful drug trial merely implies that the probability curve has been shifted to the right.

Another way of looking at the probabilistic nature of inducibility is illustrated by what the author calls the "dunk-tank model" of reentrant ventricular tachycardia (Figure 7.11). In this model, the patient with ventricular tachycardia can be visualized as sitting on a typical dunk-tank platform (except, of course, this dunk tank is filled not with water but with boiling oil). The patient's reentrant circuit is analogous to the target–platform mechanism, and the triggering electrical impulse (a PVC or paced beat) is analogous to the softballs that one throws at the target. In the baseline state

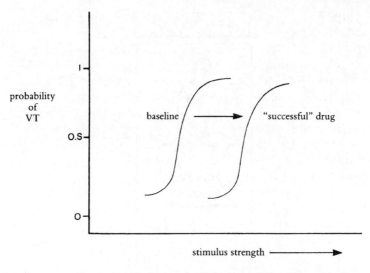

Figure 7.10 The probabilistic nature of the inducibility of ventricular tachycardia. It is postulated that the probability of inducing ventricular tachycardia (VT) follows a typical S-shaped curve, similar to the probability functions that describe most physiologic systems. In this model, a drug that prevents inducibility in the electrophysiology laboratory has merely shifted the curve to the right, so that with a fixed amount of stimulation the probability of inducing the arrhythmia is diminished.

(Figure 7.11a), the target is close enough for the thrower to have an excellent chance of hitting it with one allotment of softballs (or with one stimulation protocol). This patient would be called inducible. An "effective" antiarrhythmic drug can be visualized as moving the target farther away (Figure 7.11b), so that the probability of striking the target with one allotment of softballs has been substantially reduced (say, to 15%). This patient would be labeled noninducible. If, however, one were to keep buying more softballs to throw, the cumulative probability of hitting the target would gradually and inexorably increase.

This model fits not only our experimental data but also the clinical results seen with serial drug testing. The probability that a fatal ventricular arrhythmia will occur over any given time interval is reduced after "successful" serial drug testing—but the overall, cumulative probability of having an arrhythmia (as more and more time intervals accumulate) remains high.

185

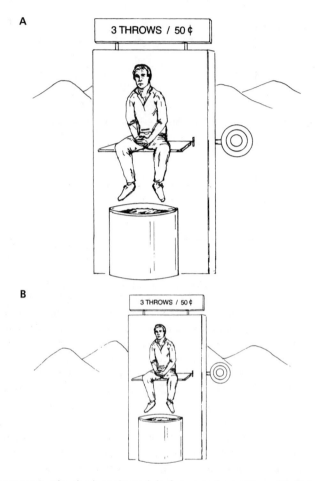

Figure 7.11 The dunk-tank model of ventricular tachycardia. This figure presents a different way of illustrating the probabilistic nature of ventricular tachycardia. The patient with ventricular tachycardia is visualized as sitting on a dunk-tank platform. The target–platform mechanism represents the reentrant circuit, and the softballs that one throws at the target represent ventricular ectopy (or the premature beats introduced by the electrophysiologist). In (a), the target is close enough to the thrower that the probability of "dunking" the patient with a single allotment of softballs is relatively high. (b) shows the proposed effect of a "successful" antiarrhythmic drug. The target is now far enough away from the thrower that it is unlikely that it will be struck with a single allotment of softballs. However, if one is persistent in throwing at the target, sooner or later the patient will wind up in the drink.

Viewing the inducibility status of a patient from this point of view does not render the electrophysiology study useless. On the contrary, it offers a more realistic perspective (than does the binary, deterministic model) from which to interpret the results of an electrophysiology study, whether that study is a serial drug test or a diagnostic procedure. As with any test performed in medicine, it is important for the doctor to understand the inherent limitations and benefits of the electrophysiology study, so as to provide more appropriate clinical recommendations.

The electrophysiology study in the treatment of reentrant ventricular tachyarrhythmias

While in the recent past, performing electrophysiologic testing was considered standard care in the management of sustained ventricular arrhythmias, this is not the case today. Nonetheless, the electrophysiology study can still be quite useful in helping to treat ventricular arrhythmias in at least two ways. First, the electrophysiology study plays an essential role in the transcatheter ablation of ventricular arrhythmias. This technique will be discussed in Chapter 8. Second, electrophysiologic testing can be useful in tailoring the way that ICDs are programmed to handle recurrent arrhythmias.

Preoperative electrophysiologic testing for ICDs Appropriately programming ICDs often requires several complex decisions. One such decision is whether and how to use antitachycardia pacing (ATP) to terminate recurrent ventricular tachycardia. In programming ATP, the physician sets a rate zone in which ATP is to be attempted. For instance, one might choose to attempt ATP for arrhythmias whose rate is between 150 and 190 beats/min. If a ventricular tachycardia of more than 190 beats/min were to occur, ATP would not be used—a DC shock would be administered instead. A shock would also be given if a preselected number of ATP attempts failed to stop a ventricular tachycardia, or if the arrhythmia were to accelerate with an ATP attempt.

Programming ATP inappropriately can lead to serious problems. Because ATP is a potentially "kinder, gentler" therapy, the physician might be tempted to try it even for rapid, hemodynamically unstable tachycardias that would otherwise be treated immediately with high-energy shocks. Because rapid tachycardias are (most electrophysiologists agree) more difficult to terminate with ATP than slower tachycardias, prolonged attempts at ATP could conceivably allow prolonged hemodynamic compromise before "definitive" therapy was finally administered.

Conversely, the availability of ATP might tempt physicians to use implantable devices to treat slow, relatively well-tolerated tachycardias that might be better treated by other means. In such cases, the ICD might be programmed to deliver therapy at slower heart rates which are often reached when the patient develops sinus tachycardia or atrial fibrillation, thus potentially triggering inappropriate ATP attempts. Not only would such inappropriate ATP sequences fail to stop the supraventricular tachycardia, but they might also induce the very ventricular tachycardias that they were supposed to terminate. In any case, once an ICD begins delivering therapy, it does not stop until the heart rate falls below the programmed rate cut-off. Thus, unless the supraventricular arrhythmia terminates spontaneously, the device gradually, inexorably, and inappropriately escalates therapy until a series of high-energy shocks are delivered.

It is for the purpose of avoiding such problems that some electrophysiologists perform electrophysiologic testing prior to ICD implantation. The purpose of such testing is to characterize the nature of the patient's sustained ventricular tachycardia—its rate, how well it is tolerated, and what kinds of pacing sequences seem to reliably terminate it. Generally in these tests, ventricular tachycardia is induced and terminated several times in order to characterize the arrhythmia and the response to ATP as fully as possible.

Some electrophysiologists feel that pre-ICD testing is extremely useful, and they do it routinely. Other electrophysiologists point out that the characteristics of a patient's induced ventricular tachycardia are often quite different from those of their spontaneous tachycardia, and that the odds of successfully pace-terminating a patient's induced arrhythmia frequently vary from day to day—and thus that the usefulness of pre-op testing is questionable. Further, this species of electrophysiologist feels that one achieves adequate (and even equivalent) success rates simply by programming ATP empirically. The author, having done scores of preoperative electrophysiology studies and observed the results, now tends to agree with the latter electrophysiologists. That being said, many electrophysiologists swear by preoperative testing, which therefore remains a common and legitimate indication for electrophysiologic testing.

Automatic ventricular arrhythmias

Abnormal automaticity accounts for a minority of lethal ventricular tachyarrhythmias. In distinction to reentrant ventricular arrhythmias, which are almost always associated with chronic, underlying disease of the myocardium, automatic ventricular arrhythmias tend to be associated with acute, reversible medical conditions, such as acute myocardial ischemia, hypoxemia, acid–base disturbances, electrolyte abnormalities (especially hypokalemia and hypomagnesemia), and high adrenergic tone. Thus, automatic ventricular arrhythmias tend to be seen in two general clinical settings: in patients who are acutely ill (e.g. in the intensive care setting) and in patients who are having acute myocardial ischemia or infarction. It can be argued that patients who are desperately ill in the intensive care unit are not candidates for truly "sudden" death, and, indeed, these patients are not included in most of the statistics on sudden death. On the other hand, lethal arrhythmias secondary to acute myocardial ischemia or infarction can and do occur "suddenly."

The automatic ventricular arrhythmias that occur during the first 24–48 hours after an acute myocardial infarction are thought to account for about 20% of the sudden cardiac deaths in the United States. The major success of the coronary care unit has been in preventing these early arrhythmic deaths (although, unfortunately, many of these arrhythmias occur within the first hour after an acute infarction—often before the patient has access to modern facilities). The automatic arrhythmias seen during the first day or two after an acute myocardial infarction are probably related to the residual ischemia seen acutely in the zone of infarction. Once the infarction heals, the substrate for these early arrhythmias disappears. Therefore, the automatic ventricular arrhythmias that occur early during an acute myocardial infarction are thought to have little long-term prognostic significance (provided, of course, that the patient survives them).

Because automatic arrhythmias generally occur secondarily to metabolic abnormalities, treatment should be aimed at identifying and reversing the underlying cause whenever possible. In many instances, intravenous antiarrhythmic drugs (particularly lidocaine, phenytoin, and amiodarone) can be helpful in temporarily suppressing automaticity while the primary problem is being addressed.

Automatic ventricular arrhythmias are not inducible in the electrophysiology laboratory and the electrophysiology study is not useful in their evaluation or treatment.

Triggered activity

As noted in Chapter 2, triggered activity is a mechanism for ventricular arrhythmias that has features of both automaticity and reentry. In recent years, the clinical features of arrhythmias mediated by triggered activity have been better characterized. Although triggered activity is a relatively uncommon cause of ventricular arrhythmias, the clinician must be alert to such arrhythmias for two reasons. First, these arrhythmias, like any ventricular tachyarrhythmia, are life-threatening. Second, the successful treatment of arrhythmias mediated by triggered activity can be uniquely different from treatment used for other forms of ventricular arrhythmia.

Two fairly distinct clinical syndromes have been identified involving triggered activity: pause-dependent arrhythmias and catechol-dependent arrhythmias. In each syndrome, patients develop the polymorphic ventricular tachycardias that have been called torsades de pointes. Although the arrhythmias tend to occur in relatively short bursts and are usually accompanied by lightheadedness or syncope, the arrhythmias can persist long enough to cause sudden death.

Pause-dependent triggered activity

Pause-dependent triggered activity is caused by afterdepolarizations that occur during phase 3 of the cardiac action potential; hence they are called *early* afterdepolarizations (EADs; Figure 7.12a). If the afterdepolarization reaches the threshold potential of the cardiac cell, another action potential can be generated. Pause-dependent triggered activity is almost always related to conditions that prolong the duration of the cardiac action potential, such as electrolyte abnormalities (hypokalemia and hypomagnesemia) or the use of class Ia or III antiarrhythmic agents. Individuals who develop triggered arrhythmias when their QT intervals are prolonged most likely have an inborn subclinical abnormality of the cardiac cell membrane, which becomes manifest only when their action-potential durations are increased.

The ventricular arrhythmias themselves (referred to as torsades de pointes) are typically polymorphic and tend to occur in short bursts. The ECG, while in sinus rhythm, usually shows

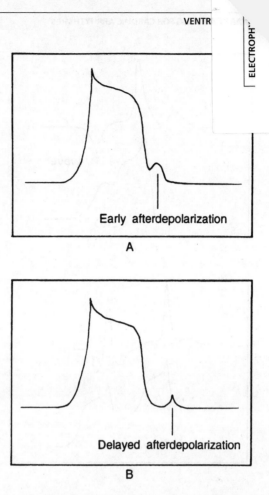

Early afterdepolarization

A

Delayed afterdepolarization

B

Figure 7.12 Afterdepolarizations. (a) An early afterdepolarization (EAD), the type of afterdepolarization associated with pause-dependent triggered activity. EADs occur during phase 3 of the action potential. (b) A delayed afterdepolarization (DAD), the type associated with catechol-dependent triggered activity. DADs occur after the end of phase 3.

prolongation of the QT interval and distortion of the T wave; often, a distinct U wave occurs. During studies using the mono-phasic action potential, Warren Jackman at the University of Oklahoma has convincingly shown that the U waves are, in fact, the ECG manifestation of the EADs themselves. When a burst of ventricular tachycardia occurs, the first beat of tachycardia is invariably superimposed on the U wave (or the distorted T

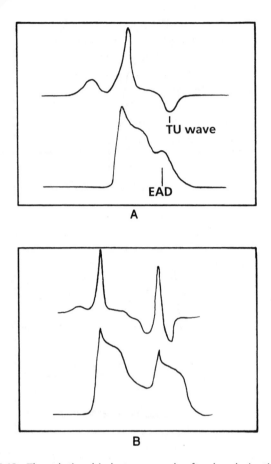

Figure 7.13 The relationship between early afterdepolarizations (EADs), TU wave abnormalities, and premature ventricular complexes. (a) The temporal association between EADs and the TU abnormalities as seen on the surface ECG. The TU wave is most likely the surface manifestation of the EADs themselves. (b) If an EAD is of sufficient magnitude to reach threshold potential, a premature complex results. Note that the timing of the premature complex is such that it occurs precisely on the TU wave of the previous beat.

wave), suggesting that the EAD (represented by that U wave) has reached the transmembrane potential for generating an action potential (Figure 7.13).

The TU wave abnormalities in this condition are usually dynamic. They tend to wax and wane, depending largely on the previous cycle length; the longer the previous cycle length, the more exaggerated the TU wave aberration of the following complex—hence, the condition is "pause dependent." Once a burst of ventricular tachycardia has been initiated, it tends to repeat in a pattern of "ventricular tachycardia bigeminy"—the burst of ventricular tachycardia causes a compensatory pause, and that pause causes the following sinus beat to develop marked U wave abnormalities (i.e. a pronounced EAD occurs). Thus, another burst of tachycardia is generated after that first sinus beat. Pause-dependent triggered activity should be strongly suspected when this ECG pattern occurs either in the setting of QT interval prolongation or in the setting of conditions that predispose to QT interval prolongation, even if overt QT prolongation is not present (Figure 7.14).

The treatment of pause-dependent triggered activity is aimed at reducing the duration of the action potential. Drugs that prolong the QT interval should be discontinued and avoided—specifically, antiarrhythmic drugs that prolong action-potential duration should not be used (drugs that cause this type of triggered activity are listed in Table 3.2). Electrolyte abnormalities should be rapidly corrected. Intravenous magnesium sulfate often ameliorates these arrhythmias, even when the serum magnesium level is not depressed. The mainstay of emergent treatment of these arrhythmias, however, is to eliminate pauses; that is, to increase the heart rate. This is usually accomplished either by atrial or ventricular pacing, or by beginning an isoproterenol infusion.

Because the conditions that lead to pause-dependent triggered activity are generally reversible, long-term therapy is aimed at avoiding conditions that cause prolongation of the QT interval.

Catechol-dependent triggered activity

Catechol-dependent triggered activity is caused by afterdepolarizations that occur during phase 4 of the cardiac action potential (Figure 7.12b). Thus, they are called *delayed* afterdepolarizations (DADs). DADs occur in the setting of digitalis toxicity, in cardiac ischemia, and in some patients who have congenital QT interval prolongation. These congenital syndromes are the Romano–Ward syndrome and the Jervell–Lange–Nielson syndrome (in which QT prolongation is accompanied by neural deafness). Patients with catechol-dependent triggered activity have been postulated to have an imbalance in sympathetic innervation of the heart, with predominant input from the left stellate ganglion, stimulation of which can reproduce DADs.

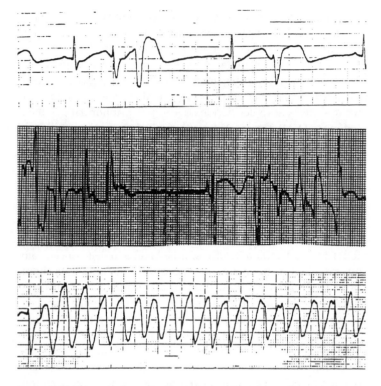

Figure 7.14 Ventricular arrhythmias caused by pause-dependent triggered activity (torsades de pointes). Features of pause-dependent ventricular arrhythmias are shown in a patient with QT prolongation from quinidine. In the top panel, "late" premature ventricular complexes (coincident with the onset of the U wave) arise immediately after a relatively long interval (i.e. a "pause") between QRS complexes. In patients prone to developing these arrhythmias, the pause itself induces afterdepolarizations (*see text*), thus triggering ectopic complexes. The bigeminal pattern seen here is typical, because each ectopic complex tends to produce a compensatory pause, which, in turn, produces another ectopic complex. In the middle panel, the ectopy has become more sustained. Compensatory pauses still follow each burst of ventricular tachycardia, so that the patient now displays "ventricular tachycardia bigeminy." In the bottom panel, the arrhythmia has become even more prolonged and now displays a more typical "torsades de pointes" morphology. The key to recognizing torsades de pointes is to recognize the pause-dependent nature of the arrhythmia; the key to treating these arrhythmias is to eliminate the pauses. Thus, overdrive pacing reliably suppresses these arrhythmias.

Catechol-dependent triggered activity generally is not dependent on pauses (although pause-dependent features are seen in some patients). Instead, it is brought out in conditions of high sympathetic tone. Thus, patients experience ventricular tachycardia (manifested by syncope or cardiac arrest) during times of exercise or of emotional stress. Often, the QT interval is normal at rest. During stress testing, QT prolongation occurs, and often ventricular tachycardia is seen. Left stellate sympathectomy has eliminated arrhythmias in some patients.

Treatment of catechol-dependent triggered activity usually consists of β-blockers and, because DADs are thought to be mediated by calcium-dependent channels, calcium channel blockers. In addition, more and more clinicians are using ICDs in these patients.

Miscellaneous types of ventricular arrhythmia

Clinical syndromes involving unusual ventricular arrhythmias have been described in which the arrhythmias do not fit clearly into any of the categories described so far. In many cases, these arrhythmias occur in the setting of a structurally normal heart, and in most cases, their mechanisms are not well understood. The literature is confusing regarding their classification and nomenclature, which is merely a reflection of our incomplete understanding of these arrhythmias. The following is a brief description of these syndromes.

Idiopathic left ventricular tachycardia

This arrhythmia tends to occur in younger patients without structural heart disease. The arrhythmia has a right bundle branch block (RBBB) morphology with a left, superior axis. It is inducible with programmed stimulation, and each QRS complex is preceded by a distinct His spike. The arrhythmic focus maps to the inferior aspect of the septum, and in several patients it has been successfully ablated. It tends to respond to therapy with β-blockers and calcium channel blockers. Both reentry and triggered activity have been advanced as the mechanism of this arrhythmia.

Outflow tract ventricular tachycardia

This arrhythmia, which has also been termed "repetitive monomorphic ventricular tachycardia," originates in the right ventricular outflow tract. It manifests as a nonsustained left bundle branch

block (LBBB) tachycardia with an inferior axis and is often provoked by exercise. Although the arrhythmia is often not inducible
with programmed extrastimuli, pacing the heart at a rapid rate or
instituting an isoproterenol infusion (i.e. simulating the heart-rate
response with exercise) can often induce the arrhythmia. It is usually seen in younger patients without structural heart disease. The
arrhythmia tends to be responsive to therapy with β-blockers and
calcium channel blockers, but the treatment of choice is usually
transcatheter ablation, which has a high success rate in completely
eliminating the arrhythmia. Whether this arrhythmia represents
automaticity or triggered activity is unknown.

Right ventricular dysplasia

Right ventricular dysplasia is a rare condition, usually seen in younger patients, in which a variable amount of right ventricular myocardium is replaced by fatty and fibrous tissue. This condition
appears to be genetic in origin; recently, a genetic mutation has
been identified that accounts for up to 30% of cases. The ventricular tachycardia seen in right ventricular dysplasia usually has a left
bundle branch morphology, and is almost invariably inducible with
programmed stimulation. The treatment of this arrhythmia is similar to treatment for the reentrant ventricular tachycardias that are
seen in the setting of coronary artery disease. Surgery to cause electrical isolation of the dysplastic areas of the right ventricle has been
tried, and although it has been successful in controlling the
arrhythmia, right ventricular failure commonly follows. Transcatheter ablation of arrhythmogenic foci has been used with only limited success In general, patients with this condition who have had
episodes of sustained ventricular tachycardia or ventricular fibrillation should be offered an ICD.

Bundle branch reentry

Bundle branch reentry is a distinct form of ventricular tachycardia
seen rarely in patients with idiopathic cardiomyopathy who also
have intraventricular conduction disturbances. Most of these
patients present with rapid monomorphic ventricular tachycardia
that has an LBBB morphology. The reentrant circuit uses the right
bundle branch in the downward direction and the left bundle
branch in the upward direction. Its significance lies in the fact that
it can be cured with the transcatheter ablation of the right bundle
branch. The ablation of bundle branch reentrant ventricular tachycardia is discussed in Chapter 8.

Brugada syndrome and sudden unexpected nocturnal death syndrome (SUNDS)

Brugada syndrome was first recognized as a clinical complex consisting of ventricular tachyarrhythmias—often presenting as sudden death, cardiac arrest, or syncope—in patients who have unusual baseline ECGs displaying nonischemic ST segment elevation in leads V1–V3, as well as pseudo-RBBB. These patients are now thought to have genetic abnormalities involving the cardiac sodium channel (the channel that is mostly responsible for depolarization—phase 0—of the cardiac action potential). Brugada syndrome affects males far more often than females, and the arrhythmias seen with it frequently occur during sleep. This condition is related to (and may be the same as) the sudden unexpected nocturnal death syndrome (SUNDS) that has been described in apparently healthy Asian males.

There are several variants of the Brugada syndrome, probably reflecting various mutations in the cardiac sodium channel gene. In some patients, baseline ST changes are transient, in which case the characteristic ST changes can often be brought out by administering class I antiarrhythmic drugs (the drugs that operate on the sodium channel) or by pacing or vagal maneuvers. The arrhythmias associated with this syndrome are often inducible with programmed pacing, so a diagnostic electrophysiology study may be useful if Brugada syndrome is suspected. A history of prior cardiac arrest or syncope or a family history of sudden death greatly increase the risk of sudden death in a patient with Brugada syndrome.

The only treatment demonstrated to reduce the risk of sudden death in patients with Brugada syndrome is the ICD. β-blockers and amiodarone have not been shown to protect these patients. The generally accepted approach to treatment is to use clinical parameters to assess the patient's risk of sudden death and, if the risk is deemed to be relatively high, to insert an ICD.

Catecholaminergic polymorphic ventricular tachycardia

Catecholaminergic polymorphic ventricular tachycardia is a congenital disorder manifesting as rapid, polymorphic ventricular tachycardia or ventricular fibrillation, which is triggered by exercise or emotional stress. This condition presents as stress-induced sudden death or stress-induced syncope, usually in children or teenagers. There is often a family history of similar events. Notably, there is no prolongation of the QT interval in this condition.

Catecholaminergic polymorphic ventricular tachycardia has been associated with two specific genetic mutations (the cardiac ryanodine receptor and calsequestrin 2). These mutations are often inherited, but can occur spontaneously. The mechanism of the polymorphic arrhythmia itself is not clear, but generally the arrhythmia is not inducible during electrophysiologic testing.

The polymorphic arrhythmias in this condition are often reduced in frequency by the use of β-blockers. Patients who have survived cardiac arrest, or who have had a recurrence of symptoms on β-blockers, should be offered an ICD.

Ventricular tachyarrhythmias associated with mitral valve prolapse

Ventricular tachyarrhythmia associated with mitral valve prolapse is mentioned only to point out its minimal significance. Although there are many case reports in the medical literature that attribute sudden death to mitral valve prolapse, there is no epidemiologic study showing that patients with prolapse are any more susceptible to ventricular tachyarrhythmias than the general population. The purported association between sudden death and prolapse is probably related to the fact that between 5 and 10% of the general population have mitral valve prolapse, so that 5–10% of patients with unexplained sudden death are found to have prolapse on autopsy.

An overview of the treatment of ventricular arrhythmias

The optimal treatment of ventricular arrhythmias has changed radically since the first edition of this book was published over 20 years ago. Today, thanks to advances in technology and the new knowledge gained from large randomized clinical trials, thousands of patients are being offered therapies they could not have received in earlier decades, and they are being kept alive as a result. The progress has been remarkable.

The following discussion offers an overview of what we have learned over the last 20–30 years on the treatment of ventricular arrhythmias, as well as a perspective on what the future might hold.

Four general truths we have learned about treating ventricular arrhythmias

(1) Suppression of ventricular ectopy with antiarrhythmic drugs does not reduce risk

As we have noted, in the setting of underlying cardiac disease, complex ventricular ectopy is one of the risk factors for sudden death.

For years, it was assumed that antiarrhythmic drugs aimed at suppressing such ectopy would reduce the risk. The medical community was finally disabused of this benign view of ectopy suppression in 1989, with the results of the Cardiac Arrhythmia Suppression Trial (CAST; Echt DS *et al.*, N Engl J Med 1991; 324:781). CAST was designed to study whether suppressing ventricular ectopy in patients with recent myocardial infarctions reduced the risk of death. What it showed instead was that the successful suppression of ectopy with two of the three drugs studied (encainide and flecainide) actually *doubled or tripled* the risk of death or cardiac arrest, while successful suppression of ectopy with the third drug (moricizine) provided no survival benefit. There were plenty of other reasons at the time to suspect that using antiarrhythmic drugs to suppress ectopy was risky, but CAST drove home the point—suppression of ambient ventricular ectopy with antiarrhythmic drugs does not lead to a reduction in mortality and in fact may increase mortality.

In contrast, the other major method for choosing antiarrhythmic drug therapy—serial drug testing in the electrophysiology laboratory—assessed the effect of antiarrhythmic drugs on the reentrant circuit itself and not merely on ambient ectopy. Drugs selected for chronic administration in this manner rarely produced the sort of proarrhythmia seen in CAST, since most proarrhythmic effects could be identified in the laboratory, before committing the patient to chronic therapy. Indeed, because such proarrhythmic effects were so frequently identified during serial drug testing, many electrophysiologists who did this kind of testing were not at all surprised by the results of CAST.

Nonetheless, while antiarrhythmic drugs chosen by serial electrophysiologic testing allowed clinicians to avoid most of the proarrhythmic effects of these drugs, the overall survival of patients whose lethal ventricular arrhythmias were treated in this way proved to be very disappointing.

The bottom line is that the use of antiarrhythmic drugs, whether the therapy is aimed at suppressing ventricular ectopy or at inhibiting the induction of ventricular tachyarrhythmias in the electrophysiology laboratory, is not an effective method of reducing the risk of sudden death.

(2) Empiric treatment with amiodarone does not sufficiently reduce risk

Amiodarone is a uniquely effective antiarrhythmic drug and, in addition, has the virtue of not causing very much proarrhythmia.

On the negative side, it has complex pharmacokinetic properties (its half-life is between 30 and 100 days, and it does not achieve its peak efficacy until it has been loaded for several weeks) and it has an extraordinarily impressive side-effect profile (refer to Table 3.4). Because amiodarone must be administered for weeks before it becomes fully effective, and because, when it is discontinued, measurable amounts of amiodarone will be present in a patient's serum for a very long time, the drug is most often used empirically. Still, despite these drawbacks, its relative efficacy leads electrophysiologists to using amiodarone fairly often.

Several randomized clinical trials have now tested the hypothesis that empiric treatment with amiodarone is an adequate method of reducing the risk of sudden death in high-risk patients. Some of the more important studies that have examined this issue are listed in Table 7.6. The bottom line is that, while amiodarone may improve mortality in some subsets of patients (a conclusion that has by no means been firmly established), it is not nearly as effective as the ICD. The use of amiodarone in high-risk patients should generally be limited to those who are not eligible for (or refuse) the ICD, or to adjunctive therapy to an ICD in order to reduce the frequency of recurrent arrhythmias.

(3) Ablation of reentrant foci is an effective way of treating some patients with ventricular tachycardia

Because ablation can eliminate the reentrant substrate for ventricular arrhythmias, for patients whose ventricular tachycardia is suitable, ablation should be strongly considered as a treatment option. Unfortunately, only a small minority of patients with ventricular arrhythmias are currently good candidates for this approach. Transcatheter ablation of ventricular tachycardia will be discussed in Chapter 8.

(4) In the great majority of high-risk patients, the ICD is the only treatment that reliably reduces the risk of death from ventricular arrhythmias

The ICD automatically and reliably terminates the ventricular tachyarrhythmias responsible for sudden death. Except for those few cases in which ablation is a good option, no other therapy approaches the level of efficacy achieved with the ICD. Indeed, when deciding on the best therapy for a patient who is at high risk of sudden cardiac death from ventricular arrhythmias, the main question is typically not whether the ICD will be effective, but

Table 7.6 Major clinical trials using amiodarone empirically in different groups of patients at increased risk for sudden death from ventricular arrhythmias. There is no evidence of a survival benefit with amiodarone in patients with ischemic heart disease. While two earlier trials (GESICA and CHF-STAT) showed a trend toward benefit in patients with nonischemic cardiomyopathy, the much larger SCH-HeFT trial subsequently revealed no such trend

Study	Patient population	Randomization	Results
GESICA[a]	516 pts, NYHA class II/IV, cardiac enlargement	Amiodarone vs placebo	Benefit with amiodarone at 13 months (33.5 vs 41.4%) Significant survival
CHF-STAT[b]	674 pts, LVEF < 0.4, complex ectopy, cardiac enlargement	Amiodarone vs placebo	No significant survival benefit, but pts with nonischemic cardiomyopathy showed a trend toward amiodarone benefit
CAMIAT[c]	1202 MI survivors, complex ectopy	Amiodarone vs placebo	No significant survival benefit
EMIAT[d]	1500 MI survivors, LVEF < 0.4	Amiodarone vs placebo	No significant survival benefit
SCD-HeFT[e]	2521 pts, LVEF ≤ 0.35, NYHA class II/III	ICD vs amiodarone vs conventional therapy	No reduction in mortality with amiodarone Significant survival benefit with ICD

GESICA, Study Group on Survival of Heart Failure in Argentina; CHF-STAT, Survival Trial of Antiarrhythmic Therapy in Congestive Heart Failure; CAMIAT, Canadian Amiodarone Myocardial Infarction Trial; EMIAT, European Myocardial Infarction Trial; SCD-HeFT, Sudden Cardiac Death in Heart Failure Trial; LVEF, left ventricular ejection fraction; MI, myocardial infarction; NYHA, New York Heart Association Functional Class; pts, patients.
[a]Doval HC et al., Lancet 1994; 344:493.
[b]Singh SN et al., N Engl J Med 1995; 333:77.
[c]Cairns JA et al., Lancet 1997; 349:675.
[d]Julian DG et al., Lancet 1997; 349:667.
[e]Bardy GH et al., N Engl J Med 2005; 352:225.

instead whether one is "allowed" to use the ICD in that particular patient.

Which leads us to the real question regarding the treatment of ventricular arrhythmias: when is it OK to use the ICD?

The evidence-based approach to using the ICD

Today, the use of ICDs—and the physicians who use them—has come under significant scrutiny, and clinicians are best advised to apply this therapy under close adherence to formal, approved guidelines. Because the guidelines for using ICDs are changeable, and because the variable emphasis which payers give to certain aspects of those guidelines may occasionally appear at least somewhat arbitrary, the author will not attempt to reproduce formal ICD guidelines here, or prescribe how a clinician ought to behave in light of them.

Rather, it would be more useful to briefly review the current state of clinical evidence regarding ICDs, as derived from the randomized clinical trials that form the basis for those guidelines.

The randomized clinical trials assessing the benefits of ICDs can be divided into two general categories: the secondary prevention trials (in which ICDs were studied in patients who already experienced life-threatening ventricular arrhythmias) and the primary prevention trials (which studied patients judged to be at elevated risk but who had not yet experienced life-threatening arrhythmias). Because the secondary prevention trials were the first to be conducted, we will begin with those.

Secondary prevention trials

Results from three randomized clinical trials have now demonstrated that therapy with the ICD can significantly prolong the survival of patients presenting with sustained ventricular tachyarrhythmias, as compared to other therapies (most specifically, amiodarone)—see Table 7.7. The designs of these studies were relatively straightforward, and so are the subsequent indications. The ICD is now generally recognized as the treatment of choice for patients presenting with sustained ventricular tachyarrhythmias.

Primary prevention trials

While the secondary prevention trials with the ICD were aimed at confirming the correctness of ICD usage in patients with manifest ventricular arrhythmias, the primary prevention trials were aimed instead at testing the ICD in high-risk patients who had not yet had

Table 7.7 The three major randomized clinical trials conducted with the ICD in patients presenting with sustained ventricular tachyarrhythmias (i.e. the secondary prevention trials). These trials confirmed the effectiveness of the ICD in patients presenting with life-threatening, sustained ventricular tachyarrhythmias

Study	Patient population	Randomization	Results
AVID[a]	1016 pts with life-threatening sustained VT/VF	ICD vs amiodarone or sotalol	Survival benefit with ICD
CASH[b]	288 survivors of cardiac arrest	ICD vs one of three drug treatment arms	Survival benefit with ICD
CIDS[c]	659 pts with sustained VT/VF	ICD vs amiodarone	Trend toward survival benefit with ICD

AVID, Antiarrhythmics vs Implantable Defibrillators; CASH, Cardiac Arrest Study Hamburg; CIDS, Canadian Implantable Defibrillator Study; ICD, implantable cardioverter–defibrillator; pts, patients; VT/VF, ventricular tachycardia or ventricular fibrillation.
[a]The Antiarrhythmics versus Implantable Defibrillators (AVID) Investigators, N Engl J Med 1997; 337:1576.
[b]Kuck KH et al., Circulation 2000; 102:748.
[c]Connolly SJ et al., Circulation 2000; 101:1297.

sustained ventricular arrhythmias. As one might predict, the designs of these studies (and therefore resulting ICD indications) were much less straightforward than those of the secondary prevention trials. Table 7.8 lists the major primary prevention trials that have affected indications for the ICD and their most relevant design features.

MADIT I (Multicenter Automatic Defibrillation Implantation Trial) was the first primary prevention trial to be completed. In this study, patients with prior myocardial infarctions, left ventricular ejection fractions of less than 0.35, spontaneous nonsustained ventricular tachycardia, and inducible sustained ventricular tachycardia that was not suppressed with drug testing in the electrophysiology laboratory were randomized to receive either the ICD or the "best" antiarrhythmic drug therapy (in most cases, amiodarone). At the end of the trial, patients randomized to the ICD had significantly improved overall survival. Subsequently, ICD indications were expanded to include patients who met *all* the MADIT I

Table 7.8 The major randomized clinical trials conducted with the ICD in patients with an increased risk of sudden death but who had never experienced sustained ventricular tachyarrhythmias (i.e. the primary prevention trials). Each of these trials except DINAMIT showed a survival benefit with the ICD. Owing to the varied subsets of patients entered into these trials, the resulting indications for the ICD are also somewhat complicated (*see text*)

Study	Patient population	Randomization	Results
MADIT I[a]	196 MI survivors, NSVT, LVEF < 0.35, inducible VT, failed drug trial	ICD vs drug (mainly amiodarone)	Survival benefit with ICD
MUSTT[b]	704 MI survivors, NSVT, LVEF ≤ 0.4, inducible VT	No therapy vs EP-guided therapy	Survival benefit in EP-guided therapy pts who received ICD
MADIT II[c]	1232 MI survivors, LVEF ≤ 0.3	ICD vs conventional therapy	Survival benefit with ICD
SCD-HeFT[d]	2521 pts, LVEF ≤ 0.35, NYHA class II/III	ICD vs amiodarone vs conventional therapy	Survival benefit with ICD; none with amiodarone
DINAMIT[e]	674 pts, recent acute MI, LVEF ≤ 0.35, sympathetic overdrive	ICD vs conventional therapy	Reduced arrhythmic deaths with ICD, but no overall survival benefit
IRIS[f]	898 pts, recent acute MI, LVEF <=0.4, sympathetic overdrive	ICD vs conventional therapy	Reduced arrhythmic deaths with ICD, but no overall survival benefits

MADIT, Multicenter Automatic Defibrillator Implantation Trial; MUSTT, Multicenter Unsustained Tachycardia Trial; SCD-HeFT, Sudden Cardiac Death in Heart Failure Trial; DINAMIT, Defibrillator in Acute Myocardial Infarction Trial; EP, electrophysiology study; ICD, implantable cardioverter–defibrillator; LVEF, left ventricular ejection fraction; MI, myocardial infarction; NSVT, nonsustained ventricular tachycardia; NYHA, New York Heart Association Functional Class; VT, ventricular tachycardia.
[a]Moss AJ *et al.*, N Engl J Med 1996; 335:1933.
[b]Buxton AE *et al.*, N Engl J Med 1999; 341:1882.
[c]Moss AJ *et al.*, N Engl J Med 2002; 346:877.
[d]Bardy GH *et al.*, N Engl J Med 2005; 352:225.
[e]Hohnloser SH *et al.*, N Engl J Med 2004; 351:2481.
[f]Steinbeck G *et al.*, N Engl J Med 2009; 361:1427.

requirements (including electrophysiologic testing and at least one drug trial).

MUSTT (Multicenter Unsustained Tachycardia Trial) was even more complex in design than MADIT I, and it was in fact not specifically designed as an ICD trial at all. But for our purposes, this trial can be thought of as being similar to MADIT I, except that it was more liberal in terms of its ejection-fraction entrance criterion (patients were allowed into MUSTT with ejection fractions of >0.4). In this trial, the ICD again significantly improved survival.

MADIT II randomized patients with prior myocardial infarctions and left ventricular ejection fractions of <=0.3 to either ICDs or conventional medical therapy. The requirements for nonsustained ventricular tachycardia and electrophysiologic testing were dropped in this trial. The results of MADIT II showed the group receiving ICDs having significantly improved survival.

SCD-HeFT (Sudden Cardiac Death in Heart Failure Trial) enrolled patients with heart failure due to either prior myocardial infarction or nonischemic cardiomyopathy (this is the first primary prevention trial to include nonischemic patients). Enrollees were required to have left ventricular ejection fractions of <=0.35 and NYHA class II or III heart failure. They were randomized to ICD implantation, empiric amiodarone, or placebo. At the end of the trial, the ICD produced a significant reduction in overall mortality compared to either amiodarone or placebo, while amiodarone itself offered no survival benefit as compared to placebo.

DINAMIT (Defibrillator in Acute Myocardial Infarction Trial) randomized patients to receive either an ICD or conventional medical therapy an average of 18 days after an acute myocardial infarction. All patients had left ventricular ejection fractions of <=0.35 and evidence of sympathetic overstimulation (either reduced heart-rate variability or an increased resting heart rate) but no overt congestive heart failure. The ICD reduced arrhythmic death by 50% but did not reduce overall mortality. The "excess" in nonsudden deaths in the ICD group—deaths that cancelled out the reduction in arrhythmic deaths—was due to pump failure and mainly occurred in patients who earlier had been rescued from arrhythmic death by their ICDs.

The *IRIS* (Immediate Risk Stratification Improves Survival) trial, like DINAMIT, also enrolled patients within a month of an acute myocardial infarction, and randomized them to ICD versus medical therapy. IRIS patients all had left ventricular ejection fractions of 40% or less, and also had episodes of nonsustained ventricular tachycardia. Further, they all had heart rates at rest of at least 90 beats per minute. After a mean follow-up of about 3 years, there was no difference in overall mortality. The ICD group had a lower risk of sudden death, but a higher risk of nonsudden cardiac death.

The conclusion generally drawn from the DINAMIT and IRIS trials is that any decision on implanting an ICD should be delayed for 4–6 weeks following an acute myocardial infarction, since ICD implantation during this interval has not been shown to be of benefit. It is noteworthy, however, that all patients enrolled in these two studies had evidence of impending heart failure, manifested by elevated resting heart rates or reduced heart-rate variability. Given that a rapid resting heart rate is, prognostically, the worst heart rhythm one can have after a heart attack, it is likely that these two trials selected patients who had a particularly high risk of developing pump failure as their hearts remodeled. Patients who were similar but had normal resting heart rates might well have enjoyed an overall survival benefit with the ICD—but neither of these studies enrolled any such patients. And since they were not studied, subsequent guidelines do not allow for ICD implantation in such patients.

Evidence-based indications for the ICD

So, after collecting all this evidence from randomized clinical trials, where do we stand? The following is an attempt to summarize what might be considered logical clinical behavior based on current clinical evidence, and is not an attempt to precisely duplicate the formal clinical guidelines against which physicians' behaviors will be judged in courts of law and other intimidating venues.

Regarding patients presenting with sustained ventricular tachyarrhythmias, the answer is simple. These patients generally ought to receive the ICD.

It gets a bit more complicated when considering high-risk patients who have not yet had sustained ventricular arrhythmias (i.e. primary prevention patients). Given the results of currently-available randomized clinical trials, however, the indications for using the ICD for the primary prevention of sudden death ought to look something like the following. You should be considered for an ICD if:

1. You have an ejection fraction ≤ 0.35 from a cardiomyopathy that is either ischemic or nonischemic in origin, you have not had an acute myocardial infarction in the last 4–6 weeks (see Note 1), and you have NYHA class II/III heart failure (from SCD-HeFT).

2. You do not have NYHA class II/III heart failure, but you have had a prior myocardial infarction more than 4–6 weeks ago and you have an ejection fraction ≤0.3 (from MADIT II).

3. You do not meet criteria 1 or 2, but you have had a prior myocardial infarction more than 4–6 weeks ago and you have an ejection fraction of <0.4 (from MUSTT) or <0.35 (from MADIT I), nonsustained ventricular tachycardia, and inducible sustained ventricular tachycardia that is not suppressed with drug testing.

Figure 7.15 reduces these conclusions to a hypothetical treatment strategy for patients who are at a high risk of sudden death from ventricular tachyarrhythmias. This treatment strategy generally reflects (but likely does not perfectly duplicate) formal guidelines for using the ICD.

Under this strategy, two general forms of therapy are available: the ICD and "conventional" arrhythmia therapy. Such conventional arrhythmia therapy would consist of whichever treatment the physician chose short of the ICD, possibly including empiric amiodarone, antiarrhythmic drugs selected by serial drug testing or some other methodology, or no specific antiarrhythmic therapy. It is assumed that all patients will receive any indicated conventional cardiac therapy (such as β-blockers, ACE inhibitors, and ischemia control), as well as any necessary risk factor modification, whether they receive the ICD or not.

Under this treatment strategy, patients presenting with sustained ventricular tachycardia or ventricular fibrillation generally are offered the ICD. All other high-risk patients should be evaluated to determine whether they fall into one of the subsets of patients who appear to have benefitted from an ICD in one of the primary prevention randomized clinical trials discussed above.

Those who have either ischemic or nonischemic cardiomyopathy with ejection fractions of <=0.35, and who also have NYHA class II or III heart failure, but who have not had a myocardial infarction within the past 4–6 weeks, should be offered an ICD. The evidence for this treatment node comes from SCD-HeFT.

Any patients with nonischemic cardiomyopathy who do not meet the SCD-HeFT criteria should be offered "conventional" therapy.

Patients with ischemic heart disease not meeting SCD-HeFT criteria may be offered an ICD if they have not had myocardial infarctions within the past 4–6 weeks, have ejection fractions of <=0.3, and are NYHA class I. The evidence for this treatment node comes from MADIT II.

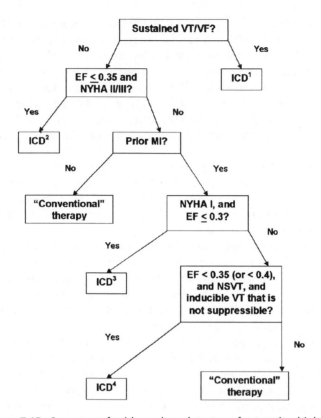

Figure 7.15 Summary of evidence-based strategy for treating high-risk patients. This treatment strategy is derived from the results of the randomized trials discussed in Chapter 7 (*see text for details*). "Conventional" antiarrhythmic therapy consists of any arrhythmia therapy the physician chooses, short of an ICD. ICD[1], evidence base for this treatment node comes from the secondary prevention trials with the ICD; ICD[2], evidence base for this treatment node comes from SCD-HeFT; ICD[3], evidence base for this treatment node comes from MADIT II; ICD[4], evidence base for this treatment node comes from MADIT I (for ejection fractions <0.35) and MUSTT (for ejection fractions <0.4). Note: for any primary prevention indication, the general consensus is that ICDs should not be implanted for 4–6 weeks following an acute myocardial infarction (from DINAMIT). EF, ejection fraction; ICD, implantable cardioverter–defibrillator; NYHA, New York Heart Association Functional Class; MI, myocardial infarction; VT/VF, ventricular tachycardia or ventricular fibrillation.

If patients with ischemic heart disease fail to meet either the SCD-HeFT or the MADIT II criteria, they may still be eligible for the ICD if they have not had myocardial infarctions within the past 4–6 weeks, have ejection fractions of <=0.35 (or possibly <=0.4) and nonsustained ventricular tachycardia, and, when sent for electrophysiologic testing, are found to have inducible ventricular tachycardia that is not suppressed during at least one trial with an antiarrhythmic drug. This treatment node is supported by MADIT I (for ejection fractions of <=0.35) and by MUSTT (for ejection fractions of <=0.4).

All other patients will be eligible for "conventional" treatment only.

Note 1: The imperative to wait 4–6 weeks following an acute myocardial infarction before implanting an ICD for the primary prevention of sudden death comes from the DINAMIT and IRIS trials.

Note 2: The only NYHA class I patients with a primary prevention indication for an ICD are those who meet MADIT II criteria (i.e. patients with prior MI who have ejection fractions of =<0.3). Very few patients with these low ejection fractions can be expected to be in NYHA class I.

Note 3: The Centers for Medicare & Medicaid Services (CMS) have now ruled that patients who meet CMS requirements for cardiac resynchronization therapy (CRT) and are NYHA class IV can receive a CRT device that also provides defibrillation therapy. This is the only group of patients in NYHA class IV that currently has an indication for implantable defibrillation therapy; the rationale here is that class IV patients who receive CRT therapy often experience a significant improvement in their functional class—and would thus find themselves eligible for an ICD a few weeks or months after receiving CRT. (CRT devices are discussed in Chapter 9.)

8 Transcatheter Ablation: Therapeutic Electrophysiology

Over the past two decades, the most important advance in the field of electrophysiology has been the rapid transformation of the electrophysiology study from a largely diagnostic procedure to a largely therapeutic one. Many cardiac arrhythmias that formerly required the use of potentially toxic drugs or cardiac surgery now can be routinely cured (or at least palliated) in the electrophysiology laboratory by means of transcatheter ablation techniques.

The basic idea behind transcatheter ablation is to position a catheter at a critical area within the heart, and to apply damaging energy through the catheter in order to create a discrete scar. Strategically placed scar tissue can disrupt the pathways necessary for pathologic tachyarrhythmias, since it is electrically inert. In this chapter, we will briefly review the techniques used to ablate cardiac arrhythmias in the electrophysiology laboratory and the present-day applications of these techniques.

The technology of transcatheter ablation

Successful transcatheter ablation requires three things. First, a thorough understanding of the arrhythmia being treated—specifically, a precise understanding of the location and physiology of the electrical pathways involved. Second, an understanding of the cardiac anatomy associated with those pathways. Finally, the technology to enable the precise positioning of a catheter and to create the right kind of lesion at a critical location within the pathway. The rapid advance of transcatheter ablation as a therapeutic technique has hinged on steady progression in all three of these requirements.

We will begin by briefly reviewing the technology of lesion generation, and then we will survey the electrophysiology and anat-

Electrophysiologic Testing, Fifth Edition. Richard N. Fogoros.
© 2012 John Wiley & Sons, Ltd. Published 2012 by John Wiley & Sons, Ltd.

omy of the arrhythmias that have proven amenable to transcatheter ablation.

Direct-current (DC) shocks

The use of direct-current (DC) shocks for transcatheter ablation is now mainly of historical interest, as DC energy has been entirely supplanted for this use by radiofrequency (RF) energy. From the first successful ablation in a human in 1982 until approximately 1989, however, DC shocks were the most commonly used energy source for the performance of transcatheter ablation.

To ablate with DC energy, a standard electrode catheter is connected to a conventional defibrillator and a shock is delivered to the distal electrode of the catheter, using a surface electrode as the energy sink. DC shocks delivered in this way generate very high voltages (2000–4000 V) and high currents at the catheter tip. The temperature of the tip electrode instantaneously rises to thousands of degrees Farenheit. The resultant vaporization of blood creates a virtual explosion within the heart, manifested by a rapidly expanding and collapsing incandescent gas globe that generates instantaneous pressures of up to 70 lb/in^2 and produces a flash of light and a disquieting popping noise. Thus, transcatheter DC shocks result in several forms of potentially damaging energy—light, heat, pressure, and electrical current. The only "useful" damage created by DC shocks is thought to result from the electrical current; all the other forms of energy tend only to increase the possibility of complications.

The extent of the lesions created by DC energy is related to the amount of energy used. With energies in excess of 250 J, transmural lesions of 2–4 cm^2 are common. Unfortunately, the periphery of the lesions created with DC shocks is often patchy—and therefore potentially arrhythmogenic.

Because of the traumatic nature of intracardiac DC shocks and because of the nonideal lesions created, DC energy proved to be of limited utility. Ablation with DC shocks was largely limited to ablation of the His bundle to produce complete heart block. Meanwhile, researchers sought an alternative means of creating intracardiac lesions that would be less dangerous and more effective.

Radiofrequency (RF) energy

As it turned out, such a means was readily available. RF energy had been used for many years in operating rooms (in the form of Bovie machines) to cauterize small bleeding vessels within the surgical wound. It wasn't long before electrophysiologists recognized that attaching an RF generator to an electrode catheter would permit the creation of a discrete, well-demarcated intracardiac lesion.

RF energy consists of alternating current (AC) with a frequency range of 100 kHz to 1.5 MHz. In the electrophysiology lab, relatively low frequencies are used in order to avoid the sparking seen with the higher frequencies used in the operating suite. The RF current flow causes localized heating at the tip of the catheter and leads to desiccation and coagulation necrosis of the underlying tissue. The voltage created during RF ablation is relatively low (40–60 V), thus avoiding the barotrauma (i.e. the explosion) seen with DC shocks.

RF generators specifically designed for electrophysiology procedures are now widely available. These RF generators allow instantaneous monitoring of the energy being delivered to the cardiac tissue. The voltage, current, wattage, and impedance can be tracked, permitting the operator to carefully titrate the applied energy. In addition, some ablation systems allow monitoring of the temperature at the catheter tip, thus allowing the operator to more easily avoid coagulation of blood (temperatures in excess of 100 °C are associated with formation of a coagulum at the catheter tip, thus dramatically decreasing the energy delivered to the target tissue).

Special catheters have also been developed for use during RF ablation procedures. These come in a variety of shapes and sizes, and allow the operator to apply variable amounts of "bend" to the distal end, in order to facilitate accurate manipulation of the tip of the catheter. Ablation catheters also come equipped with enlarged tip electrodes (usually 4 mm, instead of the "standard" electrode size of 1 mm). The enlarged surface area provides for a more efficient application of RF energy.

RF energy has several advantages over DC shocks. First, RF energy does not produce an explosion. It can thus be applied, in judicious amounts, to thin-walled structures such as the coronary sinus and cardiac veins without producing rupture. Second, RF energy produces very little stimulation of muscle or nerve, so it can be applied without using general anesthesia. Third, because the energy applied can be titrated, graded amounts can be delivered to cause partial tissue damage. Fourth, RF energy produces small, homogeneous lesions, which are less arrhythmogenic.

There are also two disadvantages to the use of RF energy. First, the lesions it produces are small (4–5 mm in diameter and approximately 3 mm in depth). Extremely precise mapping is thus required in order to damage the target area sufficiently, and target tissue that is relatively broad or deep (e.g. a bypass tract that is located epicardially) might not be readily amenable to RF ablation. Further, the delivery of RF energy is not instantaneous. This means that stable contact between the catheter tip and the tissue must be maintained for the entire 5–120 seconds during which RF energy is applied. Monitoring of the impedance in the ablation system during the application of energy is helpful in ensuring adequate tissue contact.

Several other kinds of energy are being developed for the transcatheter ablation of arrhythmias—including laser energy, microwave energy, and cryoenergy (i.e. freezing). While each of these forms of energy is being used clinically today in ablation procedures, and while one or more of these may end up largely supplanting RF ablation, RF energy remains by far the most commonly used method of ablating cardiac arrhythmias.

Ablation of the AV junction

The original indication for transcatheter ablation was to produce complete heart block in patients with chronic atrial fibrillation and persistently rapid ventricular rates.

AV junction ablation

Ablation of the AV junction is aimed at producing complete heart block at the level of the AV node. While insertion of a permanent pacemaker is always required after this procedure, in most cases the patient is left with a relatively stable escape rhythm after AV nodal ablation.

To perform ablation of the AV junction, a temporary pacemaker is first placed into the right ventricle. The ablation catheter is then used to map the His bundle. Once the largest His deflection is carefully localized, the catheter is gradually withdrawn, while recording from the distal (ablating) electrode, until the His and ventricular deflections become relatively small and the atrial deflection becomes relatively large. This position indicates that the catheter tip is in the region of the compact AV node. Excellent contact of the catheter tip with the cardiac tissue must be seen, and the catheter position must be entirely stable. When optimal positioning has been confirmed, RF energy is applied to the tip electrode (usually 20–35 W for 30–60 seconds). Successful AV nodal ablation is often heralded by the development of an accelerated junctional tachycardia during application of the RF energy (hence, junctional tachycardia during RF application is a "good sign"). If the attempt is unsuccessful, the catheter is repositioned and RF ablation is repeated. In the hands of an experienced operator, RF ablation of the AV junction is possible in over 98% of cases, although in 5–10% of cases a second procedure is required to assure permanent block.

Occasionally, ablations of the AV junction using this technique will be unsuccessful, and in these cases ablation of the His bundle from the left ventricle may be required. Ablating the His bundle from the left ventricle is accomplished by positioning the ablation catheter just inferiorly to the aortic valve along the septal wall of the left ventricle. The intracardiac electrogram during left-sided ablation should show a His-bundle deflection at least 110 msec earlier than the ventricular deflection (a closer spacing between the His deflection and the ventricular deflection means that the catheter is not actually recording the His bundle, but instead is recording the left bundle branch).

A few cases of sudden death have been reported within several days of ablation of the AV junction. It is thought that these deaths are likely due to torsades de pointes, most likely provoked in susceptible patients by a sudden, relative bradycardia. The risk for this event appears to be transient, and can be avoided by pacing patients relatively rapidly (i.e. 90–100 beats/min) for a few days to a few weeks after AV junction ablation.

Ablation of AV nodal reentrant tachycardia

RF ablation is now the treatment of choice for AV nodal reentrant tachycardia.

Successfully ablating AV nodal reentrant tachycardia has required a change in the way electrophysiologists visualize the AV node. In the past, most electrophysiologists thought of the AV node simply as a compact, button-like structure, as depicted in Figure 8.1a. It has now become apparent that the AV node behaves more as depicted in Figure 8.1b. The AV node does indeed appear to have a compact distal component (i.e. the part of the node that gives rise to the His bundle), but the more proximal portion of the AV node appears to be "diffuse."

To visualize what this means, it is helpful to imagine the course of the electrical impulse as it approaches the AV node from the atria. We have seen that the electrical impulse arises in the sinus node and then travels across the atria in a radial fashion. Recent findings suggest that as this electrical impulse approaches the AV node, it is gathered into bands of conducting fibers, which coalesce into "tracts", which in turn coalesce to form the compact AV node. At

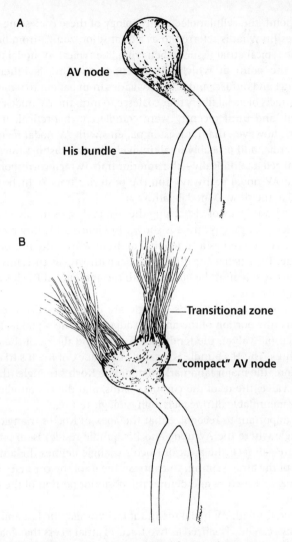

Figure 8.1 "Old" and "new" concepts of AV node anatomy and physiology. (a) The AV node as it commonly used to be conceived, namely as a compact "button" of specialized tissue. (b) The AV node as it is currently conceptualized by electrophysiologists. In this "new" model, tracts of conducting fibers coalesce to form the compact AV node. The transition from atrial electrophysiology to AV nodal electrophysiology probably occurs proximal to the compact node. Anatomists have been describing this for years, but until ablationists arrived on the scene there seemed to be no good reason to believe them.

some point, the cellular electrophysiology of these coalescing tracts changes (in what is referred to as a "transition zone") from behaving like typical atrial tissue to behaving like typical AV nodal tissue. Thus, the point at which the AV node "begins" is inherently indistinct and diffuse, and probably varies from patient to patient.

The tracts of atrial fibers that coalesce to form the AV node are ill-defined, and until recently were completely theoretical. It now appears, however, that (at least in patients with AV nodal reentrant tachycardia, and probably in all individuals) two distinct tracts can be localized anatomically—the anterior tract (which corresponds to the fast AV nodal pathway) and the posterior tract (which corresponds to the slow AV nodal pathway).

The "classic" way of visualizing the two pathways involved in AV nodal reentrant tachycardia is shown in Figure 6.11, in which the two tracts are seen as a functional division within the button-like AV node. To visualize the dual AV nodal pathways as currently conceptualized, one must be familiar with the anatomy of Koch's triangle (Figure 8.2).

The three sides of Koch's triangle are defined by the tricuspid annulus (the portion of the annulus adjacent to the septal leaflet of the tricuspid valve), the tendon of Todaro, and the os of the coronary sinus. The His bundle is located at the apex of Koch's triangle. Therefore, the major landmarks that define Koch's triangle (the tricuspid valve, the os of the coronary sinus, and the His bundle) are readily identifiable during electrophysiologic testing.

It is important to recognize that the apex of Koch's triangle (i.e. the angle where the AV node and His bundle reside) is an *anterior* structure—in fact, the apex of Koch's triangle defines the anterior aspect of the atrial septum. In contrast, the os of the coronary sinus is a *posterior* structure and defines the posterior portion of the atrial septum.

In patients with AV nodal reentrant tachycardia, the fast and slow pathways can be visualized as two tracts of atrial fibers that coalesce to form the compact AV node (Figure 8.3). The fast pathway is an *anterior* and *superior* tract of fibers, located along the tendon of Todaro. The slow pathway is a *posterior* and *inferior* tract of fibers, located along the tricuspid annulus near the os of the coronary sinus. Thus, the anatomic correlates of the "functional" dual AV nodal pathways have now been identified. Because the two pathways can be discretely localized, they can be discretely ablated.

When the anatomy of dual AV nodal pathways was first recognized, most attempts at curing AV nodal reentry focused on ablating

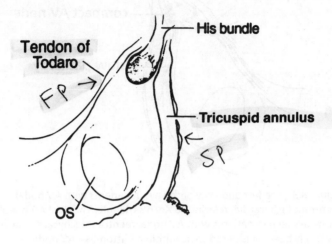

ANTERIOR

POSTERIOR

Figure 8.2 The triangle of Koch. Long described by anatomists and long ignored by electrophysiologists, Koch's triangle has become vitally important in performing transcatheter ablations. Koch's triangle is defined posteriorly by the os of the coronary sinus. The apex of the triangle is defined anteriorly by the His bundle. The tendon of Todaro and the tricuspid valve annulus compose the other two sides of the triangle. In the electrophysiology laboratory, the landmarks of Koch's triangle are identified by one catheter recording the His deflection and by another placed in the os of the coronary sinus. Koch's triangle lies between these two catheters.

the fast pathway. These attempts were generally successful, but unfortunately they yielded a relatively high incidence of complete heart block (up to 20%). The heart block most likely resulted from the fact that the fast pathway and the compact AV node are in close proximity (i.e. both structures are anterior).

The ablation of AV nodal reentry in recent years has been generally accomplished by ablating the slow pathway. Since the slow pathway is posterior, it is relatively distant from the AV node, and thus ablation of this structure yields a low incidence of complete heart block (generally less than 1%).

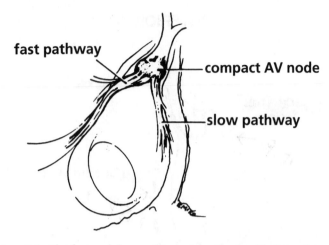

fast pathway

compact AV node

slow pathway

Figure 8.3 The fast and slow pathways in patients with AV nodal reentrant tachycardia, relating to Koch's triangle. The dual AV nodal pathways seen in patients with AV nodal reentrant tachycardia have classically been considered to lie within a button-like AV node. Electrophysiologists performing RF transcatheter ablation, however, have now clearly shown that the fast and slow pathways are readily discernible and can be distinctly localized within Koch's triangle. Both pathways appear to be located proximally to the compact AV node. The fast pathway is an anterior and superior structure and lies near the compact AV node along the tendon of Todaro. The slow pathway is a posterior and inferior structure and can usually be identified along the tricuspid annulus near the os of the coronary sinus. Because the slow pathway is farther away from the AV node than the fast pathway, the slow pathway can usually be selectively ablated without causing complete heart block.

In general, two approaches are commonly used for ablation of the slow AV nodal pathway—the "mapping" approach and the anatomic approach. Both approaches begin by first identifying the anatomic limits of Koch's triangle, by placing one catheter in the His position and another in the os of the coronary sinus. The ablation catheter is then advanced from the femoral vein to the tricuspid annulus, near the os of the coronary sinus.

With the "mapping" approach, the ablation catheter is carefully manipulated along the tricuspid annulus, searching for discrete "slow potentials" that presumably represent depolarization of the slow pathway itself (Figure 8.4). These slow potentials are located

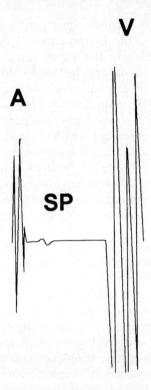

Figure 8.4 Slow AV nodal pathway potential. Mapping of the slow pathway in patients with AV nodal reentrant tachycardia is accomplished by seeking the slow potential (SP) along the tricuspid annulus within Koch's triangle. See text for details. A, atrial deflection; V, ventricular deflection.

between the atrial and ventricular deflections in the intracardiac electrogram. Mapping of AV nodal reentrant tachycardia is thus best accomplished during sinus rhythm and not during tachycardia, so that the atrial and ventricular deflections during mapping remain separate and distinct. When the slow potentials are identified, an RF lesion applied at their location almost always ablates the slow pathway.

With the anatomic approach to slow pathway ablation, no attempt is made to map the slow potentials. Instead, ablation sites are identified by fluoroscopic means. Generally, the length of the tricuspid annulus between the os of the coronary sinus and the His bundle is visually divided into three equal sections—posterior (closest to the os of the coronary sinus), middle, and anterior (closest to the His bundle). The ablation catheter is positioned across the tricuspid valve in the posterior section and gradually withdrawn until both atrial and ventricular deflections are recorded, with the ventricular deflection being larger than the atrial deflection. An RF lesion is made, and if the slow pathway has not been successfully ablated, the catheter is moved further anteriorly and the procedure is repeated. Lesions are placed in each of the three sections serially, from posterior to anterior, until the slow pathway has been ablated.

Many electrophysiologists have evolved an integrated approach which begins with ablations posteriorly and moving anteriorly (as with the anatomic approach), but which adds at least a brief search for slow pathway potentials within that anatomic zone prior to applying RF energy.

Accelerated junctional tachycardia occurs during RF application in virtually 100% of successful slow pathway ablations. Therefore, if no tachycardia occurs after 10–15 seconds of RF application, the RF should be terminated and the catheter repositioned. If tachycardia does occur, 30–60 seconds of RF energy should be applied. Successful ablation is documented by confirming that the physiology of dual AV nodal pathways is no longer present (see Chapter 6).

When one or both of these techniques for slow pathway ablation is used, successful treatment of AV nodal reentrant tachycardia can be achieved in over 98% of patients, with a very low risk of producing complete heart block.

Ablation of bypass tracts

In the late 1980s, RF ablation of bypass tracts was considered a difficult and somewhat mystical technique performed by only a few adventurous shamans. During the 1990s, however, it evolved into a widely available and highly effective procedure. For most patients with significantly symptomatic or life-threatening bypass tracts, RF ablation is now the therapy of choice.

Characteristics of bypass tracts

As noted in Chapter 6, bypass tracts are tiny bands of myocardial tissue that form a bridge across the AV junction, connecting atrial tissue to ventricular tissue. They can occur anywhere along the AV groove, except along the portion directly between the mitral and aortic valves. Because they are composed of bands of myocardial tissue, bypass tracts tend to exhibit the electrophysiologic features of myocardial tissue instead of AV nodal tissue; that is, their refractory periods tend to shorten instead of lengthen with decreases in cycle length, and they tend to develop second-degree block in a Mobitz II pattern instead of a Mobitz I pattern.

Localization of bypass tracts begins by studying the surface ECG and continues with intracardiac mapping.

ECG localization of bypass tracts

Bypass tracts are divided into five general categories according to their location (Figure 8.5). These categories are left free wall, right free wall, posterior septal, anterior septal, and midseptal. The general approach to mapping in the electrophysiology laboratory is different for each of these categories, so it is important to have some idea as to the location of a bypass tract before the ablation procedure begins. In most cases, the surface ECG fortunately gives a very good indication of where the bypass tract is located.

Table 8.1 lists the ECG criteria for grossly localizing bypass tracts. *The "key" is to look for the leads with the negative delta wave, because the negative delta wave "points" to the bypass tract* (Figure 8.6).

Consider the delta waves in ECG lead I, which is a "left-sided" lead. Delta waves in lead I are negative for left free-wall tracts, are

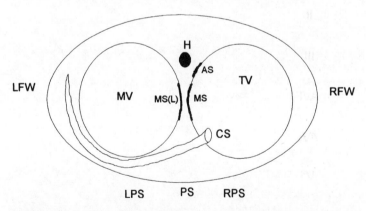

Figure 8.5 Location of bypass tracts. The anatomic structures shown in this figure are the mitral valve (MV), the tricuspid valve (TV), the coronary sinus (CS), and the His bundle (H). LFW, left free-wall tracts; LPS, left paraseptal tracts; PS, posteroseptal tracts; RPS, right paraseptal tracts; RFW, right free-wall tracts; AS, anteroseptal tracts; MS, midseptal tracts; MS(L), left-sided midseptal tracts. See text for details.

Table 8.1 Electrocardiographic localization of bypass tracts

Location of tract	Characteristics of preexcited QRS
Left free wall	Negative delta wave in AVL and often in lead I. Positive delta wave in inferior and precordial leads. Normal QRS axis.
Right free wall	Negative delta wave in leads III and AVF. Positive delta waves in leads I and II. Normal QRS axis.
Posteroseptal	Negative delta waves in inferior leads. Positive delta waves in leads I and AVL. R/S ratio in $V_1 < 1$; left superior axis.
Anteroseptal	Negative delta wave in leads V_1 and V_2. Positive delta wave in leads I and II. Normal QRS axis.
Midseptal	ECG similar to anteroseptal, except that in inferior leads, delta waves are not positive.

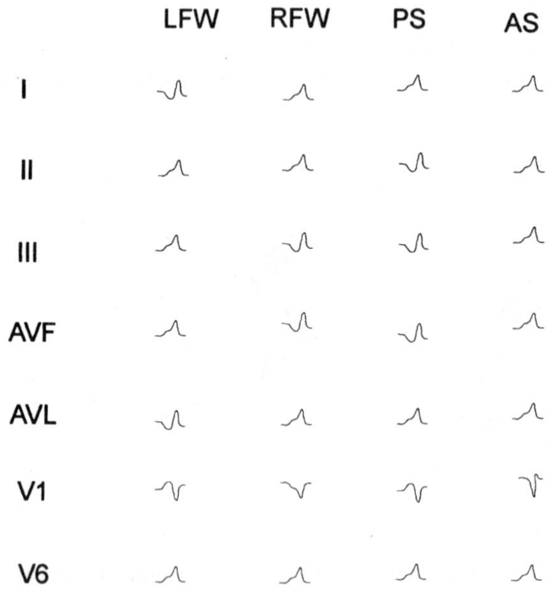

Figure 8.6 Electrocardiographic manifestations of the major categories of bypass tract. Typical electrocardiographic patterns are shown for left free-wall tracts (LFW), right free-wall tracts (RFW), posteroseptal tracts (PS), and anteroseptal tracts (AS). See text and Table 8.1 for details.

biphasic (or isoelectric) for left posterior to right posterior tracts, and are positive for right free-wall tracts.

The delta waves in lead V_1 (a right-sided lead) are positive for left free-wall and posterior septal tracts and negative for right free-wall tracts. They are biphasic (or isoelectric) for anteroseptal tracts.

The delta waves in leads II, III, and AVF (inferior leads) are negative for posterior septal tracts and become positive as the tracts move anteriorly toward the anteroseptal regions.

Based on this general concept, and on the more specific criteria listed in Table 8.1, a very good idea of the location of a bypass tract can be ascertained before the electrophysiologic procedure is begun—and thus, before an accurate preliminary action plan is made.

Considerations for successfully mapping and ablating bypass tracts

Before outlining specific approaches to various types of bypass tract, let us review some general considerations for successfully mapping and ablating these tracts:

1. Mapping can be conducted on either the atrial or the ventricular aspect of the AV groove. In general, when mapping on the ventricular aspect, antegrade conduction over the bypass tract (i.e. the delta wave) is mapped. Maximal preexcitation is helpful in mapping the delta wave. This can be accomplished by pacing the atrium at a rate that maximizes preexcitation, or by administering drugs (such as verapamil) that increase refractory periods in the normal conducting system. When mapping on the atrial aspect of the AV groove, or when mapping concealed bypass tracts, retrograde conduction over the bypass tract is studied. This is best accomplished during orthodromic macroreentrant tachycardia (i.e. tachycardia that uses the bypass tract for retrograde conduction and the normal conducting system for antegrade conduction) or with ventricular pacing at a rate that optimizes retrograde conduction via the bypass tract.

2. When the mapping catheter is located near the bypass tract (whether on the atrial or the ventricular aspect of the AV groove), the interval between the atrial and ventricular depolarizations (assuming that either antegrade or retrograde conduction of impulses is occurring across the bypass tract) will be short. Generally, the localized AV interval is no more than 60 msec, and

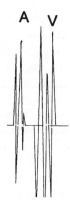

Figure 8.7 Depiction of the narrow AV interval seen when the mapping catheter is in proximity to the bypass tract. Compare this to the more "usual" AV interval shown in Figure 8.4. When mapping bypass tracts, the optimal localized AV interval is generally less than 60 msec.

sometimes the atrial and ventricular depolarizations are virtually continuous (Figure 8.7).

3. When the mapping catheter is near the bypass tract and preexcitation is occurring, the local ventricular depolarization should be earlier than the earliest ventricular depolarization seen on any surface ECG lead.

4. Loss of preexcitation (i.e. disappearance of the delta wave) when pressure is applied with the tip of the mapping catheter is an excellent indication that the site of the bypass tract has been localized.

5. In many patients, a localized potential from the bypass tract itself can be recorded (Figure 8.8). These bypass-tract potentials tend to be relatively low in amplitude, but to have discrete, sharp onsets. They generally resemble His-bundle electrograms more than they do the slow pathway potentials seen when mapping the slow AV nodal pathways. Sometimes it can be difficult to differentiate between a bypass-tract potential and a part of the atrial or ventricular depolarizations. Pacing techniques can often be used to demonstrate that the bypass-tract potentials are distinct from either the atrial or the ventricular potentials. A clear-cut bypass-tract potential is an excellent indication that RF ablation at that site will be successful.

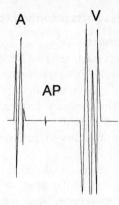

Figure 8.8 Recording of a bypass-tract potential. Often, a localized potential from the bypass tract itself (AP, "accessory pathway" potential) can be recorded from a well-positioned mapping catheter.

6. Unipolar recordings from the tip of the mapping catheter can be extremely helpful in localizing the bypass tract, as unipolar recordings give information about the direction of the cardiac impulse being recorded (a positive deflection means the impulse is moving toward the unipolar electrode, while a negative deflection means it is moving away). When the QRS complex is preexcited, the unipolar ventricular electrogram should be predominantly negative (i.e. a QS complex should be recorded). A negative unipolar ventricular electrogram indicates that the electrical impulse during ventricular depolarization is always moving away from the catheter tip—which is possible only if the catheter tip is located at the site of earliest ventricular activation. A negative ventricular deflection on the unipolar electrogram is entirely analogous to a negative delta wave seen on the corresponding surface ECG leads.

7. Finally, once the bypass tract has been carefully mapped and it is time to perform the ablation, catheter stability is critical, since RF energy must be continuously applied to the target tissue for a sustained period of time (often 60 seconds or longer). The catheter is considered to be sufficiently stable when the ratio of the amplitudes of atrial to ventricular deflections on the local intracardiac electrogram varies by less than 10%.

The approach to bypass tracts according to location

Left free-wall bypass tracts

More than 50% of bypass tracts referred for RF ablation have been located in the left free wall. These tracts cross the AV groove along the anterolateral, lateral, posterolateral, or posterior aspects of the mitral valve annulus. The coronary sinus also courses along the same portion of the mitral annulus, and thus provides a convenient means of mapping the annulus in patients with left free-wall pathways.

Standard electrode catheters are placed in the high right atrium, His position, and right ventricular apex. A multipolar electrode catheter is placed into the coronary sinus (often a 10-lead catheter is used) and multiple bipolar recordings are established along its length. After the earliest sites of antegrade and retrograde preexcitation are approximated using the electrodes within the coronary sinus, the mapping and ablation catheter is inserted.

There are two general approaches for ablating left free-wall pathways: the retrograde approach and the transseptal approach.

The retrograde approach is the most commonly used and usually yields favorable results. The mapping catheter is inserted through a femoral artery and advanced across the aortic valve into the left ventricle. The catheter tip is then maneuvered into the AV groove beneath the mitral valve leaflets and the bypass tract is localized.

The transseptal approach is also very effective in skilled hands. The mapping catheter is inserted through a femoral vein and advanced across the intraatrial septum into the left atrium. In most cases, crossing the intraatrial septum requires that a puncture be made through the septal wall, using a catheter-based tool designed specifically for that purpose. When the transseptal approach is used, the atrial aspect of the mitral annulus is mapped.

With either approach, the multipolar coronary sinus catheter is used as a stable reference for guiding mapping maneuvers. Also with either approach, successful ablation of left free-wall bypass tracts can be achieved in more than 95% of cases.

Right free-wall bypass tracts

Right free-wall tracts are seen in approximately 10% of patients with bypass tracts referred for ablation. These tracts are more difficult to map and ablate than left free-wall tracts because a stable catheter position is more difficult to attain and there is no anatomic structure analogous to the coronary sinus to aid in mapping.

Standard electrode catheters are placed in the high right atrium, His position, right ventricular apex, and coronary sinus. The mapping and ablation catheter is usually inserted via a femoral vein, advanced across the tricuspid valve, and then withdrawn so that the mapping electrodes are positioned along the tricuspid annulus in such a way that both atrial and ventricular deflections are recorded. Mapping is often conducted using the left anterior oblique (LAO) projection, which allows the tricuspid annulus to be visualized as the face of a clock (Figure 8.9). In this projection, the His bundle is located at approximately 1 o'clock, and the os of the coronary sinus at approximately 5 o'clock. If the bypass tract proves to be difficult to map, or if catheter stability is a problem, alternative approaches can be tried. Introducing the mapping catheter via the superior instead of the inferior vena cava is sometimes helpful. Long intravascular sheaths can also be used to lend stability to the mapping catheter.

In experienced hands, right free-wall pathways can be successfully ablated in over 90% of cases.

Mahaim bypass tracts

Mahaim bypass tracts, as originally described, supposedly connect the AV node either to the right bundle branch (nodofascicular

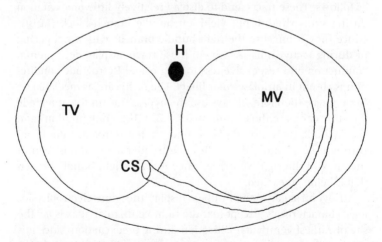

Figure 8.9 Orientation of the tricuspid annulus (TV) in the left anterior oblique (LAO) projection. In the LAO projection, the tricuspid annulus can be visualized as the face of a clock, with the His bundle (H) in the 1 o'clock position and the os of the coronary sinus (CS) in the 5 o'clock position. MV, mitral valve annulus.

fibers) or to ventricular muscle (nodoventricular fibers). Recently, it has been determined with careful mapping that Mahaim tracts actually do not arise within the AV node itself, but instead within atrial muscle. Thus, these bypass tracts actually form connections between atrial muscle and the right bundle branch (atriofascicular fibers) or ventricular muscle (atrioventricular fibers).

The original confusion as to their site of atrial insertion arose from the fact that atriofascicular and atrioventricular tracts display the same sort of decremental conduction usually associated with AV nodal tissue; that is, with atrial pacing, faster pacing rates *increase* the stimulus–delta wave interval, unlike in a more typical bypass tract, where faster pacing rates decrease the stimulus–delta wave interval. Further, Mahaim bypass tracts tend to respond to adenosine similarly to AV nodal tissue. For practical purposes, therefore, while Mahaim fibers turn out to be anatomically distinct from the AV node, they are electrophysiologically similar to the AV node. Conceptually, Mahaim fibers can be visualized as strands of slow AV nodal fibers (i.e. the fibers that course along the tricuspid annulus within Koch's triangle) that abnormally veer off, bypassing the AV node and connecting directly to the right bundle branch or right ventricular myocardium.

The electrophysiologic characteristics of atriofascicular tracts are as follows. These tracts tend to display relatively little preexcitation during sinus rhythm but yield left bundle branch block (LBBB) (since they connect to the right bundle branch) with atrial pacing or during tachycardia. As noted, these tracts display decremental conduction and responsiveness to adenosine. Retrograde conduction is absent in atriofascicular fibers. The tachycardias mediated by these tracts, therefore, always use the bypass tract in the antegrade direction (and are thus manifested by an LBBB configuration) and the AV node (or a second bypass tract) in the retrograde direction. During preexcitation, the earliest ventricular activation is seen in the apex of the right ventricle, since it is the right bundle branch that is being preexcited.

Atrioventricular Mahaim fibers display the same electrophysiologic characteristics, except that the right ventricular apex is *not* the site of earliest ventricular activation during preexcitation, since it is the ventricular muscle adjacent to the tricuspid valve that is being preexcited and not the right bundle branch.

Mapping and ablation of atriofascicular and atrioventricular fibers is performed in a manner similar to that described for other right-sided bypass tracts, except that antegrade mapping must always be performed, since these tracts do not display retrograde conduction. This generally requires mapping either during tachycardia or at an atrial pacing rate that maximizes preexcitation. Mapping is conducted along the tricuspid annulus between the His bundle and the os of the coronary sinus.

Posterior septal (and paraseptal) bypass tracts

Posterior septal and paraseptal bypass tracts account for over 20% of bypass tracts referred for ablation (Figure 8.10).

Posterior septal tracts cross the AV groove near the os of the coronary sinus, where the right atrium and left ventricle are in proximity. Thus, the atrial insertion of a posterior septal tract is in the *right atrium*, while the ventricular insertion is in the *left ventricle*. In contrast, right paraseptal bypass tracts cross the AV groove just to the right of this region and connect the right atrium with the right ventricle. Left paraseptal bypass tracts cross the AV groove just to the left of this region and connect the left atrium with the left ventricle.

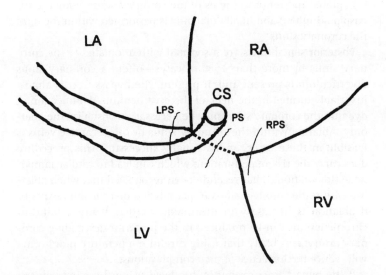

Figure 8.10 Insertions for bypass tracts located in the posterior septal region. The anatomic structures shown are the left atrium (LA), right atrium (RA), left ventricle (LV), right ventricle (RV), and coronary sinus (CS). Posterior septal tracts (PS) connect the right atrium with the left ventricle. Right paraseptal tracts (RPS) connect the right atrium with the right ventricle. Left paraseptal tracts (LPS) connect the left atrium with the left ventricle. See text for details.

Because the connections of posterior septal, left paraseptal, and right paraseptal tracts are all different from one another, the response to bundle branch block that occurs during macroreentrant tachycardia can be useful in differentiating among these three types of posterior bypass tract. Recall that when bundle branch block occurs during macroreentrant tachycardia and the block is on the same side as a bypass tract, the cycle length of tachycardia increases (see Figure 6.11). Accordingly, with left paraseptal bypass tracts, the onset of LBBB will increase the cycle length of the tachycardia, whereas for right paraseptal tracts, only right bundle branch block (RBBB) will increase the cycle length. Finally, with posterior septal tracts (which connect the left ventricle with the right atrium), LBBB will prolong the cycle length but RBBB will not.

When ablating posterior septal or paraseptal tracts, the mapping catheter is inserted first into the right atrium. Mapping is begun anteriorly in Koch's triangle, along the tricuspid annulus near the bundle of His. Gradually, the mapping progresses posteriorly to the os of the coronary sinus. Then the right posterior paraseptal region is explored (posterior to the os of the coronary sinus along the tricuspid annulus), and finally mapping is performed within the os of the coronary sinus.

Posterior septal tracts are associated with anomalies of the coronary sinus in more than 15% of cases—often, a coronary sinus diverticulum is present and, if present, the bypass tract is almost invariably located in the neck of the diverticulum. An injection of dye into the coronary sinus may be necessary to visualize the anatomy. Ablating within the coronary sinus or other cardiac veins is feasible in these cases, and is usually successful. This procedure does carry the risk of perforation, which can lead to cardiac tamponade. In addition, it has recently been recognized that when ablating within the coronary sinus (especially if a diverticulum exists or if ablation is necessary in the middle cardiac vein), significant chronic lesions can be produced in the posterior descending coronary artery. It is likely that using careful temperature monitoring will reduce the incidence of such complications.

If the bypass tract cannot be localized using these maneuvers, mapping of the left posterior paraseptal region may be necessary— this requires insertion of a mapping catheter retrogradely across the aortic valve. Generally, at least one attempt at ablating the "earliest" site on the right side is made before moving to the left side.

Successful ablation of posterior septal and paraseptal tracts can be achieved in 85–90% of patients.

Anteroseptal and midseptal bypass tracts

In the preablation era, anteroseptal and midseptal pathways were lumped together as "anteroseptal bypass tracts," owing to their similar electrocardiographic manifestations. These tracts are now known to be quite distinct. They require different approaches during ablation procedures, so their differentiation is important. Bypass tracts arising in the region anterior and superior to the His bundle are termed *anteroseptal tracts*. Bypass tracts arising in the area between the His bundle and the os of the coronary sinus (i.e. in the triangle of Koch) are termed *midseptal pathways* (see Figure 8.5).

On the surface ECG, anteroseptal pathways display positive delta waves in leads I, II, III, and AVF; normal QRS axis; biphasic or positive delta waves in lead V_1; and positive delta waves in V_2–V_6 (see Figure 8.6).

The electrocardiographic manifestations of midseptal pathways are similar to those of anteroseptal pathways, with the following exceptions: for midseptal tracts close to the AV node, the delta wave is isoelectric (instead of positive) in leads III and AVF; for midseptal tracts closer to the coronary sinus, the delta wave is predominantly negative in leads III and AVF, and isoelectric in lead V_1 (Figure 8.11).

The techniques used in ablating anteroseptal and midseptal tracts are similar to those used for any other bypass tract. In either case, reference electrodes are placed in the right atrium, His position, coronary sinus, and right ventricular apex. The mapping and ablation catheter is inserted from the jugular or subclavian vein (for anteroseptal tracts) or from the femoral vein (for either anteroseptal or midseptal tracts).

For anteroseptal bypass tracts, mapping can be accomplished from either the atrial or the ventricular aspect of the tricuspid valve. In general, a careful attempt should be made to record the anteroseptal bypass tract potential itself, and to carefully differentiate it from the His potential (since anteroseptal tracts are often in close proximity to the His bundle). To differentiate the bypass tract from the His bundle, mapping during macroreentrant tachycardia is often very helpful, since during tachycardia the bypass tract is depolarized retrogradely and the His bundle antegradely. Administering adenosine to selectively block AV conduction via the normal conducting system is also helpful in differentiating between the two.

The procedure for ablating midseptal pathways is similar to the procedure for performing slow pathway ablation in AV nodal reentrant tachycardia. Mapping is performed on the tricuspid

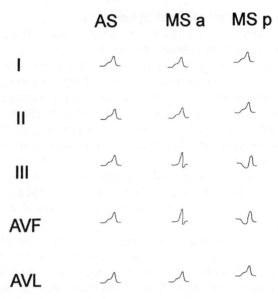

Figure 8.11 Electrocardiographic differentiation between anteroseptal and midseptal bypass tracts. Midseptal tracts are more posterior than anteroseptal tracts, and thus tend to have some of the electrocardiographic manifestations of posterior septal tracts. The more posterior the midseptal tracts, the more negative the delta waves in the inferior ECG leads (i.e. leads II, III, and AVF) (*see text*). AS, anteroseptal; MS a, midseptal tracts located relatively anteriorly; MS p, midseptal tracts located relatively posteriorly.

annulus, between the His bundle and the os of the coronary sinus. If ablation cannot be accomplished from the right side, left-sided mapping (along the mitral annulus between the His bundle and the os of the coronary sinus) may be required.

For both midseptal and anteroseptal bypass tracts that are in close proximity to the AV node or His bundle, ablation should be conducted while the patient is in macroreentrant tachycardia, so that the integrity of the normal conducting system can be closely monitored. In general, successful ablation of these bypass tracts can be accomplished in more than 90% of patients. The incidence of inadvertent, complete heart block is generally reported as being less than 5%, but RBBB has occurred in up to 40% of patients who have ablation of anteroseptal tracts.

Ablation of atrial tachyarrhythmias

Ablation of focal atrial tachycardias

Focal atrial tachycardias can be paroxysmal or incessant, and, depending on their frequency, duration, and rate, they can produce symptoms that are anywhere from mild to severe. These arrhythmias can be caused by automatic foci, foci of triggered activity, or microreentrant circuits.

Because they are focal, atrial tachycardias can often be mapped and are thus amenable to RF ablation. The site of atrial tachycardia is often associated with particular anatomic structures, most commonly the crista terminalis in the right atrium (see the next subsection), the ostia of the pulmonary veins in the left atrium, the os of the coronary sinus, and the tricuspid annulus.

Ablating atrial tachycardia requires activation mapping—the earliest atrial deflection is sought that precedes the P wave on the surface electrogram. Thus, successful mapping depends on one's ability to induce atrial tachycardia during the ablation procedure or in the presence of incessant or very frequent tachycardia. Application of RF energy should also be performed during the tachycardia.

Activation mapping of atrial tachycardia is greatly facilitated by the use of modern, computerized activation mapping systems. These systems are discussed later in this chapter.

Ablation of atrial flutter

Careful mapping of the atria during atrial flutter has revealed this rhythm to be a macroreentrant arrhythmia that, in most cases, arises in the right atrium. In most patients with atrial flutter, the reentrant pathway is highly stereotypical. As a result of the particular pathway taken by this "typical" atrial flutter, this atrial flutter is an arrhythmia that can often be readily ablated.

Figure 8.12 demonstrates the typical reentrant pathway for atrial flutter. This schematic depicts the interior right atrium, demonstrating the important anatomic features that determine the reentrant pathway for atrial flutter. Two key features should be noted. First, it is the crista terminalis (a ridge of tissue running roughly from the superior to the inferior vena cava) which presents the electrical barrier that defines the reentrant circuit and allows atrial flutter to develop. Second, in typical atrial flutter, the flutter wave must pass through a narrow isthmus defined by the inferior vena cava and the tricuspid annulus.

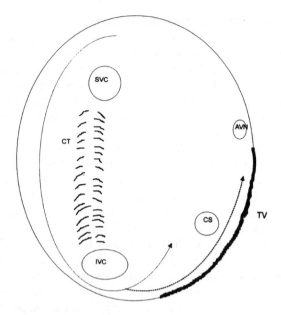

Figure 8.12 Typical reentrant pathway for atrial flutter. The right atrium is depicted, including the inferior vena cava (IVC), the superior vena cava (SVC), the tricuspid annulus (TV), the AV node (AVN), the os of the coronary sinus (CS), and the crista terminalis (CT). The CT is a ridge of tissue roughly connecting the SVC and the IVC. In most patients with atrial flutter, the CT functionally divides the right atrium into two sections. The flutter circuit (indicated by the arrows) must pass through the narrow isthmus between the IVC and the tricuspid annulus. This isthmus thus presents a favorable target for ablation. See text for details.

It is this latter feature that makes RF ablation a viable option for many patients with atrial flutter. If a linear lesion can be made, extending from the tricuspid annulus to the opening of the inferior vena cava, then electrical blockade of the necessary isthmus can be created (Figure 8.13).

To accomplish this feat, the ablation catheter is introduced from the femoral vein and advanced into the right atrium and across the tricuspid valve. The tip of the catheter is rotated so that it is inferior to the os of the coronary sinus and is then pulled back to the tricuspid annulus. RF energy is then applied as the catheter is slowly drawn back from the annulus to the inferior vena cava (moving it a few millimeters every 30 seconds or so). The linear lesion thus

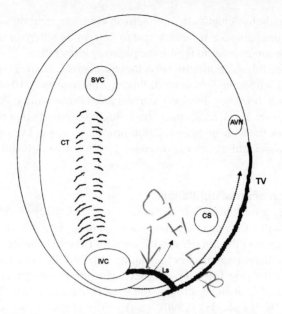

Figure 8.13 Placement of the lesion for the ablation of atrial flutter. The anatomic features shown here are the same as in Figure 8.12. The ablation lesion (the dark line indicated by "Ls") is depicted. This lesion transects the isthmus between the IVC and the tricuspid annulus, blocking the pathway necessary for typical atrial flutter. See text for details.

created must produce a complete electrical blockade between the inferior vena cava and the tricuspid annulus—even a minute discontinuity in the line of block will permit atrial flutter to continue. Complete electrical blockade is confirmed by pacing the atrium immediately adjacent to the line of block and confirming that the resultant atrial activation on the opposite side of the line of block is late. This indicates that the wave of depolarization must proceed around the entire right atrium to the opposite side of the line of block.

Some forms of atrial flutter are atypical—while they are still macroreentrant in nature, their reentrant circuits follow pathways other than the typical one described in Figure 8.12. Such atypical flutters are most often seen in patients who have had prior cardiac surgery and who have surgical scars in the atrium. In these cases, the scar (instead of the crista terminalis) serves as the line of block around which atrial flutter becomes established. The challenge to the electrophysiologist attempting to ablate these arrhythmias is to define the pathway of reentry and to determine where to make a linear lesion in order to render the pathway inoperative.

Successful ablation can be achieved acutely in over 90% of patients who have typical atrial flutter. Approximately 10–20% of these will, however, develop recurrent atrial flutter during the next 1 or 2 years. These recurrences are thought to indicate that the linear block made during the ablation procedure was not quite complete. A second ablation procedure is often successful in these patients.

Ablation of atrial fibrillation

Ablating atrial fibrillation has been a major challenge to electrophysiologists for years, and, while a lot of progress has been made, especially over the last decade, it continues to be a challenge today.

Two different approaches to ablating atrial fibrillation have been used: destroying the substrate necessary for the propagation of atrial fibrillation and destroying the triggers that initiate atrial fibrillation. During the late 1990s, most of the emphasis was on the former; since the turn of the millennium, interest has clearly shifted toward the latter.

Destroying the substrate for atrial fibrillation

Atrial fibrillation is a reentrant arrhythmia quite unlike the "typical" reentrant arrhythmias we have been talking about so far in this book. Atrial fibrillation is not generated by a fixed, localized, and mappable reentrant circuit. Instead, it is caused by multiple reentrant wavefronts, moving haphazardly across the surface of the atria like a family of tornadoes—continuously colliding with each other, extinguishing each other, and spinning off new twisters. This conceptualization of atrial fibrillation is referred to as the "atrial wavefront" model.

Just as tornadoes are frequent on the uninterrupted expanse of the Great Plains but almost unheard of in the choppy terrain of the Rocky Mountains, atrial fibrillation occurs only when the atria present a large surface area of contiguous, electrically active tissue. This is why small animal hearts cannot be made to fibrillate. It is also why procedures that divide the large, contiguous atrial surface into smaller regions can eliminate atrial fibrillation.

The "maze" procedure does just this. In the initial surgical incarnation of the maze procedure, the surgeon produced a pattern of transmural incisions within the atria, creating a series of strategically placed linear scars that resemble a maze. These scars prevented the propagation of the wavefronts responsible for atrial fibrillation—just as a series of mountain ranges discourages the formation of tornadoes. While the original surgical-maze procedure was highly invasive and was associated with significant morbidity, it did indeed prevent the recurrence of atrial fibrillation. Less-invasive surgical-maze procedures are now being developed and employed with some success, using RF energy or cryolesions instead of transmural incisions, in order to minimize morbidity. In general, however, this approach is limited to patients who are already having open-heart surgery for some other purpose such as mitral valve replacement.

Still, the ability of the surgical-maze to prevent atrial fibrillation has provided strong evidence in favor of the atrial wavefront model for atrial fibrillation, and it has stimulated the effort to develop catheter-based maze procedures in order to duplicate the success of the surgical approach. As it turns out, seven discrete linear scars (three in the right atrium and four in the left atrium) can approximate the lesions created in the surgical-maze procedure.

Efforts to develop a catheter-maze procedure that can be performed safely and reliably have until now met with only limited success. The chief problem has been the difficulty of creating effective linear lesions with a catheter. These efforts, however, have clearly proven the potential of such a technique. A substantial proportion of patients who have had catheter-maze procedures to date (most of whom had refractory arrhythmias) have indeed been rendered free of atrial fibrillation. These procedures, however, have been exceedingly tedious and lengthy, and have resulted in significant morbidity (the chief problem being systemic embolization, as a result of catheters being placed in the left heart for extended periods of time). The catheter-maze procedure has by no means been abandoned, but many electrophysiologists who were initially excited about this approach have stopped using it, awaiting technologies and techniques that will allow it to be achieved more quickly, more safely, and more simply.

Destroying the triggers of atrial fibrillation

Largely because of the frustration that electrophysiologists have experienced in their attempts at the catheter-maze approach, the ablation of atrial fibrillation has shifted in recent years to an entirely different direction, namely eliminating the ectopic foci that trigger the arrhythmia.

The reasoning behind this approach is relatively simple. Atrial fibrillation may be an extremely complex reentrant arrhythmia, but it still *is* a reentrant arrhythmia—which means it must be initiated by a premature impulse. So why not eliminate the premature impulses that trigger it? The obvious advantage here is that, if the triggering ectopic foci can be identified, the ablation procedure becomes focal instead of general, and ablation of atrial fibrillation becomes much simpler.

Initial attempts at attacking the ectopic triggers of atrial fibrillation met with poor results, mainly because it is often quite difficult to identify and map spontaneous atrial ectopic beats during an electrophysiology study (ectopic beats being notoriously random in frequency). Eventually, however, studies were conducted in a selected series of patients who had frequent episodes of atrial fibrillation (so that triggers could be more easily evaluated). To everyone's surprise, it was learned that over 90% of the episodes of atrial fibrillation in these patients were triggered from ectopic beats originating in the pulmonary veins. Further, when these foci were ablated, most of these patients had no further atrial fibrillation during follow-up. Suddenly, the pulmonary veins became the main focus of the ablation of atrial fibrillation.

Subsequent studies have confirmed that a high proportion of patients with paroxysmal atrial fibrillation have ectopic foci in the pulmonary veins (especially the left and right superior pulmonary veins). Interest quickly shifted away from trying to identify, map, and ablate specific ectopic foci in patients with atrial fibrillation, toward performing empirical ablation in or around the pulmonary veins in these patients.

After several years of trial-and-error attempts, it seems now to be well established that achieving complete electrical isolation of the pulmonary veins is much more effective in preventing atrial fibrillation than the selective ablation of specific ectopic foci. Such complete electrical isolation implies either making four complete, circumferential lesions around the opening of the four pulmonary veins or creating one circumferential lesion that encompasses all four veins.

Several techniques have been developed (and are still being developed) for achieving complete electrical isolation of the pulmonary veins. The most promising of these involve catheters that are designed to generate circumferential lesions, using one of several different energy sources and guided either by echocardiography or by newer mapping techniques, such as electromagnetic or noncontact mapping (see next section).

Using the most advanced techniques, in experienced hands electrical isolation of the four pulmonary veins in selected patients with paroxysmal atrial fibrillation has yielded success rates (i.e. a "cure" of or significant reduction in atrial fibrillation) in excess of 80%. A substantial minority of patients, however, end up with a unique form of atrial flutter—localized to the left atrium—following these procedures. Some electrophysiologists have taken to routinely "adding" a linear lesion extending from one of the inferior pulmonary veins to the mitral valve annulus after pulmonary vein isolation, just to prevent such an arrhythmia.

Obviously, the odds of success in ablating paroxysmal atrial fibrillation in this way depend on whether complete pulmonary vein electrical isolation is achieved, in patients whose triggers for atrial fibrillation are isolated to the pulmonary veins. In the best of circumstances, the success rate in preventing atrial fibrillation is not likely to greatly exceed 90% using pulmonary vein isolation alone, since between 5 and 10% of patients with paroxysmal atrial fibrillation have ectopic foci elsewhere in the heart (the superior vena cava is the next most common location). Further, while pulmonary vein isolation seems to work reasonably well in patients with paroxysmal episodes of atrial fibrillation, patients with more persistent forms of atrial fibrillation commonly have multiple ectopic sources in several locations other than the pulmonary veins, and the success rate with pulmonary vein isolation is correspondingly much lower. In other words, this is mainly a procedure for patients with paroxysmal atrial fibrillation.

Systemic embolization remains a risk of pulmonary vein isolation, although its incidence appears to be much less than with the catheter-maze approach. Pulmonary vein stenosis is a potentially devastating complication of pulmonary vein isolation—its onset can be relatively subtle, and it can be quite difficult to manage. With more advanced techniques for creating circumferential pulmonary vein lesions safely and reliably, pulmonary vein stenosis should become largely avoidable.

Chapter 6 examines the overall management of atrial fibrillation, including a discussion of when ablation might be a good option.

Ablation of reentrant ventricular tachycardias

Ablation of reentrant ventricular arrhythmias is based on the assumption that these arrhythmias have as their origin a fixed, discretely located, reentrant circuit, and that the arrhythmia can be cured if that circuit can be localized and ablated.

Mapping ventricular reentrant circuits

The localization of reentrant circuits within the ventricle can usually be accomplished using one or more of several methods: seeking areas of early ventricular activation; seeking areas of slow, fractionated conduction; pace-mapping; and entrainment.

As noted in Chapter 7, reentrant ventricular tachycardia is generally possible only when areas within the ventricular muscle become damaged, either from a myocardial infarction or from some other disease process that produces fibrosis within the ventricular myocardium. These damaged areas provide the substrate for the multiple pathways and the slow conduction that are necessary to sustain reentry.

During reentrant ventricular tachycardia, the earliest portion of the QRS complex is generally assumed to arise from the exit point of the electrical impulse as it leaves the damaged area of slow conduction and begins depolarizing normal ventricular myocardium. By recording localized electrograms during ventricular tachycardia, the earliest site of ventricular activation can be assumed to be near the "exit point" of the reentrant circuit. This technique is called "activation mapping," and is the one used most frequently in ablating ventricular tachycardia. Ideally, a localized "presystolic" signal, one that is inscribed before the onset of the surface QRS complex, indicates a critical area of the reentrant circuit itself and can pinpoint an appropriate area for ablation (Figure 8.14).

To perform such activation mapping, the following conditions should be fulfilled. First, the arrhythmia should be monomorphic ventricular tachycardia. Polymorphic arrhythmias are extremely difficult to localize because complexes of different morphologies likely have various exit points and thus tend to map to different areas. Ventricular fibrillation is impossible to localize because it is not a localized arrhythmia—it is more proper to visualize it, as in atrial fibrillation, as a series of tornadoes moving across the myocardial surface. Second, the tachycardia should be relatively slow, because for tachycardias in excess of 220 beats/min it is virtually impossible to distinguish the QRS complex from the T wave, so distinguishing the "onset" of the QRS complex becomes impossible. Third, the patient should ideally have only one type of ventricular tachycardia, because tachycardias of various morphologies tend to imply multiple reentrant circuits. Fourth, when transcatheter ablation is to be used, the patient should be able to tolerate ventricular tachycardia sufficiently to allow mapping to proceed. Fifth, the patient should ideally have a discrete myocardial scar rather than a

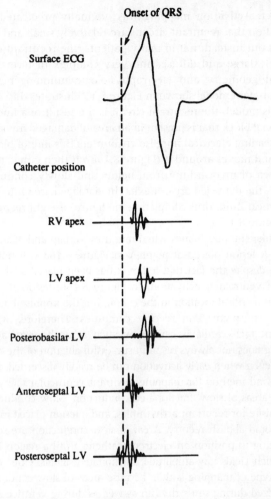

Figure 8.14 Mapping of ventricular tachycardia. By recording intracardiac electrograms from multiple ventricular positions during sustained ventricular tachycardia, the earliest site of ventricular activation is sought (in this example, in the posteroseptal left ventricle). In most individuals, the earliest site of activation corresponds to the location of the reentrant circuit. LV, left ventricle; RV, right ventricle.

diffuse cardiomyopathy. In this latter condition, the results of trans-catheter ablations have been poor.

Even if all these features are present, activation mapping is not always successful, probably because the basic assumptions that make activation mapping an attractive approach are sometimes incorrect. Activation mapping was originally predicated on the assumption that reentrant circuits are relatively small and discrete. It turns out instead that in many patients, the reentrant circuit is relatively large and diffuse, and very complex in terms of both physical geometry and electrophysiologic inhomogeneity. The figure-of-eight model shown in Figure 8.15 illustrates this.

In this model, the reentrant circuit is the result of a line of unidirectional block that is present in an area of damaged myocardium. The spreading electrical impulse encounters this line of block from above and moves around it (Figure 8.15a). It then enters the damaged area of myocardium from below and slowly conducts back through the damaged area. It exits the damaged area into the normal myocardium, thus completing the figure-of-eight reentrant circuit (Figure 8.15b).

Consider the possibilities when one tries to map and ablate such a circuit. A lesion placed at point A in Figure 8.16a will not abolish reentry, despite the fact that lesion A has been placed at the earliest point of ventricular activation. In Figure 8.16b, lesion B has been placed at a critical location in the circuit, but the impulse has found a second exit point, and reentry continues. Therefore, when the reentrant tachycardia is caused by such a mechanism, activation mapping does not always result in successful ablation of the reentrant circuit, even when early activation can be readily discerned.

A second method for mapping reentrant ventricular tachycardia is to seek areas of slow, fractionated conduction. Slow conduction is a prerequisite for reentrant arrhythmias, and a lesion placed in such an area should abolish reentry. Areas of slow conduction are sought by attempting to position an electrode catheter until a region is identified which yields low-amplitude, fractionated signals. One advantage to this type of mapping is that, because areas of slow conduction are depolarized during sinus rhythm as well as during ventricular tachycardia, mapping can sometimes be conducted during sinus rhythm.

One of the major problems with mapping areas of slow conduction is illustrated in Figure 8.17. The figure-of-eight reentrant impulse enters the area of damaged myocardium at several points, each of which yields electrograms showing low-amplitude, fractionated activity. Yet, because most of these areas do not participate in the reentrant circuit, lesions placed in them do not interrupt the circuit, and reentry continues (lesions A through D). Only lesion E abolishes reentry in this figure.

A third method of mapping reentrant ventricular tachycardia is pace mapping. With pace mapping, a 12-lead ECG is recorded while

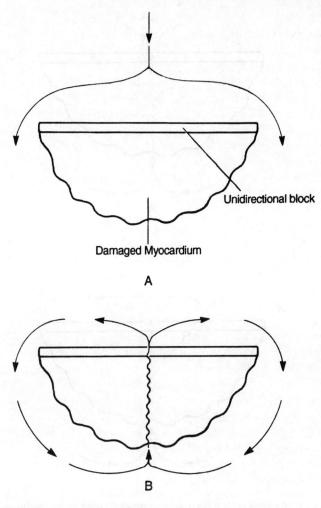

Figure 8.15 The figure-of-eight model of ventricular tachycardia. Substantial evidence now indicates that reentrant ventricular tachycardia operates according to this mechanism in many patients. This fact probably accounts for the difficulty electrophysiologists have had in performing successful transcatheter ablation of ventricular tachycardia. (a) A patch of damaged myocardium that is protected in the antegrade direction by a line of unidirectional block. An electrical impulse encountering this line of block is forced around the periphery of the damaged area. (b) The completed reentrant circuit. The electrical impulse enters the damaged area from the retrograde direction. After conducting slowly through the damaged myocardium, it exits back into normal tissue, thus completing the circuit.

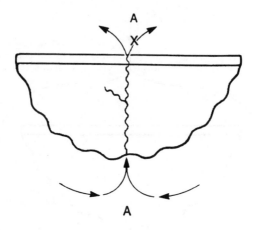

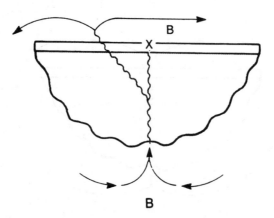

Figure 8.16 Why activation mapping may not lead to successful ablation of ventricular tachycardia. In this figure, activation mapping has successfully identified the point of "exit" from the area of damaged myocardium, and attempts at transcatheter ablation are performed (in this and the next figure, ablation lesions are denoted by "X"). In (a), the lesion that has been created is extremely close to the exit point (lesion A), but yet has not been placed in an area critical to the reentrant circuit. In (b), the precise exit point has been ablated (lesion B). Although this lesion has successfully abolished the original reentrant pathway, a second exit point has now appeared, and ventricular tachycardia (probably with a somewhat different morphology) remains.

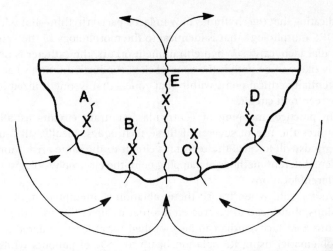

Figure 8.17 Why mapping areas of slow conduction may not lead to successful ablation of ventricular tachycardia. The circulating wavefront enters the damaged myocardium at several points, creating multiple areas that will show localized slow conduction. However, lesions placed at points A through D ablate areas of "bystander slow conduction" and do not affect the reentrant circuit. Only lesion E has the potential to ablate the arrhythmia.

pacing from various locations within the ventricle at approximately the same rate as that of the patient's ventricular tachycardia, in order to seek a location that exactly reproduces the QRS morphology seen during ventricular tachycardia. The assumption is that such sites are near the exit point of the reentrant circuit. Pace mapping often yields locations different from those obtained during activation mapping. As with activation mapping, however, pace mapping can yield points such as that shown in Figure 8.16a—these points may be near the exit point but not in a critical area of the circuit itself.

Entrainment mapping is a variation of pace mapping. The idea is to pace from various areas within the ventricle during sustained ventricular tachycardia, at a cycle length slightly shorter than that of the tachycardia. If the pacing catheter is located within the zone of slow conduction, entrainment can often be accomplished. Because conduction within the zone of slow conduction is usually functionally unidirectional (i.e. "retrograde" conduction does not occur in this zone), the pacing impulse will tend to exit the slow zone at the same point at which the reentrant impulse exits. The electrophysiologist observes an increase in the rate of the ventricular tachycardia during entrainment—equal to the rate of pacing, indicating that the rhythm is now in fact a paced rhythm—but with a QRS morphology that is identical to the morphology of the ventricular tachycardia. When entrainment occurs, the catheter is not only likely to be within the zone of slow conduction, but also at a potentially critical point within that zone—that is, one utilized by the reentrant circuit.

In practice, mapping of ventricular reentrant circuits usually requires the use of several of these techniques. Ideally, all four methods will localize the reentrant circuit to the same area. More often, different methods of mapping point the electrophysiologist to different locations.

As a result, when transcatheter ablation is attempted, multiple lesions often need to be created in order to affect the arrhythmia. Ventricular tachycardia can be abolished (or at least rendered less problematic) using RF ablation in up to 75% of patients whose arrhythmias and underlying cardiac disease are "ideal" for ablation. The rate of success falls off dramatically if the arrhythmia is not ideally suited for ablation. The morbidity of RF ablation of ventricular tachycardia appears to be relatively low, especially when compared to surgical ablation, but few large series have been published, and techniques are evolving so rapidly that published series may not reflect the current practice.

Unfortunately, many ventricular tachycardias are not ideal for ablation. In addition to lacking the "ideal" characteristics listed above, many reentrant ventricular arrhythmias are located in areas that are largely inaccessible to endocardial mapping. These areas include the mid-myocardial and subepicardial regions, and the intraseptal areas (all of which are difficult to localize endocardially, and may not be affected by endocardial RF applications).

During surgical ablation of ventricular tachycardia, the same principles of mapping are used, with the exception of pace mapping (because the open and distorted ventricle is unlikely to yield morphologies during pacing that reflect the clinical arrhythmia). Although precise intraoperative mapping is possible, in practice very large surgical lesions are usually created, mainly because one does not expect to have a second chance to surgically ablate ventricular tachycardia. One thus tends to err on the side of creating overly generous rather than overly fastidious lesions. Surgical "cures" of ventricular tachycardia are seen in up to 80% of carefully selected patients (generally patients with discrete anterior ventricular aneurysms and ideal arrhythmias). The major problem with surgical ablation of ventricular tachycardia is the perioperative mortality (usually reported as being between 5 and 15%) and morbidity.

As with atrial tachycardias, activation mapping of ventricular tachycardia is markedly enhanced when using the modern, computerized activation mapping systems discussed later in this chapter.

Ablation of unusual ventricular tachycardias

In Chapter 7, we mentioned several unusual types of ventricular tachycardia that do not fit neatly into the standard classifications of ventricular arrhythmias. As it turns out, at least three of these unusual ventricular tachycardias are often amenable to RF ablation—right ventricular outflow tract tachycardia, idiopathic left ventricular tachycardia, and bundle branch reentrant tachycardia.

Right ventricular outflow tract tachycardia

Right ventricular outflow tract tachycardia, an arrhythmia often seen in young patients with apparently normal hearts, is characterized by its LBBB configuration with a relatively narrow QRS complex (usually less than 140 msec). It often presents as repetitive monomorphic ventricular tachycardia (i.e. as extremely frequent nonsustained ventricular tachycardia).

This tachycardia originates in the right ventricular outflow area, usually just proximal to the pulmonic valve. The arrhythmia is generally not inducible with programmed pacing but can often be induced with an isoproterenol infusion. If so, activation mapping can be performed. Otherwise, pace mapping is necessary. Fortunately, because these tachycardias are quite focal in origin, pacing from the site of tachycardia produces a QRS complex that is identical to the clinical arrhythmia. Pace mapping thus tends to be much more reliable for this arrhythmia than for typical reentrant ventricular tachycardia.

Successful ablation of right ventricular outflow tract tachycardia can be achieved in over 95% of patients presenting with this arrhythmia. Complications are rare but include perforation of the right ventricle and the production of occlusive lesions in coronary arteries overlying the site of ablation. Both of these complications are related to the fact that the right ventricle is a very thin-walled structure, and both can probably be reduced in frequency by monitoring temperature during RF ablation.

Idiopathic left ventricular tachycardia

Idiopathic left ventricular tachycardia, also called left posteroseptal tachycardia, is a verapamil-sensitive arrhythmia originating in the posteroapical aspect of the left ventricular septum, in the region of the left posterior fascicle. The arrhythmia displays a right bundle branch morphology with left axis deviation. It is also seen in patients who have otherwise normal hearts.

Ablation is conducted by performing activation mapping in the distal left ventricular septum. At the site of earliest ventricular activation, the ventricular deflection is preceded (by up to 40 msec) by a distinct "fascicular" potential that resembles a His potential.

Successful ablation can be performed in approximately 75–80% of patients with idiopathic left ventricular tachycardia.

Bundle branch reentrant tachycardia

Bundle branch reentrant tachycardia, as opposed to the other forms of readily ablatable ventricular tachycardia, does not occur in patients who have otherwise "normal" ventricles. Patients with sustained bundle branch reentry generally have underlying nonischemic dilated cardiomyopathy that is relatively severe, and also have intraventricular conduction defects on their electrocardiograms. The arrhythmia is rapid, usually symptomatic (often presenting with syncope or cardiac arrest), and is most often of left bundle branch morphology.

The reentrant circuit uses one bundle branch (usually the right bundle branch) in the antegrade direction and the other bundle branch (usually the left) in the retrograde direction (Figure 8.18). Establishing a sustained bundle branch reentrant tachycardia requires a conduction delay within the bundle branches (and thus intrinsic conduction system disease). Thus, bundle branch reentry should be suspected in patients with nonischemic cardiomyopathy and intraventricular conduction delays on their 12-lead ECGs who present with ventricular tachycardia that has left bundle branch morphology.

During the electrophysiology study, each QRS complex of the tachycardia is preceded by a His bundle deflection. The HV interval during tachycardia may be the same as, slightly longer than, or slightly shorter than that during sinus rhythm, depending on the site of the recording catheter and the conduction velocity in the right bundle branch during the tachycardia. AV dissociation is usually present during bundle branch reentrant tachycardia.

During this tachycardia, the interval between the His deflection and the right bundle branch deflection is usually shorter than that during sinus rhythm. This finding helps to differentiate bundle branch reentry from supraventricular tachycardias with aberrancy (in which the His–right bundle deflection is normal or prolonged).

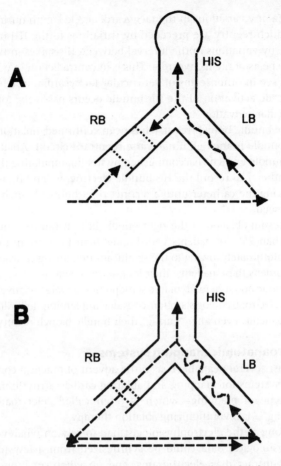

Figure 8.18 Bundle branch reentry. The His bundle and right and left bundle branches are depicted. Sustained bundle branch reentrant tachycardia requires intrinsic conduction delay in the bundle branches, most often manifested by an intraventricular conduction delay on the ECG. In (a), a premature ventricular impulse blocks retrogradely in the right bundle branch (RB), then conducts up the left bundle branch (LB), but finds the RB still refractory in the antegrade direction. Bundle branch reentry is thus not established. A more appropriately timed premature impulse (b) might encounter very slow retrograde conduction up the LB, so that antegrade penetration of the RB is now possible. A sustained reentrant arrhythmia using the RB antegradely and the LB retrogradely is now established. The resultant ventricular tachycardia will have an LBBB configuration.

Further, any variations in the tachycardia cycle length during bundle branch reentry are preceded by variations in the HH interval; that is, by variations in the interval between His spikes in two successive beats of the tachycardia. This is in contradiction to what one would see in other forms of ventricular tachycardia, in which the retrograde activation of the His bundle occurs passively, following ventricular activation.

Once bundle branch reentry has been confirmed, ablation of the right bundle branch eliminates the reentrant circuit. Ablating the right bundle branch is accomplished by first manipulating the ablation catheter to record the His bundle electrogram and then slowly advancing the catheter until a distinct right bundle branch deflection is seen.

Successful ablation of the right bundle branch can be achieved in more than 95% of patients with bundle branch reentrant tachycardia. Unfortunately, owing to the significant underlying cardiac disease that burdens these patients, their long-term prognosis—from both an arrhythmic and a hemodynamic standpoint—remains relatively poor. Many electrophysiologists often consider implanting defibrillators in these patients, even after "curing" their bundle branch reentry.

Electroanatomic mapping systems

The past several years have seen the advent of practical computer-based systems for mapping and ablating cardiac arrhythmias. This new type of mapping—which is often called "electroanatomic mapping"—is revolutionizing ablation therapy.

As long as the electrophysiologist had to rely on whatever electrophysiological data could be synthesized from a few (or even many) intracardiac electrograms, and on whatever limited anatomic data could be discerned from fluoroscopic images, ablation procedures generally had to be limited to treating the simpler arrhythmias, such as AV nodal reentry, or arrhythmias mediated by AV bypass tracts.

Electroanatomic mapping breaks both informational barriers—the electrophysiologic and the anatomic—to successful ablation. These new mapping systems allow detailed, three-dimensional maps to be constructed for an entire cardiac chamber (or chambers), which can show how the electrical impulse propagates across the heart, and where there might be areas of ectopic origin, areas of slow conduction, and areas of low voltage (i.e. scar). The 3D display delineates both electrical activation and critical anatomic landmarks (such as blood vessels and valves). The 3D maps are usually detailed enough that, once they are constructed, any further catheter maneuvering within the mapped cardiac chamber can often be accomplished without fluoroscopy.

Electroanatomic mapping permits the electrophysiologist to see the details of complex reentrant arrhythmias and to identify specific anatomic areas—such as regions of slow conduction or scarring—which may be good targets for ablating reentrant arrhythmias. The origin of ectopic arrhythmias can be readily identified and pinpointed. Some systems allow for detailed mapping even when arrhythmias are nonsustained, very rapid, or otherwise unsuitable for typical mapping procedures.

These new mapping systems are especially helpful for mapping and ablating those "nonsimple" arrhythmias that are extremely difficult or impossible with more traditional ablation procedures. Chief among these is atrial fibrillation.

Successful ablation of atrial fibrillation usually requires producing complete electrical isolation of the pulmonary veins, and in many cases also the ablation of ectopic foci. Because left atrial anatomy is so variable (with frequent variations in the number and sites of pulmonary veins, and numerous unexpected pits and ridges), it is extremely difficult to effectively isolate the pulmonary veins without a detailed anatomic map of the left atrium. By providing the electrophysiologist with that detailed anatomy and the means to maneuver within it, and by providing a mechanism for mapping any remaining atrial ectopic foci, electroanatomic mapping makes the ablation of atrial fibrillation feasible in many more patients than it has ever been before.

Several electroanatomic mapping systems are now available. None are without limitations. We will briefly discuss the three systems which are in broadest use, and compare their relative advantages and disadvantages.

CARTO mapping system (Biosense Webster)—magnetic field mapping

The CARTO mapping system uses a magnetic field to create a 3D, color-coded image of the cardiac chambers. The magnetic field is generated from a three-coil locator pad mounted beneath the catheterization table. The specialized mapping catheter used with the CARTO system (a flexible-tip quadripolar RF ablation catheter) itself contains a magnet at the distal tip, which can sense the field strength from each of the three magnetic coils. The precise location of the catheter tip can then be triangulated in real time, and the position of the catheter within the 3D image of the relevant cardiac chamber can be continuously displayed.

Because the maps made with the CARTO system are dependent on the patient's location, they can become inaccurate if the patient moves. To mitigate this issue, a special electrode is placed directly on the patient's back as a location reference. The mapping system records the original location of this location reference, so that if the patient moves (or the electrode is displaced) the original position can be found again.

It is also important to establish a timing reference, to use as "time zero" for gating the electrical signal from the mapping catheter. This is done by placing an electrode catheter in a stable position (usually in the coronary sinus).

Once everything is in place, the mapping catheter is advanced to the cardiac chamber of interest, and an electroanatomic map is generated. This is accomplished by slowly moving the mapping catheter across the endocardial surface and acquiring and processing both anatomic and electrical data from multiple points. This is called "point-to-point mapping." In the resultant map (which is continuously updated as the point-to-point mapping proceeds), the electrical data are superimposed on the anatomic map, in a color-coded fashion. These electrical data can be displayed in multiple ways—as an activation map, a dynamic propagation map, or a voltage map. Important anatomic features (such as valve rings, blood vessels, and the His bundle) can be labeled on the map. The maps can be viewed in virtually any projection.

Care must be taken in generating the map, so that all the key landmarks of the chamber of interest are identified. For instance, in mapping the right atrium, the operator usually begins by advancing the mapping catheter to the superior vena cava under fluoroscopy and, while directing the tip along the lateral wall, withdrawing it to the junction of the superior vena cava and the high right atrium. A point is acquired there. Then the catheter is slowly withdrawn down the lateral wall of the right atrium to the inferior vena cava, acquiring points every centimeter or so. The catheter is then advanced back up to the superior vena cava, and point-to-point mapping is conducted down the length of the posterior and anterior walls of the right atrium. Particular care is taken to identify points at the superior vena cava/RA junction, the inferior vena cava/RA junction, the coronary sinus ostium, and, with multiple points, the His bundle. The more points are acquired, the more detailed the electroanatomic map.

A similar procedure—dragging the mapping catheter across the surface of the endocardium to acquire numerous anatomic and electrical points throughout the chamber—is used to draw the electroanatomic maps for the other three cardiac chambers. Generally, this detailed mapping is done only for the cardiac chambers which are important in ablating the target arrhythmia.

In right ventricular mapping, key anatomic points that need to be identified are the right ventricular apex, several points in the right ventricular infundibulum near the hinge of the pulmonic valve, and the diaphragmatic aspect of the ventricle just beneath the mural leaflet of the tricuspid valve.

In left atrial mapping, key anatomic points include several locations along the mitral annulus and (especially if ablating atrial fibrillation is the goal) all of the pulmonary veins.

In left ventricular mapping, key anatomic points include the left ventricular apex, several points in the aortic outflow tract below the aortic valve, and the diaphragmatic wall of the ventricle, below the mitral annulus.

In most cases it will be important to create the electroanatomic map after inducing the arrhythmia of interest, so that cardiac activation can be observed during the arrhythmia. When superimposed on the anatomic image, activation maps acquired during the arrhythmia should allow the confirmation of the mechanism of the arrhythmia and the identification of targets for ablation.

In ablating atrial fibrillation, on the other hand, the emphasis is on the anatomy, and not on electrical activation. Because the anatomy of the left atrium is so variable, a very detailed anatomic image is sometimes necessary in order to adequately isolate the pulmonary veins. To assist in producing this detailed anatomy, the CARTO system allows the integration of the electroanatomic map with an image of the heart previously obtained using CT scanning or MRI. The CARTO system also makes available a module that superimposes the electroanatomic map on to an image derived from intracardiac echocardiography. With such anatomic tools, placement of lesions to isolate the pulmonary veins can often be carried out with remarkable precision.

The chief disadvantages of the CARTO system are that it requires the use of an expensive, proprietary, single-use mapping/ablation catheter; the point-to-point mapping required to generate the electroanatomic image can be tedious; and it is sensitive to patient movement (such that if the patient shifts position, the mapping may need to be repeated).

EnSite NavX system (St Jude Medical)—electrical field mapping

The Ensite NavX system is in many ways quite similar to the CARTO system. The main difference is that while the CARTO system uses a magnetic field to triangulate the precise real-time position of the mapping catheter, NavX uses an electrical field (specifically, the voltage and impedance recorded at an electrode within an electrical field) to do the same thing. This electrical field is generated by applying a low-level current through three skin patches placed on the patient's body in an orthogonal orientation.

The chief advantage of mapping by means of an electrical field is that the NavX system is compatible with any mapping/ablation electrode catheter and does not require the use of a proprietary, magnet-containing mapping catheter. The NavX system can also be used to localize up to 12 catheters and 64 electrodes at a time. However, an intracavitary reference electrode must be in position during the procedure, and its position needs to be stable.

The NavX system constructs a detailed, 3D, color-coded electroanatomic map, quite similar to that generated by the CARTO system. Also like the CARTO system, it does so by employing point-to-point mapping; that is, by carefully maneuvering the mapping catheter across the endocardial surface of the cardiac chamber of interest. However, since multiple catheters with multiple electrodes can be used with the NavX system, potentially the flouroscopy time can be substantially reduced. Like CARTO, NavX can also import and integrate prior CT or MRI images to facilitate anatomy-based ablation procedures.

The disadvantages of the NavX system are that it requires point-to-point mapping in order to construct the electroanatomic image and that it is very sensitive to any movement in the intracavitary reference electrode. If the reference electrode moves, mapping usually needs to be repeated.

The chief advantages of the NavX system over the CARTO system are that any mapping catheter capable of RF ablation can be used and several mapping catheters can be employed at once.

EnSite Array system (St Jude Medical)—noncontact mapping

Because both the CARTO and the NavX systems require time-consuming point-to-point mapping to generate an electroanatomic map, neither of them is likely to be very useful in mapping arrhythmias that are hemodynamically unstable, difficult to induce, or nonsustained.

The EnSite Array system specifically addresses this problem. The EnSite Array uses a 64-electrode array on an inflatable balloon catheter to achieve high-density noncontact mapping of a cardiac chamber. A low-level current applied between an electrode at the tip of the balloon array catheter and two ring electrodes on its shaft is used to generate an anatomic image of the chamber. The balloon-array catheter is deployed in the appropriate cardiac chamber, and acts as a 64-electrode reference. A standard electrode catheter can then be swept around the chamber to establish the endocardial borders. Once this geometry is established, far-field electrical potentials are recorded, and 3360 "virtual" unipolar electrograms are created to generate an anatomic image of the chamber.

The image generated by the EnSite Array becomes inaccurate for anatomic positions which are more than 34 mm from the balloon array, so the anatomic details provided by this system are often inferior to those obtained with point-to-point mapping systems.

Within this anatomic image, any electrode catheter capable of RF ablation can be used as a mapping catheter. The real-time localization of the mapping electrode is accomplished by a current applied between the distal mapping electrode and the ring electrodes on the balloon array.

The major advantage of the EnSite Array system is that once the anatomic image is generated, a single cycle of an arrhythmia can be used to generate an activation map. So this system is suited to mapping nonsustained arrhythmias, including premature atrial and premature ventricular complexes, and arrhythmias that are hemodynamically poorly tolerated.

The chief disadvantages of the Ensite Array are that cardiac chambers which are too large or too small may yield inaccurate anatomic images, and in small cardiac chambers the presence of the balloon catheter may limit the maneuverability of the mapping catheter. The Array system is also generally inferior to the CARTO system and the NavX system for creating the detailed anatomic images necessary for the ablation of atrial fibrillation.

Table 8.2 lists the main characteristics, including the relative advantages and disadvantages, of these three types of electroanatomic mapping system.

Complications of RF ablation

RF ablation carries the same risks as a standard electrophysiology study (discussed in Chapter 4), plus the added risks related to performing the RF ablation itself.

Table 8.2 Comparison of three electroanatomic mapping systems

	CARTO	EnSite NavX	EnSite Array
Location method	Magnetic field	Electrical field	Electrical field
Mapping technique	Point-to-point	Point-to-point	Noncontact (balloon array)
Compatible with multiple mapping catheters and electrodes	No	Yes	Yes
Compatible with any electrode catheter	No (requires proprietary mapping catheter)	Yes	Yes
Sensitive to patient motion	Yes	No	No
Requires intracavitary reference electrode	No	Yes	Yes (balloon array)
Can integrate CT or MRI images	Yes	Yes	No
Can integrate intracardiac echocardio-graphy (ICE) images	Yes	No	No
Easy mapping of single beat or nonsustained arrhythmia	No	No	Yes
Major advantages	Accurate anatomic display, integrates CT or MRI images, integrates ICE	Accurate anatomic display, allows multiple mapping catheters, integrates CT or MRI image	Activation mapping on single beat

Major disadvantages	Proprietary single-use catheter, sensitive to patient motion, point-to-point mapping	Sensitive to movement of reference electrode, point-to-point mapping	Anatomic display can be inaccurate, mapping challenging in small cardiac chambers

The two most common of these are the risk of creating inadvertent, complete heart block (usually when ablating in proximity to the normal conducting system) and the risk of causing cardiac perforation and tamponade (usually when ablating from the atria, the right ventricle, or within the coronary sinus or other cardiac veins). These complications each occur in less than 2% of patients treated with RF ablation.

Even rarer complications include the creation of arrhythmogenic foci (uncommon, since RF energy tends to create homogeneous lesions); production of mitral or tricuspid regurgitation (when ablating at or near the valvular apparatus); systemic embolization (when mapping and ablating in the left heart); pulmonary vein stenosis (when ablating for atrial fibrillation); and the creation of fixed lesions within the coronary arteries.

The creation of fixed coronary artery lesions is apparently due to disruption of the media of the coronary artery when RF energy is applied to an adjacent area. Its true incidence is unknown, but it may be of more than passing concern when ablating within the coronary sinus or the cardiac veins. It has also been reported to occur when ablating in the right ventricular outflow area. The coronary artery lesions thus created tend to be silent and are therefore likely to be unrecognized, even though they may produce a significant degree of obstruction. It is likely that temperature-monitoring during ablation will be helpful in avoiding this problem. Its incidence and its long-term significance still need to be elucidated.

Overall, the risk associated with RF ablation is low. For arrhythmias that are life-threatening or significantly symptomatic, and that have a high probability of being successfully treated with RF ablation, this is an extremely attractive option. In the author's opinion, if a patient has an arrhythmia that is readily amenable to RF ablation then ablation should be strongly considered whenever daily antiarrhythmic drug therapy would otherwise be required.

9 Cardiac Resynchronization: Pacing Therapy for Heart Failure

Electrophysiologists have always been intrigued with the notion that, somehow, pacemakers can improve the function of the failing heart. When permanent pacemakers were first developed, many thought that they would be able to improve cardiac function in patients with heart failure simply by increasing the heart rate. Since cardiac output equals stroke volume times heart rate, they reasoned, pacing the heart a little faster ought to increase cardiac output. What they failed to realize (hemodynamics never being the strong suit of most electrophysiologists) was that the heart does not determine the cardiac output; the body does. The heart merely responds to the metabolic demands of the body. So, unless a patient is in overt low-output failure at rest, increasing the resting heart rate does not appreciably increase cardiac output. Instead, since the heart can only pump whatever volume of blood the body returns to it, the stroke volume falls; the cardiac output remains the same, only now at the cost of an increased heart rate and higher cardiac workload. If anything, patients with heart failure feel worse with pacemaker-induced rapid heart rates.

Then, a few years later, when dual-chambered pacemakers became available, many electrophysiologists decided to goose the other determinant of cardiac output—the stroke volume—by figuring out how to optimize the AV delay. This goal proved elusive. Attempts at optimizing the AV delay generated a confusion of literature—some experts proposing shorter AV delays, others proposing longer ones—that successfully boosted a few academic

Electrophysiologic Testing, Fifth Edition. Richard N. Fogoros.
© 2012 John Wiley & Sons, Ltd. Published 2012 by John Wiley & Sons, Ltd.

careers but not in any reliable way the cardiac function of patients with heart failure.

So we can readily understand why, when yet another attempt at improving heart failure with pacing therapy was proposed in the mid 1990s, it was initially viewed with great skepticism. This time, however, the pacing therapy worked.

Cardiac resynchronization therapy (CRT)

How it works

Cardiac resynchronization therapy (CRT), also referred to as biventricular pacing, is aimed at improving the disordered patterns of ventricular contraction—referred to as ventricular dyssynchrony—seen in some patients with heart failure. CRT is accomplished, in general, by pacing both ventricles simultaneously, thus improving the coordination of dyssynchronous left ventricular contraction.

CRT pacemakers have three pacing leads instead of two: a right atrial lead, a right ventricular lead, and a left ventricular lead. They work similarly to DDD pacemakers except for two things. First, with CRT pacing, *both* ventricles are paced instead of just the right ventricle. Second, biventricular pacing itself, rather than rate support, is the primary desired therapy—CRT pacemakers are thus programmed to pace virtually 100% of the time, under all conditions.

CRT pacemakers are used to correct ventricular dyssynchrony. Ventricular dyssynchrony is most obviously present in patients with wide QRS complexes. Since the QRS complex reflects the activation sequence of the ventricular muscle, a wide QRS complex indicates that the ventricles are being activated abnormally. Specifically, a bundle branch block implies that one ventricle is being activated before the other—that is, the ventricles are being activated sequentially instead of simultaneously.

This sort of ventricular dyssynchrony does not produce any noticeable hemodynamic consequences in people with otherwise normal hearts. But in patients with systolic dysfunction, ventricular dyssynchrony can produce enough inefficiency in ventricular contraction to cause or worsen symptoms of heart failure and, potentially, can exacerbate ventricular remodeling and a reduction in the ventricular ejection fraction. In these cases, by pacing both ventricles simultaneously one can often resynchronize ventricular contraction sufficiently to improve ventricular efficiency, reduce symptoms, and improve clinical outcomes.

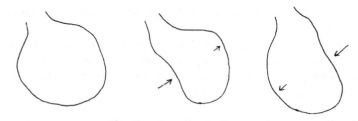

Figure 9.1 How ventricular dyssynchrony causes reduced ventricular function. The three panels in this figure illustrate ventricular systole in a patient with cardiomyopathy and LBBB. The panel on the left shows the dilated left ventricle at end-diastole. The middle panel shows the first 60 msec of systole. Here, the septum (which is activated along with the right ventricle) is already contracting, but the left ventricular free wall has not yet been activated. In fact, the free wall bulges outward. The panel on the right shows the last 60 msec of systole. The left ventricular free wall is now finally being activated, but now the septum, which has already finished contracting, is pushed outward. As a result of this dyssynchrony, with each systole much of the energy expended by this diseased ventricle is applied toward creating a useless, swaying, "hula"-type movement, instead of toward ejecting blood into the aorta.

Figure 9.1 illustrates how left ventricular dyssynchrony caused by left bundle branch block (LBBB) can affect ventricular function in a patient with heart failure. The panel on the left shows a dilated left ventricle at end-diastole. The middle panel shows the first 60 msec of systole. Here, the septum (which is activated along with the right ventricle) is already contracting, but the left ventricular free wall has not yet been activated (due to the bundle branch block). In fact, the left free wall bulges outward. The panel on the right shows the last 60 msec of systole. The left ventricular free wall has finally been activated and is contracting, but now the septum, which has already finished contracting, is pushed outward. As a result, with each systole, much of the precious energy being expended by this diseased ventricle is used to create a useless, swaying, "hula"-type movement, swishing blood around inside the cardiac chamber instead of ejecting it out into the aorta.

Figure 9.2 illustrates how CRT might benefit such a ventricle. The panel on the left again shows the same dilated left ventricle at end-diastole. The panel on the right shows what happens when biventricular pacing is activated. Here, the right and left ventricles are

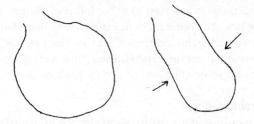

Figure 9.2 How biventricular pacing improves ventricular function. The two panels in this figure illustrate how biventricular pacing improves the function of the dyssynchronous, cardiomyopathic left ventricle illustrated in Figure 9.1. The panel on the left shows the dilated left ventricle at end-diastole. The panel on the right shows what happens when biventricular pacing is activated. Here, the right and left ventricles are paced simultaneously; both the septum and the left ventricular free wall contract at the same time. The energy expended by the ventricle now goes toward ejecting the blood, instead of merely swishing it around inside the cardiac chamber. Ventricular contraction becomes much more efficient and effective.

paced simultaneously; both the septum and the left ventricular free wall contract at the same time. The energy expended by the ventricle now goes toward ejecting blood. Ventricular contraction becomes much more efficient and effective.

Between 20 and 30% of patients with congestive heart failure have intraventricular conduction delays, and in most of these it is left ventricular activation that is delayed.

The effects of CRT
Several clinical studies have documented the benefits of CRT in appropriately selected patients.

Hemodynamic effects
CRT has consistently yielded improved hemodynamic function in patients with heart failure and LBBB, including improved cardiac output and cardiac index, increased aortic pulse pressure, and reduced pulmonary capillary wedge pressure.

Contractility
Measures of left ventricular contractility improve with CRT, including enhanced global contraction and increased left ventricular

ejection fractions. In contrast to other forms of therapy that have boosted ventricular contractility in patients with heart failure (such as the inotropic agents amrinone and milrinone), CRT actually *reduces* myocardial energy expenditures. Thus, ventricular contraction is not only more effective but also more efficient.

Reverse remodeling

Remodeling of the left ventricle—manifested by ventricular dilation, increased ventricular mass, and reduced ejection fraction—is a fundamental response to reduced systolic function. In essence, the cardiac enlargement that occurs with remodeling is a compensatory mechanism which allows the ventricle to eject a near-normal stroke volume despite reduced contractility. Aside from the fact that remodeling itself is ultimately harmful, the degree of remodeling reflects the degree of systolic dysfunction.

CRT has been demonstrated to reverse left ventricular remodeling. Specifically, it has been shown to reduce the end-systolic and end-diastolic dimensions of the left ventricle, as well as the left ventricular mass. This reverse remodeling is thought to reflect a fundamental improvement in ventricular systolic function.

Clinical studies with CRT

Numerous clinical trials have now been completed to assess the benefits of CRT in patients with heart failure due to systolic dysfunction. The results of these trials can be summarized as follows.

Patients with moderate to severe heart failure

The earliest clinical trials with CRT generally enrolled patients who had significant heart failure symptoms—generally, patients with NYHA class III or IV heart failure. In addition, these patients had QRS prolongation (at least 120–140 msec) and left ventricular ejection fractions of 0.35 or less. The major clinical trials in such patients are summarized in Table 9.1. In general, these trials strongly suggest that CRT in appropriately selected patients with severe heart failure can significantly reduce heart-failure mortality and hospitalizations, improve left ventricular ejection fractions, and improve quality of life.

In addition, a meta-analysis of 14 controlled, randomized trials that included over 1400 patients with moderate to severe heart failure has been published (McAlister FA *et al.*, JAMA 2007; 297:2502). This meta-analysis suggests that patients receiving CRT, when compared to optimal medical therapy, have a much higher chance of

Table 9.1 Major randomized trials with CRT in patients with moderate to severe heart failure due to systolic dysfunction and wide QRS complexes. These trials confirmed the effectiveness of CRT in improving functional capacity, quality of life, need for hospitalization, and survival. From the COMPANION trial, the addition of an ICD to CRT therapy greatly improves on the survival benefit seen with CRT alone

Study	Patient Population	Randomization	Results with CRT
MIRACLE[a]	435 pts, NYHA III, LVEF $\leq$ 0.35, QRS $\geq$ 130	BiV vs no BiV walk, NYHA class, LVEF, and reduced hospitalization	Improved 6-minute walk
MIRACLE ICD[b]	369 pts, same as for MIRACLE but with indication for ICD	BiV + ICD vs ICD alone, NYHA class, peak O_2 consumption, and exercise duration	Improved QOL
MUSTIC[c]	48 pts, NYHA III, QRS $\geq$ 150, no pacing indication	BiV vs no BiV for 3 months, then cross over for 3 months	Improved 6-minute walk, QOL, peak O_2 consumption, decreased hospitalization 85% of patients preferred BiV mode
COMPANION[d]	1520 pts, NYHA III–IV, LVEF $\leq$ 0.35, QRS $\geq$ 120, recent hospitalization for CHF	OPT vs BiV and vs BiV + ICD (1 : 2 : 2)	*BiV vs OPT*: significant 20% reduction in all-cause mortality or all-cause hospitalization; nonsignificant 24% reduction in mortality *BiV + ICD vs OPT*: significant 30% reduction in all-cause mortality or all-cause hospitalization; (continued)

Table 9.1 (*continued*)

Study	Patient Population	Randomization	Results with CRT
CARE-HF[e]	813 pts, NYHA III–IV, QRS ≥ 120	BiV vs no BiV	significant 36% reduction in all-cause mortality Significant reduction in death or hospitalization due to cardiovascular event (primary endpoint) Significant reduction in death from any cause (secondary endpoint)

BiV, biventricular pacing; BiV + ICD, CRT device that also has the functionality of an implantable defibrillator; LVEF, left ventricular ejection fraction; NYHA, New York Heart Association functional class; OPT, optimized pharmacological therapy; pts, patients; QOL, quality of life.
[a]Abraham WT *et al.*, N Engl J Med 2002; 346:1845.
[b]Young JB *et al.*, JAMA 2003; 289:2685.
[c]Linde C *et al.*, J Am Coll Cardiol 2002; 40:111.
[d]Bristow MR *et al.*, N Engl J Med 2004; 350:2140.
[e]Cleland JGF *et al.*, N Engl J Med 2005; 352:1539.

improving at least one NYHA class (59 vs 37%), a heart-failure hospitalization rate that is reduced by more than 35%, improved exercise capacity and quality-of-life measures, and reduced heart-failure mortality and overall mortality.

Patients with mild to moderate heart failure

Two major randomized clinical trials have now been published evaluating the effects of CRT in patients with systolic dysfunction and intraventricular conduction delays but who have only NYHA class I or II heart-failure symptoms.

The REVERSE trial (Linde C *et al.*, J Am Coll Cardiol 2008; 52:1834) enrolled 610 patients with NYHA class I or II heart failure,

QRS duration ≥120 msec, left ventricular ejection fraction <40%, and left ventricular end-diastolic diameters ≥55 mm. The patients all received CRT devices, but they were randomized as to who had biventricular pacing turned on or off. After 12 months, patients randomized to CRT had reduced hospitalizations and improved ejection fractions, but the proportion of patients who clinically worsened was not reduced by CRT pacing.

However, the 262 REVERSE patients who had been enrolled in Europe remained in their randomized pacing modes for 24 months, rather than 12. Among this subset of patients, clinical worsening was significantly reduced in those assigned to CRT pacing.

The MADIT-CRT trial (Moss AJ *et al.*, N Engl J Med 2009; 361:1329) compared ICD therapy to ICD combined with CRT pacing in 1820 NYHA class I or II patients who had reduced left ventricular ejection fractions (30% or lower) and QRS durations of at least 130 msec. After a follow-up averaging 29 months, those who received CRT pacing had a significant reduction in the primary endpoint, which was death from any cause or a nonfatal heart failure event—though the main benefit appears to have been a reduction in heart-failure episodes. In this trial, patients with LBBB and QRS duration >150 msec received the most benefit from CRT.

Indications for CRT
In general, CRT is indicated in patients who have heart failure from systolic dysfunction and significant ventricular dyssynchrony. Guidelines from medical societies to this point have defined "dyssyncrhony" solely by QRS duration, and different sets of guidelines have used different cutoffs for QRS duration.

Guidelines published in 2008 by the American College of Cardiology, American Heart Association, and Heart Rhythm Society (Epstein AE *et al.*, Circulation 2008; 117:e350) give the major indications for CRT as follows:

- CRT is recommended in patients in NYHA class III or IV, despite optimal medical therapy, who have left ventricular ejection fractions of 35% or less, and QRS durations of 120 msec or more.
- CRT is reasonable in patients in NYHA class III or IV, despite optimal medical therapy, who have left ventricular ejection fractions of 35% or less, and are largely dependent on ventricular pacing—whatever their native QRS duration might be.

- CRT can be considered in patients in NYHA class I or II, on optimal medical therapy, who have left ventricular ejection fractions of 35% or lower, who will be receiving a permanent pacemaker or ICD, and who are expected to require frequent ventricular pacing.

Guidelines published by medical societies have not yet taken into account the results of REVERSE and MADIT-CRT. However, considering the results of these trials, it seems reasonable to implant defibrillators that provide CRT pacing (referred to as CRT-D devices) in patients with NYHA class I or II heart failure, left ventricular ejection fractions of 30% or less, and QRS durations of 150 msec or more.

In fact, it ought to be noted that the vast majority of patients with an indication for CRT therapy will also have an indication for an implantable defibrillator; so the great majority of patients with heart failure who are candidates for CRT should receive CRT-D devices.

Implanting CRT devices

The only significant difference between implanting a CRT device and a pacemaker (or between implanting a CRT-D device and an ICD) is the need to place an additional lead for left ventricular pacing.

In the early days of CRT, left ventricular pacing was accomplished either with epicardial leads (requiring a limited thoracotomy) or with standard transvenous pacing leads—leads not designed for this purpose—placed into the coronary sinus. Left ventricular lead placement, in those days, was a lengthy, tedious, difficult, and often risky procedure. Nowadays, a variety of tools have been developed specifically for placement of specially designed pacing leads in the coronary venous system. These tools allow the electrophysiologist to rapidly and safely insert left ventricular pacing leads via the coronary sinus. In most cases, these leads can be placed, positioned, and tested in 30 minutes or less.

In placing left-sided leads, the os of the coronary sinus is generally first engaged with an introducer designed specifically for this purpose. Dye is injected to visualize the cardiac venous system. A "target" vein is identified. (Most patients seem to do best with CRT when the left-sided lead is placed in the mid-lateral left ventricle, so the operator looks for a vein that reaches that area.) A pacing lead is chosen whose handling characteristics are likely to suit the anatomy of the target vein, and is then inserted and positioned.

In testing the left-sided lead, the operator looks not only for adequate R wave voltage, pacing threshold, and impedance measurements, but also for evidence of diaphragmatic stimulation—the most common problem with pacing from the coronary veins. If diaphragmatic stimulation is seen, the lead needs to be repositioned. Coronary sinus leads are now available that can be "electronically repositioned" by changing the vector configurations of available electrodes. Diaphragmatic stimulation can usually be circumvented in this way without having to physically reposition the lead.

Coronary sinus perforation and subsequent pericardial tamponade is the most feared procedural complication unique to left-sided lead placement. Additional complications with CRT implantation include diaphragmatic pacing, pneumothorax, and infection.

Adequate placement of a left ventricular lead can be accomplished today via the coronary sinus approach in well over 90% of patients. Occasionally, however, pacing the left ventricle still requires an epicardial lead. Tools are being developed to make epicardial lead placement much less invasive and more reliable than it is today; it is likely that within several years, placing epicardial leads will be conducted routinely in the electrophysiology laboratory.

Unresolved issues with CRT

Responders versus nonresponders

From the very earliest days of CRT therapy, doctors took note of the fact that many patients with heart failure who received these devices had very dramatic responses. These patients improved rapidly from NYHA class III to I, or from class IV to II, and were able to accomplish physical tasks they had not been able to perform for months or years. These patients were exceedingly grateful for their new lease on life and, accordingly, the doctors were exceedingly gratified. Such patients were quickly deemed to be "responders." Roughly 40–60% of patients who receive indicated CRT devices for heart failure fall into this category.

Naturally, patients who did not have such dramatic improvements in well-being began to be regarded as "nonresponders." This designation is probably unfortunate.

The tendency to consider the lack of a dramatic response to CRT as equivalent to a lack of any meaningful response is shortsighted. It seems very unlikely that CRT will produce an "all-or-nothing" effect, where either patients have remarkable, raising-the-dead-style symptomatic improvement or no improvement at all. More likely, some patients are benefited by CRT in a more subtle way, such that, while they may not feel dramatically better, the "trajectory" of their illness improves, so that they have fewer hospitalizations over a given period of time or an improvement in mortality.

As it turns out, these more subtle benefits of CRT are the very benefits that the randomized trials (discussed earlier) were designed to measure. From these trials, the magnitude of over-all benefit to the population probably cannot be explained by the 40–60% of patients who (if the "responder"/ "nonresponder" parameter had been tabulated) would have been classified as "dramatic responders". For instance, in the CARE-HF study, mortality in the CRT group was reduced by 33%, a magnitude that would be very difficult to attribute to the 50% or so who likely responded "dramatically" to the therapy. More likely, this impressive benefit in CARE-HF was dis-tributed among both "dramatic responders" and "nondramatic responders."

And finally, evidence is accumulating that the more subtle mea-sures of CRT efficacy—such as reverse remodeling—may continue to improve for at least 12 months after CRT is initiated, even in so-called "nonresponders." This reverse remodeling suggests that some fundamental improvements in ventricular systolic function are occurring over time, and may be present whether or not a dramatic reduction in symptoms has been seen.

If we clinicians follow our understandable tendency to define "responders" by the presence or absence of a dramatic response to CRT, we will create unreasonable expectations on the parts of patients, payers, and ourselves. If we must identify certain individu-als as nonresponders, we at least ought to be circumspect about how we do so. We should define "nonresponder" in a way that allows for the more subtle but still substantial benefits of CRT. Doing so will improve our chances of actually figuring out how to maximize the benefits of CRT. It will also reduce the temptation we otherwise cre-ate for payers to withhold CRT from anyone who doesn't seem likely to turn cartwheels within 48 hours of implantation.

Optimization of CRT

Beyond the original notion that pacing the ventricles simulta-neously will help to resynchronize dyssynchronous ventricular contraction, relatively little has been accomplished so far in system-atically studying how the benefits of CRT might be optimized in each individual patient. Several methods for optimizing CRT have been proposed, and, if developed sufficiently, one or more of these might improve the overall benefits of CRT.

AV Interval

Despite the spotted history (described earlier) of AV-interval optimization in improving the hemodynamics of failing hearts, there is reason to believe that AV optimization may be an important factor in CRT.

Specifically, the chief concern is with the left atrial to left ventricular (LA–LV) interval. Since pacemakers—even CRT pacemakers—sense only the right (and not the left) atrial electrogram, any intraatrial conduction delay (i.e. a conduction delay from the right to the left atrium) is not taken into account. In other words, the "A" in "AV interval" comes from the right atrium—the left atrium is ignored. Therefore, in the setting of an intraatrial conduction delay, during CRT the programmed AV delay may result in an effective LA–LV interval that is "too short," such that left ventricular pacing may occur before left atrial contraction is completed. As a result, left ventricular stroke volume may be systematically reduced during CRT.

Whether this is more than a theoretical problem, and whether optimization of LA–LV intervals would improve the effects of CRT in some or all patients, has not been sufficiently studied. It is certainly one area of concern in the optimization of CRT.

VV Interval

Classically, CRT is accomplished by pacing the left ventricle simultaneously with right ventricular activation (or pacing). It may, however, be the case that different timing sequences between the two ventricles (the VV interval) would improve the efficacy of CRT in some patients. Data exist, for instance, suggesting that in some patients, pacing only the left ventricle (in advance of any right ventricular activation) might be better than biventricular pacing.

The VV interval ought to be viewed as a continuum of potential ventricular activation sequences, all the way from right-ventricular-only pacing (i.e. the pacing mode used in all "standard" pacemakers) to left-ventricular-only pacing. For all we know, the optimal VV interval may vary from patient to patient.

CRT devices exist today that allow the physician to vary the VV interval—but this feature is marketed with few instructions. The clinician has no objective guidance on how to choose the most appropriate VV interval. Systematic studies are needed to assess whether varying the VV intervals makes a substantial difference, and, if so, how exactly to optimize this parameter in individual patients.

Lead placement and lead number

When one stops to think about it, it begins to seem remarkable that we have seen such impressive results with CRT when positioning the left ventricular pacing leads "empirically," often in whichever location is most readily achievable.

Could the results of CRT be improved by objectively assessing which specific region within the left ventricle ought to be paced in each individual, and then taking pains to position the lead in the optimal spot? Some evidence exists (from MRI studies) suggesting that this may be so. Specifically, there may exist in at least some dyssynchronous left ventricles a "sweet spot"—generally the area of the left ventricle with the most delayed activation. Placing the pacing electrode in that spot might yield much better resynchronization than placing it just a few centimeters away. Perhaps some patients have more than one "sweet spot," and perhaps two or more left ventricular electrodes would need to be positioned, quite precisely, in order to truly optimize CRT. Optimal lead placement—and the optimal number of leads to use—is another area in need of systematic investigation.

Measuring dyssynchrony

The methodology we currently use to detect left ventricular dyssynchrony—looking for the presence or absence of an intraventricular conduction delay—is neither particularly sensitive nor specific. Substantial ventricular dyssynchrony can exist in the absence of an obvious conduction delay, and some patients with conduction delays may not have much dyssynchrony at all.

If CRT truly works by resynchronizing the contraction of a dyssynchronous left ventricle, then it seems obvious that to really optimize CRT we need to have an objective, reproducible way to measure dyssynchrony, both before and during CRT pacing. Unfortunately, we do not. Cardiac MRI shows much promise in this area but is not readily available—and it is problematic to perform MRI scans in patients with CRT devices. Tissue Doppler echocardiography (TDE) is also promising, but remains poorly standardized, and its results sometimes appear to be quite operator-dependent. Accordingly, in 2008 (Gorcsan J 3rd *et al.*, J Am Soc Echocardiogr 2008; 21:191) the American Society of Echocardiography (in what has to have been a painful process) released a consensus statement urging that patients who otherwise have an indication for CRT should *not* have CRT therapy withheld because of the results of an echocardiographic dyssynchrony study; and further, that echocardiography reports should *not* include a recommendation regarding whether CRT is likely to be beneficial or not.

While current methods fall short of the goal, the clinical need for a method of reproducibly measuring ventricular dyssynchrony has now been widely recognized. A lot of work currently aims at accomplishing this, and it is probably only a matter of time before this need is met. When that happens, we can expect improved tools for fully optimizing CRT to follow rapidly.

Should CRT be the standard mode of pacing?

If spontaneous LBBB produces ventricular dyssynchrony, and is thus detrimental to patients with systolic heart failure, then wouldn't iatrogenic LBBB created by right ventricular pacing also be detrimental to these patients? Is it really a good idea for patients who require pacing most or all of the time to have LBBB-inducing right ventricular pacing—especially patients with systolic dysfunction?

At least three trials suggest that chronic right ventricular pacing is detrimental in patients with systolic dysfunction. In the DAVID trial (Wilkoff BL *et al.*, JAMA 2002; 288:3115), patients who needed ICDs and who also had depressed left ventricular function were randomized to DDDR pacing with a lower rate limit of 70 beats/min (in order to increase the use of dual-chambered pacing) or to VVI pacing at a lower rate of 40 beats/min (to decrease the use of any pacing at all). The hypothesis of this study—which was initiated before CRT and its implications regarding ventricular dyssynchrony were widely known—was that chronic AV pacing would be beneficial in these patients. Instead, the investigators discovered the opposite. Patients randomized to frequent DDDR pacing had a significantly higher incidence of death or hospitalization for heart failure than patients randomized to minimal pacing. Most observers attribute these negative results to the dyssynchrony produced by almost constantly pacing the right ventricle in patients with underlying left ventricular dysfunction.

Similarly, the MOST trial (Sweeney MO *et al.*, Circulation 2003; 107:2932) examined clinical outcomes, using various pacing modes, in patients with sinus nodal dysfunction. In this trial, patients with higher cumulative percentages of right ventricular pacing also had more hospitalizations for heart failure.

Most telling of all is the PAVE trial (Doshi RN *et al.*, J Cardiovasc Electrophysiol 2005; 16:1160), in which 184 patients with atrial fibrillation and NYHA class II or III heart failure who received AV node ablation for rate control were randomized to standard RV pacing or to CRT pacing. Those who received CRT pacing had better 6-minute walking duration, better peak O_2 consumption during exercise, better exercise duration, and better preservation of left ventricular ejection fractions than those receiving standard right ventricular pacing. Subsequently, the US Food and Drug Administration approved CRT pacing for patients with NYHA class II or III heart failure and atrial fibrillation who undergo AV node ablation for rate control.

So what we have learned in the last few years is that CRT pacing is almost certainly superior to right ventricular pacing in patients with moderate heart failure who are likely to be in a paced rhythm all the time.

Whether CRT pacing would also yield more favorable long-term results even in patients who did not have systolic dysfunction is an intriguing question. In the PACE trial (Yu CM *et al.*, N Engl J Med 2009; 361:2123), 177 patients with normal ventricular function were randomized to RV pacing versus CRT pacing. At 12 months, those receiving CRT had significantly higher left ventricular ejection fractions and lower left ventricular end-systolic volumes than those receiving RV pacing.

However, in order for CRT pacemakers to be used routinely in patients who require pacing, we will need not only more clinical evidence to prove that CRT is significantly better than RV pacing in nearly all pacemaker-dependent patients, but also improvements in the ease and safety of implanting left-sided leads. Accordingly, several manufacturers of CRT pacemakers are working hard to improve the tools for placing left-sided leads.

10 The Evaluation of Syncope

The evaluation of patients with syncope (sudden transient loss of consciousness) has classically been difficult. This difficulty stems from the very nature of syncope itself: syncope occurs most often in a sporadic and relatively unpredictable fashion, and between episodes, patients with syncope often appear to be (and frequently are) quite normal.

For two reasons, electrophysiologists are now regularly involved in the evaluation of patients with syncope. First, cardiac arrhythmias are often either a direct cause or a prominent feature of syncope. Second, techniques developed in the electrophysiology laboratory have often proven helpful in revealing the etiology of syncope. In this chapter, we review the causes of syncope and discuss the evaluation of syncope in light of the lessons that have been learned in the electrophysiology laboratory over the past few decades.

Causes of syncope

Table 10.1 lists the major causes of syncope, divided into five major categories. Diagnosing syncope associated with the first four categories depends on taking a careful history and performing a careful physical examination. The majority of patients with syncope, however, fall into the fifth category: syncope associated with cardiac arrhythmias. In most cases, therefore, the clinician is left with having to assess whether the patient has syncope directly caused by cardiac arrhythmias (bradyarrhythmias or tachyarrhythmias) or a variant of vasodepressor syncope, in which bradycardia is often a prominent feature.

Electrophysiologic Testing, Fifth Edition. Richard N. Fogoros.
© 2012 John Wiley & Sons, Ltd. Published 2012 by John Wiley & Sons, Ltd.

Table 10.1 Major causes of syncope

Syncope from neurologic disorders	
Vertebrobasilar transient ischemic attacks	Normal pressure hydrocephalus
Subclavian steal syndrome	Seizure disorders
Syncope from metabolic disorders	
Hypoxia	Hyperventilation
Hypoglycemia	
Syncope from psychiatric disorders	
Panic disorders	Hysteria
Syncope from mechanical cardiac disease	
Aortic stenosis	Obstructive cardiomyopathy
Mitral stenosis	Left atrial myxoma
Pulmonary stenosis	Prosthetic valve dysfunction
Global ischemia	Pulmonary embolus
Aortic dissection	Pulmonary hypertension

Syncope associated with cardiac arrhythmias
Bradyarrhythmias—sinus node dysfunction, AV conduction disease
Tachyarrhythmias—supraventricular and ventricular tachyarrhythmias
Vasodepressor syncope

Bradyarrhythmias that cause syncope

Although bradyarrhythmias have been claimed as a common cause of syncope, they actually cause less than 5% of syncopal episodes. Nonetheless, bradyarrhythmias must be regarded as an important cause of syncope because they are always completely treatable. The evaluation of patients with bradyarrhythmias has been discussed in detail in Chapter 5. In this section, we review the causes and evaluation of bradyarrhythmias only briefly.

Sinus nodal dysfunction

Abnormalities of the sinus node are common in elderly patients and are most often caused by idiopathic fibrous degeneration of the sinus node. Sinus nodal dysfunction is frequently associated with a similar fibrous degeneration of the AV conduction system, producing AV block, or of the atrial tissue, producing atrial tachyarrhythmias. Although sinus nodal disease is most often benign, the potential for sudden death is real in patients whose sinus nodal dysfunction is severe enough to produce syncope.

In most patients with syncope due to sinus nodal dysfunction, abnormalities of the sinus node are overt, and are usually seen during simple cardiac monitoring. Occasionally, however, electrophysiologic testing is needed to diagnose sinus nodal dysfunction even in these patients. Therefore, electrophysiologic testing should be considered in patients with syncope when the etiology remains unknown after a full evaluation, especially in elderly patients.

AV block

On one hand, AV nodal disease is a rare cause of syncope. On the other, block in the His–Purkinje tissue is the most common cause of syncope due to bradyarrhythmias. When syncope is due to AV block, the ECG and cardiac monitoring most often reveal clues as to the etiology of syncope. Obviously, complete heart block in a patient presenting with syncope is an indication for pacing. Second-degree AV block should also be regarded as a strong clue. Even more subtle findings that can usually be safely ignored, such as intraventricular conduction disturbances or first-degree AV block, should be regarded with a high degree of suspicion in patients presenting with syncope. In such patients, electrophysiologic testing should be strongly considered, especially if no other etiology for syncope presents itself.

Tachyarrhythmias that cause syncope

Supraventricular tachycardias

Although supraventricular tachycardias are relatively frequent arrhythmias, they only rarely cause syncope. In most cases in which syncope is associated with supraventricular tachycardia, a second condition is responsible for it. Most commonly, this second condition is sinus nodal dysfunction. In a patient with sinus nodal dysfunction, supraventricular tachycardia (usually atrial fibrillation or flutter) causes exaggerated overdrive suppression of the diseased sinus node. When the arrhythmia terminates, there is a prolonged sinus pause, leading to loss of consciousness. Less commonly, syncope can accompany supraventricular tachycardias that occur without concomitant sinus nodal dysfunction. In these cases, recent evidence suggests that syncope is the result of a vasodepressor reflex, and that the tachycardia itself may simply be the triggering stimulus for the vasodepressor response that produces syncope.

When syncope is associated with supraventricular tachycardia, loss of consciousness is almost always preceded by a prominent and unambiguous sensation of palpitations. Such a history should lead the physician immediately to suspect tachycardia as an etiology.

Electrophysiologic testing should be considered early in the evaluation of such patients.

Ventricular tachyarrhythmias

Although ventricular arrhythmias were not generally recognized until the mid 1980s as a major cause of syncope, it is now apparent that these arrhythmias are frequently responsible for syncope, especially in patients with underlying cardiac disease. Ventricular tachycardia or fibrillation probably represents the cause of syncope in up to 40% of patients with heart disease who present with this symptom. Because syncope due to ventricular tachyarrhythmias is a sign of impending sudden death, the new onset of syncope in patients with significant underlying heart disease should be treated as a medical emergency.

Syncope caused by ventricular tachyarrhythmias usually occurs suddenly and without warning, although in some patients with sustained ventricular tachycardia the sensation of a rapid heart rate may precede loss of consciousness. The syncope can be quite fleeting, lasting only for moments, or it may present as dramatically as a self-terminating cardiac arrest. No other cause of syncope is likely to produce the type of pulseless, apneic, cyanotic patient produced by a ventricular arrhythmia. Many patients referred to electrophysiologists for syncope of unknown etiology are reclassified as having had an aborted cardiac arrest after careful interrogation of witnesses.

Because most ventricular tachyarrhythmias are reentrant in nature, and because most reentrant circuits require the substrate produced by myocardial fibrosis, ventricular arrhythmias are unlikely to be the cause of syncope unless a disorder of the ventricular myocardium is present. When such myocardial disease is present, however, ventricular arrhythmias must be considered as being the most likely cause of syncope until proven otherwise. When evaluating a patient with syncope of unknown etiology, one of the first questions the physician must answer is whether the patient has underlying cardiac disease. If so, the physician's focus must immediately shift away from merely preventing syncope and toward preventing sudden death.

Accordingly, if a careful history and physical examination do not yield the cause of syncope, a noninvasive cardiac workup to assess the status of the ventricular myocardium must be considered an essential part of the evaluation of the patient. If ventricular function is normal and there is no ventricular hypertrophy, ventricular arrhythmias can usually be dismissed as a cause for syncope. (The clinician, however, should also be mindful of the relatively uncommon forms of ventricular arrhythmia that can produce syncope in the absence of structural heart disease, including the long QT syndromes, Brugada syndrome, and catecholaminergic polymorphic ventricular tachycardia).

If the cardiac evaluation reveals segmental wall-motion abnormalities or a reduced left ventricular ejection fraction, potentially lethal ventricular arrhythmias must be strongly considered.

The signal-averaged ECG may also help to determine the likelihood that ventricular arrhythmias are the cause of a patient's syncope. The sensitivity of the signal-averaged ECG has generally been reported as being 73–89%, and the specificity as 89–100%, in predicting whether a patient presenting with syncope will have a positive electrophysiologic study.

Ambulatory monitoring should play a very small role in diagnosing ventricular arrhythmias as a cause of syncope, for three reasons. First, ventricular arrhythmias producing syncope are sporadic and unpredictable. The odds of capturing a syncope-producing ventricular arrhythmia while monitoring for a few days or a few weeks are small, and in a patient with underlying cardiac disease, the absence of such arrhythmias on ambulatory monitoring is meaningless. Second, the presence or absence of asymptomatic ventricular ectopy in such patients has extremely small specificity (so finding ectopy on ambulatory monitoring does not bring the clinician any closer to making a diagnosis). Third, once a patient with significant underlying heart disease has syncope of unclear origin, that patient must be presumed to be in imminent danger of sudden death, and the time for leisurely outpatient monitoring has passed. The patient should be evaluated as if he or she had suffered not "just" syncope, but an aborted cardiac arrest.

Once it has been determined that ventricular arrhythmias are reasonably likely to be the cause of a patient's syncope, that patient should immediately be admitted to a monitored bed until lethal ventricular tachyarrhythmias have been either definitively ruled out or adequately treated. In such patients, the electrophysiology study is often the most direct way of determining the cause of syncope and deciding on appropriate therapy.

Vasodepressor syncope

Vasodepressor syncope is by far the most common cause of syncope. The fact that vasodepressor syncope is known by so many names (including vasovagal syncope, cardioneurogenic syncope, and reflex syncope) is a reflection of the fact that its mechanism is poorly understood. To make matters worse, clinical syndromes that are almost certainly subcategories of vasodepressor syncope (Table 10.2) have usually been discussed in the literature as if they were completely unique and unrelated entities. This practice has led clinicians to the widespread misconception that there must be scores of causes of syncope, and accordingly, to a widespread attitude of hopelessness when faced with a patient who has syncope. In fact, patients who are prone to vasodepressor syncope often have a history of multiple syncopal episodes, and their episodes frequently match several of the syndromes listed in Table 10.2. Recognition that these different syndromes are merely variants of the same basic mechanism leads the physician immediately to the diagnosis in the majority of cases, and is a major step toward prescribing effective treatment.

The common denominator in all varieties of vasodepressor syncope is most likely the stimulation of the medullary vasodepressor region of the brain stem. The pathways that stimulate the vasodepressor region (afferent pathways) can arise from numerous locations—the resultant clinical syndrome has most often been named by the event that results in afferent stimulation of the medullary vasodepressor region (see Table 10.2). Once the vasodepressor

Table 10.2 Syndromes of vasodepressor syncope

Presumed afferent pathways	Syndromes	
Gastrointestinal/genitourinary mechanoreceptors	Micturition	Postprandial
	Defecation	Peptic ulcer
Cerebral cortex	Panic or fright	Noxious stimuli
	Pain	
Cranial nerves	Glossopharyngeal neuralgia	Oculovagal
Cardiopulmonary baroreceptors	Carotid sinus	Tussive
Cardiac C fibers	Valsalva	Postexercise
	Upright tilt	Volume depletion
	Jacuzzi	Pacemaker syndrome
	Weight-lifting	Supraventricular tachycardia
	Trumpet-playing	

region has been stimulated, that region generates efferent signals that cause both increased vagal tone (via the vagus nerve) and vasodilation (by pathways that are not well understood). Diminished cardiac filling and bradycardia follow, leading to syncope.

It should be recognized that although bradycardia is therefore often a prominent feature of this type of syncope, it is only rarely as important as vasodilation in producing symptoms. This is why therapy with pacemakers is usually not of significant benefit to patients suffering from vasodepressor syncope. It is also why the author has chosen to use the term "vasodepressor syncope" from the available menagerie of names.

In many of the syndromes listed in Table 10.2, stimulation of the cardiac C fibers (mechanocardiac receptors in the left ventricle) appears to be the origin of afferent stimulation of the vasodepressor region. The C fibers are stimulated when a volume-depleted ventricle is contracting vigorously, a situation that most commonly occurs when the venous return is decreased and the sympathetic tone is high.

Vasodepressor syncope tends to have characteristic clinical features that should lead the physician directly to the correct diagnosis. Many individuals have a predisposition to vasodepressor syncope, so that episodes recur periodically during a patient's lifetime. The initial episode of syncope often occurs during the patient's teen years. Over time, such individuals have episodes that match several of the syndromes listed in Table 10.2. Vasodepressor syncope is most often preceded by at least a few seconds of prodromal symptoms (lightheadedness, ringing in the ears, visual disturbances, diaphoresis, and nausea are the most prominent) and almost always occurs when the patient is upright (sitting or standing). Syncope resolves almost immediately when the patient assumes the supine position (often by falling). The vasodilation tends to persist for several minutes, so that if the patient tries to get up immediately after such an episode, a second syncopal episode often occurs. A prolonged feeling of being "washed out" and unable to function is common after vasodepressor syncope and is probably related to a residual autonomic imbalance triggered by the episode; unfortunately, these postdromal symptoms are often mistaken by clinicians for a "postictal" state. Patients who are predisposed to vasodepressor syncope will often have episodes of syncope when they are in a warm environment, when they have a viral illness, when they are dehydrated, or when they are under significant stress. The syndromes related to cardiac C fiber stimulation are relatively uncommon in patients with significant cardiac dysfunction, possibly because the C fibers are affected by myocardial disease. Not uncommonly, patients prone to vasodepressor syncope will experience a *flurry* of syncopal events over a period of days or weeks. Usually the reason for these flurries is unclear. In some instances, however, a flurry may be a clue that a patient has developed an occult peptic ulcer or a urinary tract infection that predisposes to vasodepressor episodes.

Obviously, given these prominent clinical features of vasodepressor syncope, taking a careful history is vitally important in making the correct diagnosis. As can be seen by studying Table 10.2, a patient's activity at the time of syncope yields strong clues as to the mechanism. Syncope that occurs while micturating, defecating, coughing, or swallowing is almost always vasodepressor in origin. The same holds for syncope associated with fright, pain, noxious stimulation, or severe emotional stress. These syncopal episodes rarely cause a diagnostic dilemma, but obtaining a history of such episodes in the past may yield clues as to the etiology of more recent and less clear-cut episodes of vasodepressor syncope. Syncope that occurs immediately after stopping prolonged or vigorous exercise is usually vasodepressor in origin (as opposed to syncope that occurs *during* vigorous exercise). In the author's experience, syncope that occurs in church (especially during the winter holidays, when tightly packed worshippers remain bundled in layers of cold-weather raiment) is usually due to a vasodepressor response. In a related phenomenon, syncope among members of a choir is also vasodepressor in origin in most cases. No other form of syncope is as *situational* as vasodepressor syncope.

Tilt-table testing

In recent years, the upright tilt-table study has entered common usage for determining a patient's propensity to develop vasodepressor syncope. When subjected to an upright, motionless tilt, patients who have vasodepressor syncope will often develop a frank syncopal episode.

The protocol used in performing tilt-table testing varies among laboratories, but most centers tilt patients for 15–45 minutes at 60–85°. "Normal" individuals compensate for such a tilt by increasing both α- and β-adrenergic tone as a result of baroreceptor stimulation and thus compensating for the decrease in venous return. In susceptible patients, however, these compensatory mechanisms eventually collapse. In such individuals, venous return is apparently never completely compensated. Thus, sympathetic tone progressively increases until, eventually, vigorous squeezing of the relatively empty ventricles results in recruitment of the cardiac C fibers. This, in turn, causes stimulation of the medullary vasodepressor region. The result is a sudden withdrawal of sympathetic tone, a sudden increase in vagal tone, sudden vasodilation, and syncope. A positive tilt-table study therefore identifies a patient who is prone to vasodepressor syncope.

The tilt-table study is positive in 30–74% of patients with syncope of unknown origin. Occasionally, however, an isoproterenol infusion is necessary to bring out syncope during tilt-table testing, even in patients who, by history, clearly have vasodepressor syncope. Further, the reproducibility of tilt-table testing has not been demonstrated, so that serial tilt-table studies to measure the efficacy of pharmacologic treatment are of questionable value.

The tilt-table study has been reported as being positive in up to 7% of individuals who do not have a history of syncope. Whether this represents a "false-positive" response or a true propensity for vasodepressor syncope is unknown. It is likely, however, that aggressive upright tilting would eventually produce hemodynamic collapse in almost anybody—otherwise, crucifixion would never have become a popular and effective form of execution.

Treating vasodepressor syncope

The most effective form of therapy for vasodepressor syncope is educating the patient. The patient who has had one or more vasodepressor episode should be advised as to the types of situation that predispose to vasodepressor syncope. Aggressive hydration should be advised when the patient is exercising, suffering from a viral illness or other infectious condition, or working in a hot environment. The symptoms experienced by the patient before losing consciousness—the prodrome of vasodepressor syncope—should be stressed as a warning that syncope is imminent. The patient should be advised to immediately assume the supine position under such circumstances until the symptoms pass, in order to avoid losing consciousness. With such measures, especially in patients who have infrequent episodes, often no other therapy is necessary.

Pharmacologic therapy for vasodepressor syncope is occasionally effective. *β-blocking agents* have recently become popular for treating vasodepressor syncope. Such therapy may seem paradoxical in a condition in which bradycardia is often a prominent feature, but because hypersympathetic tone is necessary to engage the cardiac C fibers, there is some rationale for using β-blockers. *Disopyramide* has also been used. Disopyramide has a vagolytic effect, but it also has a direct negative inotropic effect on the heart, and thus presumably inhibits stimulation of the cardiac C fibers as well. β-blockers and disopyramide can be expected to be effective only when the patient experiences episodes of syncope that are mediated by the cardiac C fibers, however. In addition, theophylline preparations, transdermal scopolamine, midodrine, fludrocortisone, and fluoxetine and other serotonin uptake inhibitors have been used with mixed success. Often, combinations of medications must be tried. Pharmacologic therapy should be reserved for patients who have frequent episodes of syncope and in whom nonpharmacologic methods have not been helpful.

Because bradycardia alone is only rarely the proximate cause of syncope in the vasodepressor syndromes, pacemaker therapy prevents these episodes only rarely and is generally reserved for patients who have profound and prolonged bradycardia accompanying their episodes. If pacemaker therapy is to be used, a dual-chamber pacemaker should be implanted to maintain AV coordination during pacing.

Evaluation of the patient with syncope

Classically, the evaluation of syncope has centered on searching for neurologic etiologies. However, it has become apparent that most syncopal episodes have cardiovascular causes. The physician evaluating a patient with syncope should therefore search carefully for cardiovascular etiologies.

Table 10.3 outlines a three-step approach for evaluating the patient with syncope. The most important step is to obtain a careful history and perform a physical examination. Although this step is important in the evaluation of any medical condition, it is particularly important in the patient with syncope. The history yields important clues relating to the presence of neurologic conditions, underlying cardiac conditions, and vasodepressor syncope. The physical examination is important in uncovering the presence of occult neurologic lesions and cardiac disorders. When you approach the patient with syncope, your attitude must be that you will not leave the bedside until a presumptive diagnosis is clear; for, once you decide that laboratory studies must be relied upon to make the diagnosis, you've got a very difficult task ahead.

The ECG is important in the patient with syncope. The presence of Q waves, an intraventricular conduction abnormality, or ventricular arrhythmias should alert the physician to the presence of

Table 10.3 Evaluation of the patient with syncope

Step 1

History and physical examination, ECG, serum electrolytes.

Step 2

(a) If neurologic problem suspected after step 1, consider an electroencephalography (EEG), brain scan, or angiography.

(b) If vasodepressor syncope suspected, consider further work-up as necessary to rule out reversible lesions (e.g. gastrointestinal or genitourinary disease), and initiate therapy. Tilt-table testing generally not necessary.

(c) If cardiac disease is suspected or if cause remains unclear, do noninvasive cardiac work-up to assess ventricular function (echocardiogram). Where appropriate, consider treadmill testing or cardiac catheterization.

Step 3

If the cause of syncope remains unclear after step 2:

(a) if structural heart disease is present, do a full cardiac evaluation, then electrophysiologic testing (you may do signal-averaged ECG as a screening study before electrophysiologic testing);

(b) if structural heart disease is absent, consider ambulatory monitoring, treadmill testing, and observation. If syncope recurs, consider tilt-table testing and electrophysiologic testing.

---

underlying cardiac disease that may predispose to lethal ventricular arrhythmias. Heart block or the presence of sinus bradycardia or sinus pauses point to bradycardias as a potential etiology. A short PR interval or preexcitation indicate a bypass tract, which may be the cause of syncope. The ECG should also be examined for signs of left ventricular hypertrophy, Brugada syndrome, repolarization abnormalities that might indicate a propensity for torsades de pointes, or signs of underlying ischemic heart disease.

The routine performance of brain scanning or electroencephalography (EEG) has not been helpful, and these tests should not be ordered unless the history or physical examination suggests a neurologic lesion or seizures. In cases in which a seizure has occurred but the EEG is negative, tilt-table testing should be considered, because seizure-like activity can be reproduced by inducing vasodepressor syncope in some patients (thus sparing the patient the diagnosis of epilepsy).

Tilt-table testing is not necessary in patients with a classic history for vasodepressor syncope. In these patients, therapy for vasodepressor syncope is appropriate even if the tilt-table study is negative.

Exercise-related syncope is usually vasodepressor in origin in younger patients, but in older patients is more likely to be related to ventricular arrhythmias, especially if underlying cardiac disease is present. Even younger patients with exercise-related syncope should have treadmill testing, however, to look for exercise-induced arrhythmias, and echocardiograms to look for structural abnormalities that might produce syncope (especially hypertrophic cardiomyopathy).

The most important, and the most neglected, part of the evaluation of syncope is to rule out underlying cardiac disease. In middle-aged and elderly patients with syncope, especially if syncope is of recent onset, a noninvasive evaluation of ventricular function is essential. An echocardiogram is probably the most useful means of assessing cardiac function, because it also yields information relative to potential aortic outflow lesions. A signal-averaged ECG also may be performed as a screening study for ventricular arrhythmias in patients suspected of having underlying cardiac disease.

Although arrhythmias are an important cause of syncope, ambulatory monitoring has generally been disappointing as a means of diagnosing arrhythmic syncope. A cardiac loop recorder (event recorder) can be helpful when symptomatic sinus nodal dysfunction or supraventricular tachycardia is suspected. When ventricular arrhythmias are suspected as the cause of syncope, however, ambulatory monitoring is inappropriate.

Immediate electrophysiologic testing is indicated in patients with syncope of unknown origin who are found to have had a previous myocardial infarction, a depressed left ventricular ejection fraction, nonsustained ventricular tachycardia, or a positive signal-averaged ECG. These patients should be presumed to be at high risk for sudden death from ventricular arrhythmias until proven otherwise, and should be hospitalized and monitored until ventricular arrhythmias are either ruled out or controlled.

Electrophysiologic testing, usually in conjunction with tilt-table testing, should be strongly considered when a careful, noninvasive evaluation has failed to reveal a presumptive diagnosis for syncope. Such combined testing can yield a presumptive diagnosis in up to 74% of patients whose syncope was of unknown origin before testing.

The evaluation of patients with syncope has often been regarded as difficult and frustrating. Using the principles outlined in this chapter, however, a diagnosis can be made relatively quickly in the vast majority of patients presenting with syncope.

11 Electrophysiologists and Dysautonomia

In the 19th century there was a common malady called neurasthenia. Victims of this condition—usually women—would inexplicably become unable to function due to some combination of strange and apparently unrelated symptoms, most often including extreme fatigue, weakness, severe pains that would come and go, palpitations, dizziness, syncope, diarrhea, dyspepsia, and (though it was rarely mentioned in that more delicate era) flatulence. Strikingly, all these debilitating symptoms were marked by a decided absence of objective medical findings. George Miller Beard in 1869 attributed the condition to a "weakened nervous system," which he speculated was caused by the stresses of modern urban life (Beard G, The Boston Medical and Surgical Journal 1869; 217–221).

But neurasthenia did not suddenly appear in the mid 1800s on the coat tails of the industrial revolution. Both Hippocrates and Galen described it in their writings, and called it "hysteria," a word that comes from the Greek for uterus (since a misbehaving womb was felt to be the cause[1]). Many centuries later women with this condition were condemned as witches, which seems rather extreme. By the time Jane Austen wrote her novels in the early 1800s, young women with neurasthenic constitutions (invariably the beautiful but delicate ones) were regarded with much more

---

[1] Indeed, well into the 20th century this condition was attributed by many doctors to humours which, they postulated, the uterus failed to expel due to insufficient coitus—and accordingly, a common approach to treatment was uterine massage to the point of "paroxysm." This treatment (usually performed by doctors or midwives) was considered so tedious that various mechanisms were developed to automate the process. Without this background it might be difficult to understand why, in the latter stages of the repressed sexuality of the Victorian era, vibrators were among the very first (and most popular) electrical appliances sold to consumers.

Electrophysiologic Testing, Fifth Edition. Richard N. Fogoros.
© 2012 John Wiley & Sons, Ltd. Published 2012 by John Wiley & Sons, Ltd.

sympathy, and in novels of the era they were often described in quite romantic terms.

Women with neurasthenia (for men were not given a diagnosis so closely associated with having a womb, no matter what symptoms they might have had) were often confined by doctors to their beds for prolonged periods, where they would either recover or, eventually, die. And while nobody knew what caused this condition, everyone—doctors and laymen alike—took it seriously. It was considered a legitimate medical problem, and it was a serious one, and the women who had it were generally treated with sympathy and respect—which probably went a long way toward encouraging their eventual recovery.

Then, in the early decades of the 20th century, neurasthenia mysteriously disappeared, virtually overnight.

Several theories as to what might have happened to neurasthenia have been advanced, but none sounds very convincing. Since it is extremely unlikely that the condition would simply go away after being well-described in the medical literature for more than 2000 years, the most likely explanation is that doctors suddenly became reluctant to make the diagnosis. This was the time when scientific theory really began permeating medical practice, and science had fully explained many diseases previously attributed to mysterious causes. As a result, doctors most likely became embarrassed to make a diagnosis like "neurasthenia," which had no physical findings, no laboratory abnormalities, and (despite scientific advances) no plausible theory behind it.

And thanks to Freud, it became easy to write these women off as being crazy, or less unkindly, as suffering from neuroses. And that's just what most doctors proceeded to do for most of the last century. So, while it is admittedly better than burning them as witches, for decades patients suffering from what used to be called neurasthenia have been nearly completely marginalized by the medical profession.

By this point, readers are wondering why the author thinks it appropriate to give a history of an obsolete disorder like neurasthenia in a book on electrophysiology. There are two reasons. First, neurasthenics are still with us, probably in greater numbers than ever. And second, they are very often sent to electrophysiologists for evaluation.

In this chapter we will first outline some of the general information which any doctor should know about the dysautonomias (the family of conditions to which the patients formerly known as neurasthenics are now assigned). We will then examine why it is important for electrophysiologists to have a good understanding of these conditions, and describe the specific conditions that are likely to send these patients their way. We will finish with a brief discussion on treating the dysautonomias.

The dysautonomias

Patients who in 1900 would have been called neurasthenics are today saddled with one or more of a host of diagnoses. These include chronic fatigue syndrome (CFS), fibromyalgia, panic attacks, irritable bowel syndrome (IBS), post-traumatic stress disorder (PTSD), postural orthostatic tachycardia syndrome (POTS), inappropriate sinus tachycardia (IST), mitral valve prolapse (MVP) syndrome, chronic Lyme disease, and vasodepressor (or vasovagal) syncope, among others. Taken together, these conditions are referred to as the dysautonomias.

In dysautonomia, the autonomic nervous system loses its normal balance, and at various times the parasympathetic or sympathetic systems inappropriately predominate. Symptoms can include frequent, vague, but disturbing aches and pains, faintness or frank syncope, fatigue and inertia, severe anxiety attacks, sinus tachycardia, hypotension, poor exercise tolerance, gastrointestinal disturbances, sweating, dizziness, blurred vision, numbness and tingling, anxiety, and (quite understandably) depression.

Sufferers of dysautonomia can experience all these symptoms or just a few of them. They can experience one cluster of symptoms at one time and another cluster at other times. And since people with dysautonomia are usually normal in every other way, a physical exam most often does not reveal any striking abnormalities. Patients are often labeled hysterical or anxious and are accorded little of the respect they might have received with similar symptoms during the 19th century. (Fortunately, doctors no longer prescribe prolonged bed rest, so the risk of mortality is now quite low.) When patients do get an actual diagnosis, the one they receive often depends on their most recent dominant symptoms and on which specialist they are referred to. The same patient sent to two or more doctors will likely receive two or more diagnoses.

The dysautonomias are usually seen in young, otherwise healthy people of either sex (though prevalence in females is higher than in males). Prior to the onset of their frequently disabling symptoms, patients are often quite happy, robust, and well-adjusted. Their first symptoms usually have a fairly sudden onset.

The dysautonomias do not have a single cause, but they often seem to be triggered by some discrete event. Some patients inherit the propensity to develop dysautonomia syndromes, and variations of dysautonomia often run in families. Acute infectious diseases can trigger a dysautonomia syndrome (including mononucleosis, Lyme disease, and influenza, but almost any acute infection will do), as can exposure to chemicals (Gulf War syndrome is, in effect, dysautonomia—low blood pressure, tachycardia, fatigue, and other symptoms—which, government denials aside, appears to have been triggered by exposure to toxins). Dysautonomia often follows an episode of trauma, including childbirth, but especially trauma to the head and chest (it has been reported to occur, for example, after breast-implant surgery). Dysautonomia can also be triggered by periods of extreme psychic stress, such as battle fatigue or the sudden loss of a child.

With any of these precipitating causes, the dysautonomia which follows can include almost any combination of symptoms. The symptoms can be constant or intermittent, can wax and wane, and can shift from one set of complaints to another.

Diagnosing dysautonomia

Patients suffering from dysautonomia often find the pathway to a diagnosis to be an ordeal. Many patients who have the audacity to complain of severe symptoms without providing the objective physical or laboratory findings to back them up are written off as being merely anxious or hysterical. This can make finding a doctor who will make the right diagnosis quite difficult.

After patients with one of these conditions have seen a doctor or two, and have had a couple of major workups which have yielded no objective findings, and after their doctors have expressed frustration with these results and have begun broaching (overtly or by hints) the idea of a psychogenic illness, or malingering, or some other such condition in which their psychological inadequacy is offered as the root cause, they actually do often become depressed and anxious—even if they began their quest with well-adjusted self-control and a sense of abiding optimism.

Patients lucky enough to be taken seriously by their primary care physician are likely to be sent to a specialist. The particular specialist they will see depends on the predominant symptoms they complain about.

Making the correct diagnosis requires the doctor to be alert to the possibility of dysautonomia in anyone presenting with one or more of the typical symptoms and a general sparsity of objective findings. In general, the most important key to the diagnosis is a history of good health, followed by some potentially triggering event, followed by unremitting (though often waxing and waning) symptoms compatible with dysautonomia.

Some of the dysautonomia conditions present next to nothing in the way of objective findings. These include CFS, fibromyalgia, and IBS. These diagnoses are made on purely clinical grounds, with heavy reliance on the medical history.

Other dysautonomias do indeed present objective findings. These generally are the conditions that include a strong component of vasomotor instability which can be objectively documented: POTS, vasovagal syncope, and IST. Fortunately for the electrophysiologist, these are the patients with dysautonomia most likely to be referred to them.

Often, in the course of working up a patient with dysautonomia, an echocardiogram is obtained, and the echo will show evidence of mild MVP. Given the high resolution achieved with today's echocardiographic equipment, at least some evidence of MVP can be identified in 25–30% of normal patients, and this finding is all the more likely to be called out on a final report if the reason given for the examination is to "rule out MVP." Consequently, these patients are likely to be diagnosed with "MVP syndrome." There is actually little if any evidence that the symptoms of dysautonomia are any more likely if MVP is present than if it is not. So in the vast majority of cases, the "MVP" (if it is actually present at all) is an incidental finding. There's probably nothing terrible about making the superfluous diagnosis of MVP syndrome, as long as the physician understands that what's actually going on is dysautonomia. But to the extent that this diagnosis steers the doctor away from recognizing dysautonomia and treating it appropriately, it is indeed a problem.

Whichever of the dysautonomia conditions a patient might have, the doctor should be alert to the likelihood of symptom overlap. So, for instance, the patient with CFS may have some orthostatic instability, or the patient with fibromyalgia may have a mild resting sinus tachycardia or a history of vasovagal syncope. These kinds of clue can provide important corroboratory evidence as to the real nature of the patient's condition.

Why electrophysiologists need to know about the dysautonomias

Whether they like it or not, electrophysiologists end up seeing many patients with dysautonomia. Typically, these patients will be referred for palpitations, for episodes of syncope, or for tachycardia. Frequently, neither the patient nor the referring doctor will realize that dysautonomia is the real problem. Likely the referring doctor will believe, and the patient will be afraid, that they are just crazy.

So the electrophysiologist will be doing a very good thing if he or she not only provides the assessment of the symptom for which the patient is being referred, but also is able to point the referring doctor and the patient in the right direction, so they can begin taking the steps necessary to get the underlying dysautonomia under control.

Dysautonomia and palpitations

Typically, the work-up of palpitations is pretty straightforward. You simply arrange for the patient to have cardiac monitoring for whatever period of time seems necessary to capture an ECG during an episode of palpitations. Sometimes that's a 24-hour Holter study, and sometimes it's two or more 4-week event-recorder studies. But once you have recorded an ECG that tells you what the heart rhythm is at the moment the patient is experiencing their typical palpitations, you generally have your diagnosis. If there's an arrhythmia, you deal with that. If the palpitations are not associated with an arrhythmia then they are likely to be due to muscle spasms or esophageal gas or some other benign noncardiac cause, and the treatment is reassurance.

It may not be so simple in the patient with dysautonomia. These patients very often have several different symptoms, which may include actual palpitations from cardiac arrhythmias, as well as other transient sensations which they may perceive in the region of the chest. And only the rare patient with dysautonomia can reliably differentiate among the various upper-body sensations they experience when they say they are having "palpitations."

Because the patient may be experiencing several types of symptom they call "palpitations," it becomes relatively easy to write off their symptoms when they are found not to be associated with specific cardiac arrhythmias. This may cause the physician to miss symptomatic episodes of tachycardia or bradycardia, both of which are also fairly common in patients with autonomic instability. Patients with dysautonomia are typically relatively young and (except for their dysautonomia) reasonably healthy, so missing sinus bradycardia or sinus tachycardia is not likely to have devastating consequences. But capturing those heart rhythms, and correlating them with symptoms, may turn out to be an important clue that dysautonomia with a certain degree of hemodynamic instability is present. And this knowledge carries treatment implications.

So, when evaluating palpitations in a patient who is suspected of having dysautonomia, the clinician ought to be a little more circumspect than usual in declaring that there is no correlation between the symptoms and the heart rhythm. Often, this is best accomplished by continuing the monitoring for a long enough period of time to record electrograms during multiple episodes of palpitations.

Dysautonomia and syncope

Chapter 10 discussed the evaluation of syncope in detail. As we saw, by far the most common cause of syncope is vasodepressor syncope. And vasodepressor syncope, at least when it is a recurrent problem, is often a form of dysautonomia.

In the majority of patients who have vasodepressor syncope, the syncopal episodes themselves are the only sign of dysautonomia. In contrast to the kinds of dysautonomia we are talking about in this chapter (in which symptoms tend to be multiple, and, with varying degrees of intermittency, relatively persistent), patients with vasodepressor syncope most typically will present with a single episode, or perhaps a short cluster of episodes—and will be entirely normal at all other times. That is, their susceptibility to syncope is usually intermittent and fairly transient.

However, some patients with vasodepressor syncope will have a more chronic condition, in which syncope is likely almost any time a potential "triggering event" happens to occur. These patients quite often, on questioning, will describe other symptoms consistent with dysautonomia, including a definitive precipitating event that first heralded the onset of their condition. Tilt-table testing (see Chapter 10), which helps to estimate a person's relative susceptibility to vasodepressor syncope, is much more likely to be strikingly positive in these patients. These patients, not surprisingly, are typically more difficult to treat than those with only rare and sporadic syncopal events.

One additional observation might help to clarify the nature of the symptoms patients sometimes experience with dysautonomia. After a vasodepressor syncopal episode, patients will often feel extremely weak, lightheaded, and fatigued for several minutes to several hours. During this post-syncopal period, they can do little more than lie down, feeling miserable; if they try to get up, they become orthostatic and dizzy. What these patients are experiencing during this interval is a transient case of acute and fairly striking dysauto-nomia. Patients who are symptomatic with many of the dysauto-nomia conditions discussed in this chapter feel more or less just like that, much of the time.

Chapter 10 describes in more detail the evaluation and treatment of patients with vasodepressor syncope.

Dysautonomia and tachycardia

Tachycardia is fairly common in patients with dysautonomia. Gen-erally, the fast heart rate is sinus tachycardia, and presumably it is caused by autonomic imbalance in the direction of increased sym-pathetic tone.

In some patients the sinus tachycardia is quite remarkable and persistent and is the most striking feature. These patients are said to have inappropriate sinus tachycardia (IST).

Patients with IST have sinus rates that are abnormally high at rest (usually around 100 beats/min, though during sleep the rates may drop to the mid 80s, or even lower) and invariably increase rapidly with even minimal exertion. They have no identifiable reason for secondary sinus tachycardia, such as anemia, infection, hyper-thyroidism, pheochromocytoma, substance abuse, or cardio-pulmonary disease. Their sinus tachycardia is therefore "inappropriate."

While IST can occur in anybody, the typical sufferer is a woman in her 20s or 30s who has been having symptoms for months to years. Prior to the onset of IST, which often follows a viral illness or physical trauma, most of these patients will have been in excellent health, both physically and emotionally. In addition to the most common symptoms of palpitations, fatigue, and especially exercise intolerance, IST can be associated with a host of other issues, including orthostatic hypotension, blurred vision, dizziness, tin-gling, gastrointestinal disturbances, shortness of breath, and sweat-ing. In other words, they often suffer from the constellation of symptoms typical for patients with dysautonomia.

Symptoms with IST can be quite severe, sometimes to the point of being disabling. All these symptoms occur with a paucity of physical findings or laboratory abnormalities. The only consistent finding is tachycardia.

IST has been a recognized clinical condition only since 1979, and while electrophysiologists by now are very familiar with it, many other doctors remain blissfully unaware that it exists. By the time the sufferer of IST gets to an electrophysiologist, if they are lucky enough to be referred, they will have been told by at least one doctor that the culprit is "anxiety." If the IST itself isn't enough to make the patient crazy, then being told it's all "in your head" may be: by the time he or she sees an electrophysiologist, anxiety often is indeed an issue.

The cause of IST, like all the dysautonomias, is unknown. And in fact, while the author obviously classifies this condition as a dysautonomia, many electrophysiologists disagree, and believe it is a primary disorder of the SA node.

Indeed there are several lines of evidence that point to IST being a primary SA nodal disorder. First, the intrinsic heart rate (see Chapter 5) in patients with IST tends to be elevated, suggesting that even in the absence of autonomic influence the SA node displays enhanced automaticity. Second, patients with IST tend to have an abnormally enhanced heart-rate response to epinephrine, similar to their exercise response. And third, at least some evidence exists that the SA node in patients with IST is structurally abnormal.

It is important to know whether IST is a primary SA nodal disorder because if it is, ablation of the SA node ought to cure the condition. Accordingly, electrophysiologists have tested this theory by performing SA nodal ablations in hundreds of patients with IST. The outcome is very interesting. The immediate response is usually quite favorable—over 90% of patients no longer have IST immediately after SA nodal ablation. Unfortunately, in about 80% of patients who have such "successful" ablations, the IST recurs within 6–9 months.

Repeat electrophysiologic testing usually shows regeneration of SA nodal function, complete with its IST-like behavior, though this regenerated SA nodal activity is often found inferior to the original site of ablation, along the crista terminalis. Repeated ablations usually yield the same results: early success and late failure.

Thus, something—this "something" being external to the SA node itself—appears to be stimulating regeneration of SA nodal tissue, complete with its inappropriate rate of firing, after ablation. This is an important piece of evidence against the "primary SA nodal disorder" hypothesis.

There is actually quite a bit of evidence that IST may often be one of the dysautonomias. It shares many of the characteristics of dysautonomia, including that its onset is frequently preceded by a viral illness or trauma and that the patient profile is typical, and "extra" symptoms frequently occur which are consistent with other forms of dysautonomia (indeed, many IST patients might have been labeled as suffering from IBS, POTS, or CFS if they had seen someone other than an electrophysiologist). Then, of course, there's the fact that something stimulates the successfully ablated SA nodes to regenerate, suggesting a more systemic problem than intrinsic SA nodal disease. Finally, even during transiently successful SA nodal ablations, the other symptoms consistent with dysautonomia typically persist.

The treatment of IST would be straightforward if SA nodal ablation offered permanent relief from symptoms. Unfortunately, however, this is usually not the case. The mainstay of therapy for IST therefore is pharmacologic therapy with β-blockers, calcium blockers, type Ic antiarrhythmic agents, and—in countries where it is available—ivabradine (a drug that slows the automaticity of the SA node). Usually, a combination of drugs is required to achieve an adequate slowing of the heart rate. Patients also often respond to the more general measures used for dysautonomia (see next section), especially long-term aerobic-exercise training.

In patients who remain largely disabled by symptoms of IST despite noninvasive efforts at control, SA nodal ablation should be strongly considered despite its drawbacks.

Finally, simply waiting may be an option for some patients. The natural history of this disorder has not been well documented, but it seems likely that IST tends to improve over time in most individuals, as is the case with most of the dysautonomias. "Doing nothing" may not be an option for patients who are severely symptomatic, but many patients with IST can tolerate their symptoms once they are assured that they do not have a life-threatening cardiac disorder, told that the problem is likely to improve on its own eventually, and enlightened as to the other treatment options.

Treating dysautonomia

Treating a patient with dysautonomia, like making the diagnosis, is often a challenge. The keys to treatment are reassurance and patience.

The physician should keep in mind that, despite the fact that dysautonomia is an honest-to-goodness, actual medical (as opposed to psychological) condition, by the time the patient has seen two or three doctors and has been told there's actually nothing wrong, or that they're crazy, it is the rule for the patient to compound their underlying dysautonomia with a state of real anxiety and/or depression. This secondary neurosis almost always greatly exacerbates their symptoms.

So a critical step in the treatment of dysautonomia is reassurance. First, the patient needs to be told that they're actually not nuts, that they have a legitimate and well-recognized medical problem—and that there's a name for it. They should be told about the concept of autonomic imbalance, and that this state of imbalance is usually triggered by some distinct event (which most often the patient will be able to identify). They should be told that, in general, dysautonomia is seen in young, healthy patients with robust autonomic nervous systems, and that over time the dysautonomia usually goes away or improves substantially (this improvement, however, may take several years). Finally, they should be told that there are several things that can be done to help minimize their symptoms while their autonomic nervous system "resets" itself.

Just telling the patient this much often provides an immediate sense of relief. They are not crazy. They have a real medical problem, and they have a doctor who understands it. It is likely to get better, and there's something they can do about it in the meantime. These facts provide the patient with a sense of control over their own destiny, and this sense of control will often relieve a lot of their anxiety, diminish the severity of their symptoms, and help them cope with the symptoms that remain.

The "patience" component of treating dysautonomia is important because there is no direct treatment for this condition. Rather, there are a host of therapies that help relieve one symptom or another in one patient or another—and so adequately treating dysautonomia often requires a prolonged period of trial-and-error therapeutics. Recognizing this fact up front will help both the doctor and the patient avoid frustration (and symptom-exacerbating anxiety) during what is likely to be a long process of optimizing therapy.

Non-drug therapy for dysautonomia

Underlying causes

In addition to the "idiopathic" varieties of dysautonomia we are discussing here, autonomic dysfunction can also be caused by numerous underlying medical conditions. These include a host of neurological conditions (including multiple sclerosis, Shy–Drager syndrome, Parkinson's disease, Huntington's disease, and Guillain–Barré syndrome), systemic diseases (including diabetes and amyloidosis), active infectious diseases (including HIV/AIDS, diphtheria, and Chagas disease), connective tissue diseases, hepatic disease, renal failure, and many others. So an early step in diagnosing and treating dysautonomia should be to do a thorough medical evaluation looking for potential underlying causes, and if one is found, to treat it aggressively.

Exercise

It is well known that chronic exercise training produces changes in autonomic balance. Further, it has been shown that in patients with dysautonomia—particularly patients with hemodynamic instability (POTS), IST, or frequent vasovagal syncope—aerobic training can significantly reduce elevated resting heart rates, improve orthostatic symptoms, and in general improve hemodynamic stability. In these patients, however, beginning an exercise program can be a challenge, since being upright can precipitate symptoms or cause excessive elevations in heart rate.

Recently, however, investigators have reported that patients with autonomic hemodynamic instability can achieve excellent results if they begin their exercise program using a "non-upright" form of exercise, such as a recumbent bicycle, a rowing machine, or swimming (Fu Q *et al.*, Hypertension 2011; DOI: 10.1161/hypertensionaha.111.172262). The exercise has to begin slowly, a few minutes at a time, a few times per week, depending on what the patient can tolerate. But generally, after a month or two, a "training effect" becomes noticeable, whereby the patient can exercise more frequently and for longer periods of time. Most patients can eventually begin upright exercise activities such as walking, jogging, or bicycling. As their fitness improves, these patients usually experience a marked improvement in their baseline symptoms.

As a bonus, the fact that the patient is actively doing something that will lead to an improvement in their often-disabling symptoms gives them a sense of control over their own destiny that is therapeutic in itself. So an exercise program, with the physician's ongoing supervision and advice, should be the "baseline" therapeutic approach to many varieties of dysautonomia—but in particular, those varieties marked by hemodynamic instability. In contrast to the older patients for whom doctors usually prescribe exercise, the much younger patients with dysautonomia—who quite often seem to have been athletes prior to their illness—are more often highly motivated to gain control over their medical condition and their lives. Typically, they will dedicate themselves to an exercise program if one is encouraged by a doctor.

Fluid management and daily precautions

Patients whose dysautonomia includes orthostatic symptoms, inappropriate tachycardia, or vasovagal syncope ought to be coached in maintaining good hydration. They generally should not be placed on salt restriction, and in some cases might benefit from increasing sodium consumption. Patients with orthostatic symptoms must take appropriate precautions when arising from a seated or lying position. This is especially important first thing in the morning, when fluid balance is typically as negative as it ever gets. Such precautions might include sitting on the side of the bed for a few minutes and drinking a glass of water before standing, immediately walking upon arising (instead of standing in place), and wearing ankle weights for the first few minutes after getting up (to stimulate muscular action in order to improve blood return). Other "tricks" that sometimes help with hemodynamic instability include elevating the head of the bed 12 inches or so at night, taking showers while sitting down, and scheduling most daily activities in the afternoon (when symptoms tend to diminish), instead of in the morning.

Other nonpharmacologic measures

Patients with dysautonomia have responded favorably to biofeedback techniques, meditation, yoga, and other similar practices known to alter autonomic tone. Doctors taking care of these individuals should try to keep an open mind about such nontraditional options.

Drug therapy for dysautonomia

Several types of medication can help alleviate symptoms associated with dysautonomia. To a large extent, these medications are used on a trial-and-error basis, and very often several drug trials are needed before a drug or drug combination is found that provides satisfactory symptom relief without producing intolerable side effects.

Drugs that seem to offer some help, at least occasionally, include β-blockers (especially carvedilol and labetalol, which provide both α and β blockade), selective serotonin reuptake inhibitors, fludrocorisone, midodrine, methyldopa, ibuprophen, clonidine, and (in patients with severe POTS) erythropoetin.

Patients with gastrointestinal symptoms often benefit from eating frequent small meals, increasing dietary fiber, avoiding foods that seem to have caused particular problems, and using anticholinergic medication.

The bottom line on treating dysautonomia

The bottom line is that treating dysautonomia is not by any means a "once and done" affair. The right therapy always needs to be individualized, and virtually always requires establishing a long-term and trusting doctor–patient relationship. The end result, however, is often very rewarding for both parties.

Electrophyiologists, given the nature of their field, will end up seeing a lot of patients with dysautonomia, and in many cases they will be the ones who actually make the diagnosis. The electrophysiolgist who is unwilling to develop the kind of long-term relationship with these patients that adequate treatment will require ought at least to feel obligated to identify a few trusted colleagues who understand this family of conditions and are able and willing to give these patients the attention they need in order to return them to a happy and functional life.

12 Electrophysiologic Testing in Perspective: The Evaluation and Treatment of Cardiac Arrhythmias

In this final chapter, we will attempt to synthesize the information presented in the first 11 chapters into a general approach to the evaluation and treatment of cardiac arrhythmias, with emphasis on the appropriate use of the electrophysiology study.

The approach outlined in this chapter is an elementary and, indeed, almost a trivial one. Quite simply, the basic principle of our approach is to tailor the aggressiveness of the therapy to the severity of the arrhythmia being treated. Nearly all serious mistakes that are made in the management of cardiac-rhythm disturbances can be traced to a violation of this modest principle. Each year, thousands of patients die because their physicians tread lightly when faced with clearly lethal rhythm disturbances or, worse, become ninja-like in their attack on benign arrhythmias. Such fatal mistakes can be avoided by taking a logical, stepwise approach to the evaluation and treatment of cardiac arrhythmias.

The three steps in evaluating and treating cardiac arrhythmias

The appropriate management of cardiac arrhythmias involves following a predetermined plan of therapy aimed at achieving specific goals. Those goals, in turn, are determined by the severity of the arrhythmia being treated. Thus, in evaluating and treating cardiac arrhythmias, three discrete steps are implicit:

Electrophysiologic Testing, Fifth Edition. Richard N. Fogoros.
© 2012 John Wiley & Sons, Ltd. Published 2012 by John Wiley & Sons, Ltd.

Step 1. Assess the severity of the arrhythmia to be treated. The physician decides whether the arrhythmia is benign, potentially harmful, or lethal, and whether the symptoms associated with the arrhythmia require treatment.

Step 2. Decide on the therapeutic end point. The physician decides whether the primary goal of treatment is to prevent death, to minimize harm, or merely to relieve symptoms.

Step 3. Design the treatment plan. The physician devises a treatment plan that is directly aimed at achieving the primary therapeutic end point.

Step 1. Assess the severity of the arrhythmia to be treated

As already stated, the most common and most serious mistake made in the management of cardiac arrhythmias is to institute therapy that is inappropriate for the arrhythmia being treated. This error most often results from the propensity of physicians to assign specific treatments to specific arrhythmias, without considering the setting in which the arrhythmia occurs.

Example: Dr X uses flecainide or encainide to treat all patients with premature ventricular contractions (PVCs; prior to 1990, this was an extremely common practice). For Patient A, who has a normal heart and asymptomatic complex ventricular ectopy, this therapy is too aggressive. Patient A has a normal risk of sudden death, and antiarrhythmic drugs cannot be expected to improve that normal risk (they may, on the other hand, increase it). For Patient B, who is a survivor of sudden cardiac death with PVCs, this therapy is not aggressive enough. Patient B has an extremely high risk of sudden death and empiric therapy with flecainide is not likely to help—indeed, the risk of proarrhythmia is especially high in such a patient.

Physicians who treat a specific arrhythmia the same way in every patient will eventually cause serious problems because the appropriate treatment for an arrhythmia depends on more than just the arrhythmia itself. The appropriate level of aggressiveness in treating an arrhythmia can be judged only when considering the setting in which the arrhythmia occurs. In assessing the severity of a patient's arrhythmia, the physician must consider at least three factors: (1) What is the arrhythmia? (2) What symptoms are associated with the arrhythmia? (3) What is the nature and the extent of any underlying cardiac disease?

Several specialized laboratory studies are available to help assess these three factors. The studies most often used are those that help to assess the arrhythmia itself (the electrophysiology study and ambulatory monitoring) and those that help to assess underlying cardiac disease (cardiac catheterization, stress testing, echocardiography, and nuclear angiography).

The electrophysiology study, as helpful as it is in guiding the therapy of many cardiac arrhythmias, is only modestly helpful in assessing the severity of arrhythmias. Because the arrhythmias induced in the electrophysiology laboratory are produced under unnatural circumstances, the electrophysiology study is poor at helping to correlate symptoms with arrhythmias. Observing symptoms with spontaneously occurring arrhythmias is far more helpful. On the other hand, in circumstances where an arrhythmia is suspected but not documented, the electrophysiology study can be helpful in diagnosing the arrhythmia itself. The most common example would be in a patient with syncope of unknown origin (see Chapter 10). In such patients, the electrophysiology study can help to diagnose sinus node disease, distal conducting system disease, and ventricular tachyarrhythmias. It bears repeating, however, that both sinus node disease and conducting system disease can most often be diagnosed noninvasively. Regarding ventricular tachyarrhythmias, the sensitivity and specificity of induced ventricular arrhythmias in patients with syncope of unknown origin are strongly related to the presence and the extent of underlying heart disease. In general, electrophysiologic testing should be done in patients with syncope of unknown origin only when they have significant heart disease or when there is a particular reason to suspect an arrhythmic etiology for syncope. The electrophysiology study, in addition, can help to assess the potential for developing severe arrhythmias in patients with atrioventricular bypass tracts (see Chapter 6). Except in patients with syncope of unknown origin or with bypass tracts, however, the electrophysiology study is of limited usefulness in assessing the severity of arrhythmias.

Ambulatory monitoring is often more helpful than electrophysiologic testing in assessing the severity of cardiac arrhythmias. In patients who are having reasonably frequent spontaneous arrhythmias, ambulatory monitoring is excellent in helping to correlate the arrhythmia with symptoms. Further, the specificity of spontaneous arrhythmias (as opposed to induced arrhythmias) is 100%. There are four general varieties of ambulatory monitoring. The Holter monitor study typically records the cardiac electrogram for 24 hours. If patients are having arrhythmias that occur at least daily, the Holter study is often ideal for assessing the severity of these arrhythmias, because it gives information on the frequency of occurrence, potential exacerbating influences, and related symptoms. The second variety of ambulatory monitor, the cardiac event recorder, records the cardiac electrogram on a continuous tape, so that at any time only the last 30–90 seconds are available for playback. When a symptomatic arrhythmia occurs, the patient can stop the tape by pressing a button and then transmit the contents of the tape by telephone. Such a monitor is usually worn for extended periods of time, until a symptomatic episode is captured on tape. This type of monitor is best suited for a patient who has relatively infrequent symptomatic arrhythmias that have been difficult to document. The third type of ambulatory monitoring is mobile cardiac outpatient telemetry—a device that continuously monitors the heart rhythm for up to several weeks at a time, and automatically transmits arrhythmic "events" to a centralized monitoring center. Physicians are contacted whenever an important arrhythmia is identified. Finally, there is the implantable rhythm monitor. This is a tiny microprocessor-based device that is placed under the skin and records a patient's ECG for weeks or months at a time. Rhythm strips from inside the device can be downloaded periodically and reviewed. Some electrophysiologists have found this device helpful in assessing the frequency and severity of benign (but symptomatic) cardiac arrhythmias. The implantable rhythm monitor has also been used to help diagnose syncope of unknown origin—but it must be stressed that it is inappropriate to rely on this form of ambulatory monitoring (or any ambulatory monitoring) to reveal arrhythmia-induced syncope, at least until ventricular arrhythmias either have been ruled out as the cause of syncope by electrophysiologic testing or have been deemed extremely unlikely after a noninvasive cardiac workup (see Chapter 10).

The studies used to assess underlying heart disease will vary from patient to patient. Nuclear angiography and echocardiography are often used because these relatively noninvasive tests give excellent information on ventricular wall motion and left ventricular ejection fraction. The echocardiogram is especially useful when significant valvular heart disease or hypertrophic cardiomyopathy are suspected. If cardiac ischemia is suspected, stress/thallium testing and cardiac catheterization are commonly used.

What is the arrhythmia?

Diagnosing the arrhythmia of concern is an important first step. Once the arrhythmia in question is known, some attempt should be made to classify the risk for sudden death imposed by the arrhythmia as low, moderate, or high. Such a classification, based on the arrhythmia itself, is listed in Table 12.1. Note that some arrhythmias, by their very nature, should automatically be considered as imposing a high risk—namely, sustained ventricular tachycardia, ventricular fibrillation, and complete heart block with an inadequate escape mechanism. The presence of atrial fibrillation itself produces an increased risk of embolic stroke. Most other arrhythmias usually impose low or moderate risk, depending on the underlying heart disease.

What symptoms are associated with the arrhythmia?

Arrhythmias generally cause only a few types of symptom: palpitations, lightheadedness or dizziness, and loss of consciousness. Palpitations are the most common symptom and are commonly associated with ectopic beats. Most patients can tolerate palpitations if this is the only symptom they experience, especially if they can be reassured that their arrhythmia is benign. Lightheadedness and

Table 12.1 Classification of the risk for sudden death imposed by arrhythmias

High risk	Moderate risk	Low risk
Ventricular tachycardia	Complex ventricular ectopy with underlying heart disease	Premature atrial complexes
Ventricular fibrillation	Second-degree AV block	Premature ventricular complexes
Third-degree AV block with an inadequate escape	Third-degree AV block with adequate escape	Sinus node dysfunction
Wolff–Parkinson–White syndrome with rapid antegrade conduction in atrial fibrillation	Atrial fibrillation	Supraventricular tachycardias
		Complex ventricular ectopy with no underlying heart disease
		First-degree AV block

dizziness, which occur with various levels of severity, tend to be associated either with bradyarrhythmias or with tachyarrhythmias that consist of more than isolated extra beats. Although many patients can tolerate occasional mild episodes of lightheadedness, others find these symptoms to be extremely disturbing. Loss of consciousness from an arrhythmia indicates extreme hemodynamic compromise, and any bradyarrhythmia or tachyarrhythmia that produces this symptom should be considered to imply a high risk of sudden death. (An important exception to this rule: syncope accompanied by bradycardias is most often vasoactive in nature. In such cases, the bradycardia itself is usually *not* the cause of syncope (instead, vasodilation is the cause) and should not be considered a lethal arrhythmia.)

Some arrhythmias cause symptoms by producing or worsening symptoms of congestive heart failure. Any form of tachycardia that persists for weeks or months (such as persistent reentrant supraventricular tachycardia, inappropriate sinus tachycardia, or atrial fibrillation with a rapid ventricular response) can ultimately produce ventricular remodeling and dilation and thus congestive heart failure. In patients with diastolic dysfunction, whose noncompliant ventricles are dependent on atrial contraction to achieve a high end-diastolic pressure while maintaining a relatively normal mean atrial pressure, loss of that atrial contraction with the onset of atrial fibrillation can produce pulmonary congestion quite acutely.

When a patient has symptoms compatible with an arrhythmia, determining whether those symptoms are actually due to an arrhythmia is not always straightforward. Quite often, a Holter-monitor study will show arrhythmias and symptoms but will fail to show a correlation between the two. In these instances, the arrhythmia should not be construed as the cause of the symptoms. Because the appropriate treatment of many nonlethal arrhythmias depends on the symptoms they produce, every attempt should be made to document a correlation between the arrhythmia and the symptoms before any potentially toxic therapy is initiated. Further, several symptoms are often attributed to arrhythmias but in fact are only rarely due to arrhythmias. These symptoms include dyspnea, nonspecific fatigue, and seizures or localizing neurologic symptoms. Any of these symptoms, even if accompanied by cardiac arrhythmias, should prompt a thorough search for other causes.

Once it is determined that symptoms are due to the arrhythmia in question, those symptoms should be categorized in terms of their severity. The classification of the severity of symptoms described in

Table 12.2 Classification of the severity of arrhythmic symptoms

Life-threatening	Presyncope, syncope, aborted sudden death
Severely disruptive	Significant lightheadedness or dizziness, severe palpitations, worsening congestive heart failure (such as in atrial fibrillation with rapid ventricular response)
Minor/none	Mild lightheadedness, palpitations

Table 12.2 includes three categories: life-threatening symptoms, severely disruptive symptoms, and minor or no symptoms.

What is the underlying heart disease?

In general, any arrhythmia is more severe in the face of significant underlying heart disease than in a normal heart. In particular, as described in Chapter 7, underlying heart disease is the primary determinant of lethal ventricular arrhythmias. Thus, complex ventricular ectopy that has only minimal significance in a patient with no heart disease has significant implications in patients with severe left ventricular dysfunction.

By considering these three factors, one can accurately judge the severity of the arrhythmia in question. The next step is to use this information to decide on a specific goal of therapy.

Step 2. Decide on the therapeutic end point

Cardiac arrhythmias are treated because they either produce symptoms, pose a threat to health, or have the potential to cause sudden death. Thus, there are three general therapeutic end points in treating cardiac arrhythmias: to relieve symptoms, to maintain health, or to prevent sudden death. Before a treatment plan can be devised, it is vital to decide which of these goals is to be pursued and to keep that goal clearly in mind.

The appropriate goal of therapy should be chosen based on the severity of the arrhythmia, as determined in step 1. The following generalizations can be made. Low-risk arrhythmias, because they do not have the potential to produce death, should be treated only if they are producing symptoms that are disruptive to the patient's life, in which case the goal of therapy is merely to reduce symptoms. High-risk arrhythmias, on the other hand, should always be treated, and the goal of therapy with these arrhythmias is to prevent sudden death.

Moderate-risk arrhythmias are the most problematic. Two arrhythmias tend to fall in to this category: atrial fibrillation and complex ventricular ectopy in the setting of significant underlying cardiac disease.

Atrial fibrillation presents a problem (aside from the symptoms caused by the arrhythmia itself) because it poses a long-term risk of embolic stroke, and in some patients it can produce or exacerbate heart failure. Furthermore, as we have discussed, "getting rid" of atrial fibrillation (with either antiarrhythmic drugs or ablation) can be extremely difficult and risky. So, in treating this arrhythmia the clinician must decide whether to use a "conservative" approach (controlling the rate response and anticoagulating) or an "aggressive" approach (trying to restore and maintain sinus rhythm). Neither of these approaches is easy or straightforward, and both may require escalating attempts at achieving the therapeutic goal (for instance, advancing from drug-based therapy to ablation-based therapy).

Complex ventricular ectopy, in the setting of significant underlying cardiac disease, has become much less a clinical dilemma than it used to be, for two reasons. First, it is now well established that trying to abolish these arrhythmias with antiarrhythmic drugs merely increases risk, and that treating empirically with amiodarone does not improve outcomes. So the temptation to treat the ectopy itself has become much less compelling. And second, as described in Chapter 7, thanks to the results of several randomized clinical trials, we can now offer implantable defibrillators to many of these patients. So, while treatment still does not entail getting rid of the ectopy itself, we are now able to materially improve the survival of many of the patients who fall into this category.

Step 3. Design the treatment plan
The final step in the management of cardiac arrhythmias is to decide on a therapeutic plan aimed at achieving the chosen goal of therapy. Keeping the goal of therapy clearly in mind is vitally important because treatments for similar arrhythmias may vary markedly from patient to patient, depending on whether the aim of therapy is to prevent sudden death or merely to relieve symptoms. (It should be noted that in managing bradyarrhythmias, the basic therapy for both relieving symptoms and preventing sudden death is essentially the same—a permanent pacemaker. The following discussion thus pertains mainly to ectopic beats and tachyarrhythmias.)

Treating to relieve symptoms

When the primary goal of therapy is to relieve symptoms, the physician must determine what steps are necessary to achieve that goal. For most patients in whom symptom relief is the therapeutic end point, the arrhythmia being treated is benign. Thus, therapy aimed at relieving symptoms is often (and appropriately) less aggressive than therapy aimed at preventing sudden death. Empiric trial-and-error therapeutic attempts are often appropriate and are frequently performed on an outpatient basis. Generally, milder therapies are tried first, moving progressively and as necessary to more aggressive treatments. Before each escalation of therapy, careful consideration is given as to whether the symptom being treated warrants yet more aggressive therapy. Although serial ambulatory monitoring is often helpful, it should be remembered that, when the goal is merely to relieve symptoms, this goal has already been met if monitoring is necessary to tell whether the arrhythmia is still present.

The level of aggressiveness used in controlling symptoms depends on the severity of the symptoms being treated. For instance, therapy to relieve symptoms does not necessarily involve suppressing the culprit arrhythmia. Quite often, the symptoms that a patient experiences with a benign arrhythmia are magnified by the anxiety that often accompanies the knowledge that one has a cardiac arrhythmia (an anxiety that is often provoked by a physician who expresses grave concern over the arrhythmia's presence). In such cases, the symptoms often can be ameliorated simply by reassuring the patient of the benign nature of the arrhythmia. The therapeutic goal of relieving symptoms, then, can sometimes be achieved without subjecting the patient to potentially toxic drugs, and without affecting the frequency of the offending arrhythmia at all.

On the other hand, a patient may have an arrhythmia that is non-life-threatening but that produces severely disabling symptoms. In such instances, it may be entirely appropriate to attempt very aggressive therapy. As an example, consider a patient with severe cardiomyopathy who has atrial fibrillation with a rapid ventricular response, resulting in moderate decompensation of the patient's congestive heart failure. With such a patient, one might begin with attempts to control the ventricular response with digitalization, calcium blockers, or β-blockers. If this were unsuccessful, one would have to consider more radical measures, such as His bundle ablation and insertion of a permanent pacemaker. Therefore, one may arrive at aggressive therapy in relieving the symptoms of an arrhythmia, but in general only after less aggressive measures have failed.

The electrophysiology study has only a moderate role in managing arrhythmias when the suppression of symptoms is the primary goal. Although the electrophysiology can help in assessing the presence of various nonlethal arrhythmias (such as sinus node or AV node dysfunction), this study cannot supply much information on the symptoms caused by these arrhythmias.

For several types of arrhythmia, however, the electrophysiology study can be helpful in abolishing symptoms. This is especially true for most reentrant supraventricular tachycardias, which usually can be cured with transcatheter ablation.

Treating to prevent sudden death

Once the physician decides that the primary goal of therapy is to prevent the patient's sudden death, a treatment plan should be devised that reflects the urgency of the therapeutic end point. By its nature, sudden death occurs instantaneously and unexpectedly. Thus, when a patient is judged to be a candidate for sudden death, immediate and aggressive efforts should be made to prevent this event. Ideally, these efforts should include placing the patient in the hospital and on a monitor until adequate therapy is derived. Trial-and-error (empiric) methods of treatment are inappropriate. When the goal of therapy is to prevent sudden death, the initial therapy must be effective because the physician is unlikely to have a second chance should therapy prove ineffective.

With regard to patients who are at high risk for sudden death from ventricular arrhythmias, the treatment "plan" has been greatly simplified over the past few years. In contrast to the days when the electrophysiology study was used as the cornerstone of a complex therapy-selection strategy, today the "baseline" treatment strategy is almost always the same: to insert an implantable defibrillator. The electrophysiology study, when done at all, is generally used to help determine how to optimally program the implantable defibrillator—for instance, in optimizing antitachycardia pacing.

For the other major variety of arrhythmia that poses an increased risk of sudden death—a bypass tract with rapid antegrade conduction—the electrophysiology study with ablation remains the mainstay of effective treatment.

Conclusion

This final chapter outlines a general approach to, and a perspective on, the use of the electrophysiology study in the management of cardiac arrhythmias. Devising a reasonable treatment plan depends on defining the goals of therapy. Those goals, in turn, depend on the severity of the arrhythmia and of the symptoms caused by the arrhythmia. The electrophysiology study can be of moderate help in assessing the severity of cardiac arrhythmias and can be extremely helpful in abolishing both the symptoms and the risk caused by several cardiac arrhythmias.

Most fatal mistakes in treating cardiac arrhythmias stem from failing to match the aggressiveness of therapy to the severity of the arrhythmia being treated. Using a logical, stepwise approach to the evaluation and treatment of cardiac arrhythmias allows one to avoid this critical error.

Questions

1 The conduction velocity of an electrical impulse through cardiac tissue is most directly determined by:
   a. The duration of the action potential
   b. The duration of the "plateau phase" of the action potential
   c. The slope of phase 0 of the action potential
   d. Not the action potential, but sympathetic tone
2 The plateau phase of the action potential is of shortest duration in:
   a. Purkinje fibers
   b. Atrial muscle
   c. Ventricular muscle
3 The depolarization phase (phase 0) of the action potential is slowest in:
   a. Purkinje fibers
   b. AV nodal cells
   c. Atrial muscle
   d. Ventricular muscle
4 The refractory period of a myocardial cell is most directly determined by:
   a. The duration of phase 0 of the action potential
   b. The duration of the plateau phase of the action potential
   c. The slope of phase 4 of the action potential
   d. Sympathetic tone
5 Phase 4 of the action potential most directly determines:
   a. Conduction velocity
   b. Refractory period
   c. Automaticity
   d. Triggered activity
6 A reentrant arrhythmia requires all of the following *except*:
   a. Triggered activity
   b. A potential circuit

Electrophysiologic Testing, Fifth Edition. Richard N. Fogoros.
© 2012 John Wiley & Sons, Ltd. Published 2012 by John Wiley & Sons, Ltd.

c. Differences in refractory periods between different parts of the circuit

d. Differences in conduction velocities between different parts of the circuit

7 Triggered activity involves abnormal behavior in which phases of the action potential:

a. Phases 0 and 1

b. Phases 1 and 2

c. Phases 3 and 4

d. Phases 4 and 0

8 The primary effect of class Ic antiarrhythmic drugs is to:

a. Block the sodium channel and slow conduction

b. Increase action-potential duration and prolong the refractory period

c. Decrease action-potential duration and shorten the refractory period

d. Slow phase 4 depolarization and block automaticity

9 The primary effect of class III antiarrhythmic drugs is to:

a. Block the sodium channel and slow conduction

b. Increase action-potential duration and prolong the refractory period

c. Block the calcium channel

d. Slow phase 4 depolarization and block automaticity

10 In systemic doses, the primary effect of class Ib antiarrhythmic drugs is to:

a. Block the sodium channel and slow conduction

b. Increase action-potential duration and prolong the refractory period

c. Decrease action-potential duration and shorten the refractory period

d. Slow phase 4 depolarization and block automaticity

11 Distinguishing characteristics of amiodarone include all of the following *except*:

a. A remarkably long half-life

b. Association with a low incidence of proarrhythmia

c. More effective than any other antiarrhythmic drug

d. Very little organ toxicity

12 The longest coupling interval for which a premature impulse fails to propagate through cardiac tissue is:

a. The effective refractory period

b. The functional refractory period

c. The relative refractory period

13 The longest coupling interval for which a premature impulse results in slowed conduction through cardiac tissue is:
   a. The effective refractory period
   b. The functional refractory period
   c. The relative refractory period

14 The shortest coupling interval in which successive impulses can conduct through a tissue is:
   a. The effective refractory period
   b. The functional refractory period
   c. The relative refractory period

15 The type of AV nodal refractory period which most directly relates to the average rate of the ventricular response in a patient with atrial fibrillation is:
   a. The effective refractory period
   b. The functional refractory period
   c. The relative refractory period

16 The measurement of the sinus node recovery time (SNRT) is based on which electrophysiologic property of the sinus node:
   a. Automaticity
   b. Triggered activity
   c. Conduction velocity
   d. Overdrive suppression
   e. Refractory period

17 An abnormal sinoatrial conduction time (SACT) is most likely to be found during electrophysiologic testing in a patient with which finding on their electrocardiogram:
   a. A regular sinus bradycardia of 48 beats/min at rest
   b. A rhythm showing periods of sinus exit block
   c. Overdrive suppression of the sinus node after an episode of atrial fibrillation
   d. An abnormally low intrinsic heart rate

18 Which of the following statements about AV nodal block is *false*:
   a. AV nodal block is usually not life-threatening, because relatively stable subsidiary pacemakers are typically available below the site of the block
   b. AV nodal block can occur as a consequence of therapy with digoxin, calcium blockers, or β-blockers
   c. AV nodal block which occurs after a myocardial infarction usually indicates permanent damage to the AV node, and typically requires a permanent pacemaker

19 Which of the following statements about using the Mobitz classification system is *false*:
- **a.** Mobitz I AV block is usually localized to block in the AV node
- **b.** Mobitz II AV block should always be considered distal heart block
- **c.** In 2 : 1 AV block, the Mobitz classification system does not apply; block could be either AV nodal or distal, and other steps should be used to localize the site of block
- **d.** 2 : 1 AV block is a form of Mobitz II AV block

20 In a patient with heart block, signs that potentially dangerous distal heart block is present include all of the following *except*:
- **a.** The degree of block increases as sympathetic tone increases
- **b.** In second-degree block, there is no gradual prolongation of the AV interval prior to the dropped P wave
- **c.** The QRS duration is 150 msec
- **d.** The heart block is more likely to occur during periods of deep sleep

21 Each of the following is itself an indication for a permanent pacemaker *except*:
- **a.** A split His signal is found on EP testing
- **b.** The HV interval is greater than 120 msec
- **c.** Distal AV block is induced during incremental atrial pacing at 550 msec
- **d.** The corrected sinus node recovery time (CSNRT) is greater than 525 msec

22 Which type of evidence gathered during electrophysiologic testing is *not* commonly used to determine the mechanism of supraventricular tachycardia:
- **a.** Whether the rate of the induced SVT is less than or greater than 180 beats/min
- **b.** Whether the SVT is readily induced with ventricular extrastimuli
- **c.** Whether activation of the ventricular myocardium is necessary for the maintenance of the SVT
- **d.** The pattern of atrial retrograde activation during the SVT

23 An ECG during multifocal atrial tachycardia most resembles the ECG with which other supraventricular arrhythmia:
- **a.** Atrial fibrillation
- **b.** Atrial flutter
- **c.** Antidromic atrioventricular macroreentrant tachycardia

    d. Sinus tachycardia with frequent PACs and ventricular aberrancy

24 A distinguishing feature of AV nodal reentrant tachycardia is that:
    a. The cycle length of the tachycardia may lengthen if bundle branch block occurs
    b. There is a distinct discontinuity in the atrioventricular conduction curve
    c. The cycle length of the tachycardia remains unchanged if AV nodal conduction is slowed

25 A distinguishing feature of intraatrial tachycardia is that:
    a. The cycle length of the tachycardia may lengthen if bundle branch block occurs
    b. There is a distinct discontinuity in the atrioventricular conduction curve
    c. The cycle length of the tachycardia remains unchanged if AV nodal conduction is slowed

26 A distinguishing feature of bypass-tract-mediated atrioventricular macroreentrant tachycardia is that:
    a. The cycle length of the tachycardia may lengthen if bundle branch block occurs
    b. There is a distinct discontinuity in the atrioventricular conduction curve
    c. The cycle length of the tachycardia remains unchanged if AV nodal conduction is slowed

27 A patient has a regular, narrow-complex tachycardia of 155 beats/min. Careful examination of the 12-lead ECG reveals no clear P waves in any lead. The most likely mechanism of the tachycardia is:
    a. Intraatrial reentrant tachycardia
    b. AV nodal reentrant tachycardia
    c. Sinus nodal reentrant tachycardia
    d. Atrioventricular macroreentrant tachycardia

28 A patient has a regular, narrow-complex tachycardia of 155 beats/min. The 12-lead ECG shows negative P waves in the inferior leads, roughly halfway between the QRS complexes. The most likely mechanism of the tachycardia is:
    a. Intraatrial reentrant tachycardia
    b. AV nodal reentrant tachycardia
    c. Sinus nodal reentrant tachycardia
    d. Atrioventricular macroreentrant tachycardia

29 A patient has a regular, narrow-complex tachycardia of 155 beats/min. The 12-lead ECG shows biphasic P waves prior to each QRS complex, with a PR interval of 120 msec. The most likely mechanism of the tachycardia is:
   a. Intraatrial reentrant tachycardia
   b. AV nodal reentrant tachycardia
   c. Sinus nodal reentrant tachycardia
   d. Atrioventricular macroreentrant tachycardia

30 Which of the following arrhythmias is *least* likely to be induced with right ventricular pacing:
   a. Atrioventricular macroreentrant tachcardia with a left lateral bypass tract
   b. Intraatrial reentrant tachycardia
   c. AV nodal reentrant tachycardia
   d. Left ventricular reentrant tachycardia

31 A patient presents with three syncopal episodes within 2 hours, and their ECG shows frequent bursts of rapid, polymorphic nonsustained ventricular tachycardia. Each of the following clues, if present, would be suggestive of triggered activity due to early afterdepolarizations (EADs) *except*:
   a. The patient's digitalis level is in the toxic range
   b. Sinus beats on the ECG show distinct U waves
   c. The patient had been placed on sotalol 3 days earlier for paroxysmal atrial fibrillation
   d. Bursts of ventricular tachycardia invariably follow a relative pause in the underlying rhythm

32 Which of these types of ventricular tachycardia is *least* likely to be treatable with ablation therapy:
   a. Idiopathic left ventricular tachycardia
   b. Outflow tract ventricular tachycardia
   c. Brugada syndrome
   d. Bundle branch reentrant tachycardia

33 The mechanism of ventricular arrhythmia which is most commonly responsible for sudden out-of-hospital arrhythmic deaths is thought to be:
   a. Triggered activity due to EADs
   b. Triggered activity due to DADs
   c. Reentrant ventricular arrhythmias associated with ischemic or nonischemic cardiomyopathy
   d. Congenital channelopathies, such as Brugada syndrome

34 A patient's sustained, monomorphic ventricular tachycardia is readily inducible during baseline electrophysiologic testing.

After administering sotalol, the tachycardia is no longer inducible on either of two successive days. What can be said about chronic treatment with sotalol in this patient:

a. Treatment with sotalol should prevent any further recurrences of the ventricular tachycardia

b. Treatment with sotalol cannot be expected to have any effect in preventing recurrences of ventricular tachycardia

c. Treatment of sotalol will probably reduce the frequency of recurrences, but should not be expected to prevent all recurrences

35 Which of these patients probably does not have a present indication for an implantable defibrillator:

a. 58-year-old man, myocardial infarction 6 months ago, LVEF 32%, NYHA class II, no known arrhythmias

b. 58-year-old man, myocardial infarction 6 months ago, LVEF 28%, asymptomatic

c. 58-year-old man, idiopathic cardiomyopathy, LVEF 32%, NYHA class III, no known arrhythmias

d. 58-year-old man, myocardial infarction 3 weeks ago, LVEF 28%, NYHA class II, complex ventricular ectopy

36 Which of the following tachycardias typically does *not* show left bundle branch morphology?

a. Tachycardia mediated by a Mahaim bypass tract

b. Tachycardia associated with Brugada syndrome

c. Tachycardia associated with right ventricular dysplasia

d. Right ventricular outflow tract ventricular tachycardia

37 Which of these statements about AV nodal reentrant tachycardia (AVNRT) is *not* correct?

a. Each of the dual pathways in AVNRT is distinctly localizable

b. The slow pathway in AVNRT is a posterior and inferior structure, located along the tricuspid annulus between the His bundle and the os of the coronary sinus

c. The fast pathway in AVNRT is an anterior and superior structure, located along the tendon of Todaro

d. In most cases, in treating AVNRT with ablation therapy, the target of ablation is the fast pathway

38 Which of the following statements about ablating the AV junction (to produce AV block) is *true*:

a. The target of the ablation procedure should be the proximal portion of the His bundle, just as it exits the AV node

b. When positioning the ablation catheter, in the ideal position the electrogram will show a His-bundle deflection at least as large as the atrial deflection

c. If accelerated junctional tachycardia is seen during application of RF energy, that ablation attempt should be aborted immediately, and the catheter repositioned

d. Ventricular pacing at 90–100 beats/min should usually be done for a few days after AV junction ablation, to avoid ventricular tachyarrhythmias

39 All the following techniques are often used for determining the location of a bypass tract *except*:

a. Mapping on the ventricular side of the AV groove while pacing the atrium at a rate that maximizes the size of the delta wave

b. Making unipolar recordings from the tip of the mapping catheter to get an idea of the direction of the cardiac impulse at various points along the AV groove

c. Making a large series of exploratory ablation lesions along the AV groove, to see whether any of them affect the delta wave

d. Observing a loss of preexcitation when pressure is applied to the tip of the catheter at a particular location along the AV groove

40 Which of the following is a sign that a patient has a left free-wall bypass tract:

a. Negative delta wave in leads I and AVL

b. Negative delta wave in leads III and AVF

c. Positive delta waves in leads I and AVL

d. During SVT, the development of RBBB increases the cycle length of the tachycardia

41 Which of the following statements about Mahaim bypass tracts is *true*:

a. Mahaim bypass tracts are now thought to arise in the compact AV node

b. Mahaim bypass tracts are now thought not to arise in the compact AV node, but instead to be atriofascicular tracts that are composed of typical atrial myocardial tissue

c. While Mahaim bypass tracts are now thought to be atriofascicular tracts, they display many of the electrophysiologic characteristics of AV nodal tissue

d. Mahaim bypass tracts commonly produce a negative delta wave in leads III and AVF

42 Which of the following statements about typical atrial flutter is *true*:
- **a.** In typical atrial flutter, the reentrant circuit follows a large but often unpredictable pathway within the right atrium
- **b.** Typical atrial flutter can generally be ablated by placing four or five spot lesions in the region of the crista terminalis
- **c.** Typical atrial flutter is usually very difficult or impossible to ablate without sophisticated electroanatomic mapping systems to fully characterize the pathway of the reentrant circuit
- **d.** Typical atrial flutter can usually be ablated by placing a linear lesion between the tricuspid annulus and the inferior vena cava

43 Each of the following approaches has been used to ablate atrial fibrillation, *except*:
- **a.** Creating a ring of lesions to electrically isolate Koch's triangle
- **b.** Creating a series of linear lesions to divide the atrial muscle into a "maze"
- **c.** Creating a series of lesions to electrically isolate the pulmonary veins
- **d.** Carefully mapping and ablating foci of atrial ectopic beats

44 Each of the following techniques is sometimes used to map reentrant, monomorphic ventricular tachycardia, *except*:
- **a.** Entrainment mapping
- **b.** Doppler mapping
- **c.** Activation mapping
- **d.** Pace mapping

45 Which of the following statements about currently available electroanatomic mapping systems is *true*:
- **a.** All available systems use magnetic fields to create three-dimensional maps
- **b.** All available systems require the use of proprietary mapping catheters with magnets built into them
- **c.** All available systems can create an activation map after a single beat of the target arrhythmia
- **d.** All available systems can improve the feasibility of successfully ablating atrial fibrillation

46 Which of the following statements about cardiac resynchronization therapy (CRT) is *false*:
- **a.** It has been established that, because right ventricular pacing invariably causes dyssynchrony, biventricular pacing

should be used in almost anyone who needs a permanent pacemaker

b. Most patients with heart failure who are indicated for CRT therapy are also indicated for ICD therapy

c. CRT has been shown to be effective in patients with NYHA class III or IV heart failure on optimal medical therapy who have left ventricular ejection fractions of 35% or less and QRS durations of 120 msec or more

d. CRT is reasonable in patients in NYHA class I or II on optimal medical therapy who have left ventricular ejection fractions of 35% or lower and who require full-time ventricular pacing–whatever their native QRS duration may be

47 Which of the following statements about arrhythmias that cause syncope is *false*:

a. Syncope caused by sinus nodal disease is often related to exaggerated overdrive suppression of the sinus node during transient episodes of atrial fibrillation

b. Heart block due to AV nodal or His-bundle disease is a particularly common cause of syncope

c. When supraventricular tachycardia produces syncope, the loss of consciousness is often caused by overdrive suppression of the sinus node, or by a vasodepressor reaction triggered by the SVT

d. In many cases, the strongest clue that a ventricular tachyarrhythmia is the cause of syncope is when the patient's first syncopal episode occurs after the onset of significant heart disease

48 Which of the following statements about the tilt-table study is *true*:

a. In most patients with vasodepressor syncope, a positive tilt-table study is an essential step in making the correct diagnosis

b. Patients with true vasodepressor syncope very rarely have a negative tilt-table study

c. Patients without a history of vasodepressor syncope very rarely have a positive tilt-table study

d. The tilt-table study is far less important than taking a careful medical history in making the correct diagnosis in patients with syncope

49 One reason electrophysiologists should be aware of the spectrum of symptoms produced by dysautonomia is:

- **a.** The dysautonomias are often characterized by a broad range of cardiac arrhythmias
- **b.** Patients with dysautonomia are particularly prone to unusual ventricular arrhythmias
- **c.** Patients with dysautonomia are often referred to electrophysiologists for fleeting symptoms; unless they are aware of the dysautonomia syndromes, electrophysiologists are likely to write these patients off as having psychiatric problems
- **d.** Patients with dysautonomia often improve with pacemaker therapy

50 Which of the following statements about inappropriate sinus tachcardia (IST) is *true*:

- **a.** It has been firmly established that IST is a form of dysautonomia
- **b.** It has been firmly established that IST is a form of primary sinus node disease
- **c.** Ablation therapy has a high probability of curing IST
- **d.** Ablation therapy is often initially very successful in treating IST, but the arrhythmia most often recurs within a few months

Answers

1. C	26. A
2. B	27. B
3. B	28. D
4. B	29. A
5. C	30. B
6. A	31. A
7. C	32. C
8. A	33. C
9. B	34. C
10. C	35. D
11. D	36. B
12. A	37. D
13. C	38. D
14. B	39. C
15. B	40. A
16. D	41. C
17. B	42. D
18. C	43. A
19. D	44. B
20. D	45. D
21. D	46. A
22. A	47. B
23. A	48. D
24. B	49. C
25. C	50. D

Electrophysiologic Testing, Fifth Edition. Richard N. Fogoros.
© 2012 John Wiley & Sons, Ltd. Published 2012 by John Wiley & Sons, Ltd.

Index

Note: page numbers followed by f refer to figures, those followed by t refer to tables.

Electrophysiologic Testing, Fifth Edition. Richard N. Fogoros.
© 2012 John Wiley & Sons, Ltd. Published 2012 by John Wiley & Sons, Ltd.